Guidelines for Comprehensive Nursing Care in Cancer

Report of a Series of Continuing Education Seminars
in the Care of the Patient with Cancer, held at
MEMORIAL SLOAN-KETTERING CANCER CENTER

Directed by
BEATRICE A. CHASE, R.N., M.A.
and GUY F. ROBBINS, M.D.

Edited by
HELEN DUNCAN BEHNKE, R.N., M.A.

PRINGER PUBLISHING COMPANY, INC., NEW YORK

Memorial Hospital and the federal government, under Regional Medical Program grant RM-00058, jointly provided the financial support which enabled the hospital's multidisciplinary staff to develop and present these symposiums. Of major importance was the input provided by the nursing staff of Memorial Hospital. Most of the panel members had been involved in the direct care of patients with cancer for many years, and this explains their practical approaches to these serious symposiums.

GUY F. ROBBINS, M.D.
Director, Memorial Hospital
Regional Medical Program

CREDITS

Pages 90, 91, 95, 96 (Figs. 1, 2, 6, 7): From Gutowski, F., Nursing Management of the Patient with Lung Cancer: In Watson, William L., editor, *Lung Cancer*. St. Louis, 1968, The C. V. Mosby Co.

Pages 93, 94 (Figs. 3, 4, 5): Copyright © 1960 by Medical Economics Co. Reprinted with permission from *RN Magazine*, Vol. 23, No. 1, January 1960.

Page 153: Reprinted with permission from American Cancer Society, Inc. © 1971.

Page 176 (Fig. 2): Reprinted with permission from *Surgery, Gynecology & Obstetrics*, June 1970, Vol. 130:988-944.

Page 272 (Fig. 1): Reprinted with permission from *Surgical Clinics of North America*, Vol. 49, No. 2 April 1969, p. 350, W. B. Saunders Company.

Pages 276, 278 (Figs. 2, 3): From *The Ureter*, Bergman, Harry, editor, 1967, Harper & Row Publishers.

Pages 342, 363, 364, 365: The tables and figure on these pages appear as Tables 1 and 2 and Figure 2 in Krakoff, I. H.: Cancer Chemotherapeutic Agents. *Ca–A Cancer Journal for Clinicians*, 23:208-219, 1973. Pages 208, 210-211, and 215.

Printed in U.S.A.

CONTENTS

FOREWORD

Wherever cancer nursing is practiced and discussed, we hear a great deal about its formidable problems. Lest this emphasis predominate, I suggest an infusion of the other aspects of cancer nursing into our thinking—for example, the abundant privileges it affords nurses. This and other qualities have been reaffirmed by the series of seminars on oncologic nursing presented at the Memorial Sloan-Kettering Cancer Center in New York City, whose distinguished nursing department brought together the talents of members of many disciplines concerned with the care of patients with cancer. For those who could attend the meetings, as I did, the demonstrations of expert care and expressions of an extraordinary philosophy of caring were a rich experience. For others, this book offers much-needed knowledge about cancer nursing—here are the up-to-date facts, figures, and feelings of experts in the field of oncologic nursing.

VIRGINIA BARCKLEY, R.N., M.S.
National Nursing Consultant,
American Cancer Society

ACKNOWLEDGMENTS

We are grateful to the many practitioners who took part in the Regional Medical Program series of seminars on oncologic nursing. Their reports of the eager search for new knowledge challenged past concepts and offered input which not only strengthened nursing's faith in its own contribution to the advancement of cancer care, but also forced the reappraisal of current efforts to find better answers to the problems that beset those who care for patients with cancer. Some of the program speakers had had rich experience in presenting information about their work to public audiences, but many had not had previous opportunities to make formal presentation of the work they know best; we thank these practitioners particularly. We also thank the participants, whose thoughtful queries presented new challenges to Memorial Hospital personnel. To those nurses who worked many hours planning the clinical nursing content of the seminars we owe a special debt of gratitude—Bernadine Cimprich, Frances Gutowski, and Carol Reed. No less important was the contribution of the clinical instructors and nursing supervisors who in many and varied ways ensured the success of the seminars and carefully reviewed the various chapters of the manuscript after they were prepared from tape recordings. In addition, a special note of gratitude is extended to both the inpatient and outpatient head nurses who by careful scheduling made it possible for all levels of Memorial personnel to attend the seminar sessions. We also thank Katherine Nelson and Frances Kreuter, two nationally known nursing leaders, whose participation added a special richness to the seminars. A sincere tribute goes to Mary H. Brown, associate director of nursing, for her untiring efforts throughout the entire series of seminars and in the review of the material for this publication.

For their support, encouragement, and personal involvement, we wish to express our appreciation to: Drs. Giulio J. D'Angio, Edward J. Beattie, Jr., Daniel Caplin, Donald G. C. Clark, Karamat U. Choudhry, J. Herbert Dietz, Jr., William Elstein, Philip R. Exelby, Joseph G. Fortner, Alfred A. Fraccia, Paul L. Goldiner, Basil S. Hilaris, Walter B. Jones, David W. Kinne, Irwin H. Krakoff, Burton J. Lee, 3rd, James B. Lepley, John L. Lewis, Jr., M. Louise Murphy, Jesus Nahmias, Sandra L. Nehlsen, Carl K. Schmidlapp, Maus W. Stearns, Jr., Elliot W. Strong, Willet F. Whitmore, Jr.

The American Cancer Society's Reach to Recovery volunteers and staff members from the Visiting Nurse Service of New York contributed much to the value of the panel discussions.

We would like to acknowledge the cooperation of the Mary Manning Walsh Home and Rockefeller University in providing meeting space for some of the seminars. In addition, it would have been impossible to conduct this kind of educational effort without the assistance of every department of the hospital, particularly the dietary, housekeeping, medical illustration, and engineering departments.

Finally, we must express our deep appreciation to the several patients who served as panel members and whose contributions strongly influenced the discussions and the positive outcome of the seminars.

BEATRICE A. CHASE, R.N., M.A.
GUY F. ROBBINS, M.D.

PREFACE

The world stands today at the threshold of major progress in the understanding, prevention, surveillance, treatment, and cure of cancer. Hence dissemination of the steadily increasing knowledge about this disease constitutes a responsibility for all health professionals. This is particularly true for professional nurses who are generally "doers" rather than writers about the innovative things they do. Consequently, much of the knowledge acquired by nurses who care for cancer patients remains in their personal repertoire of nursing activities or, at least, is not disseminated beyond the institutions that utilize their expertise in the care of oncologic patients.

This book reports the ten oncologic nursing seminars (19 sessions in all) that were conducted at Memorial Sloan-Kettering Cancer Center between September 1970 and March 1972. The program was unique in a number of ways. First, it demonstrated that it is feasible to conduct a continuing education program for professional nurses in a setting that is not primarily academic.

Second, although the program focused chiefly on nursing knowledge and nursing skills, the multidisciplinary approach about which we hear so much but rarely see in operation, gave our colleagues in other health care disciplines opportunities to share newly acquired information on cancer and the care of cancer patients. Among the 86 seminar speakers, there were five patients, 27 physicians, and 8 social workers in addition to 39 professional nurses. Further, there were representatives from such disciplines as physics, radiation therapy, recreational therapy, special education, and rehabilitation.

Third, the total registration, 4,923, suggests that the program had far-reaching appeal. There were 1,923 session registrants from the professional nursing staff of Memorial Hospital (an average of four sessions per nurse). The other 3000 registrants (most of whom were registered nurses) were representatives from 179 other health care agencies and institutions in metropolitan New York and from as far south as Philadelphia and as far north as New Haven, Connecticut.

Why and how did it come about that the department of nursing at one of the world's largest and busiest cancer centers undertook to arrange this series of multidisciplinary seminars on oncologic nursing? The answer to this question was very clear to members of this department who receive an ever increasing number of inquiries about cancer nursing. These inquiries come from student nurses, nurse practitioners, nurse instructors and other faculty members in all parts of the United States, as well as many foreign countries, and the number has grown dramatically in recent years. The need to share Memorial Sloan-Kettering's steadily growing body of knowledge of cancer and cancer nursing was perceived as a community responsibility, and as a social and professional responsibility as well.

The general purpose of the Regional Medical Program series of oncology seminars was to disseminate the newest concepts, techniques, and information about cancer. Implicit in this purpose was the objective of demonstrating how Memorial Sloan-Kettering Cancer Center utilizes the collaborative efforts of many disciplines to the end that patients with cancer may receive the most effective nursing care while hospitalized, and continuity of care after they are discharged. Another objective of this series was to promote oncologic nursing as a specialty, since this type of nursing has not advanced as rapidly as has oncologic medicine. It is incumbent upon professional nurses and other health care personnel to close this gap by developing an awareness of the depth and breadth of the disease entity known as cancer and to learn about new and bold therapeutic measures which, when reinforced with strong rehabilitative efforts, may restore many patients to useful lives. Nurses should take the lead in this educational effort so that personnel from all the various agencies and situations involved in patient care will know more about not only the medical aspects of cancer, but about the nursing, rehabilitative, and psychosocial aspects also.

It was fortuitous that the seminars were planned for exactly the time they were, because the program was initiated just prior to the formulation and passage of the National Cancer Act of 1971. Thus without planning it that way, the seminars aroused additional interest among leaders at several university hospitals where cancer centers were being developed and the seminar content had direct practical application immediately.

Perhaps one of the most fruitful results of the seminars was that they served as a dramatic demonstration of the kind of interpersonal and interdisciplinary relationships that are necessary for advancement in the care of the patient with cancer. As we prepare for the day when cancer will be cured, nursing must continue to improve the quality of life for those who suffer this catastrophic disease. The directors of the seminar program believe that it provided for dissemination of knowledge that will result in such advancement. They also believe that the program provided something further—that is, it extended the potential for maximizing the quality of nursing care to nurses and health care facilities far beyond the walls of Memorial Sloan-Kettering Cancer Center.

BEATRICE A. CHASE, R.N., M.A.
Chairman, Department of Nursing

Pediatric Oncology

Regional Medical Program — Oncology Nursing Seminar

on

NURSING MANAGEMENT IN PEDIATRIC ONCOLOGY

Seminar Leader

M. Lois Murphy, M.D.

Seminar Participants

Harriet Colvin, M.S.W., Social Worker

Barbara Dalton, R.N., Head Nurse

Mary DeMarzo, R.N., Head Nurse

Ruth Edelstein, B.A., Public School Teacher of Health
  Conservation in Hospitals

Philip R. Exelby, M.D., Chief, Pediatric Surgical Service

Ruth Johnston, R.N., Head Nurse

Kit Kimpritis, Recreation Specialist

M. Lois Murphy, M.D., Chairman, Department of Pediatrics

Jesus Nahmias, M.D., Child Psychiatrist

Annamay Ricco, R.N., Clinical Nursing Instructor

Although likenesses of children who appear to have had cancer are found among many ancient drawings, the first collection of cases of cancer in children was published in 1806. It consisted of descriptions of 20 children with cancer of the orbit. By 1900 the total number of published cases was only about 600. Therefore, one may be prompted to ask, "Just how common is cancer in children?"

In one report it was estimated that in the area in England serviced by the Manchester hospitals where there are about one million children, the general practitioner diagnoses one childhood malignancy for each 29 years of practice, and the general surgeon operates on one child with Wilms' tumor in each ten years of practice. In all of England and Wales, deaths among children from non-leukemic cancer numbered 3,759 during one ten-year period. And these cases were divided among 601 hospitals—an average of 0.6 tumors per hospital per year. How, then, can cancer be so important?

The American Cancer Society has published statistics showing that the death rate for cancer in children between one and 14 years (in the United States) is currently 7.1 per 100,000 children per year. In 1935, the 11 leading causes of death in children were accidents, pneumonia, diarrhea, appendicitis, tuberculosis, diphtheria, diseases of the heart, measles, scarlet fever, and whooping cough—in that order. Cancer was twelfth with five deaths per 100,000 children per year. Gradually, the public health requirements for immunization in infancy against the preventable diseases, and the discovery of specific chemicals and antibiotics for many infectious diseases, have reduced the frequency of these causes of death in children in 1935. Accidents still remain the leading cause of death in children, but cancer has moved up to second place. That is why it is so important.

Total cancer deaths (in the United States) anticipated for 1972, adults and children, was 345,000. Leukemia constitutes 4 percent of all cancer but 40 percent of the childhood cancers. Overall, of the 57 million children in the 1970 census, approximately 4,000 would be expected to develop fatal cancers each year, and half of them would be in the newborn to five-year age group.

Between the ages of one and five, the incidence of leukemia and malignant tumors of the brain and nervous system is high compared with other types of cancer. Neuroblastoma accounts for a peak in the central nervous system category at about two to three years. Wilms' tumor occurrence gradually falls off at the age of seven or eight, and then levels off to a very low point. Lymphoma begins to rise at about age 11. Bone tumors are infrequent in early childhood, but beginning at about age seven or eight and through the second decade, the incidence of Ewing's tumor and osteogenic sarcoma—the malignant bone tumors—goes up. The peak years for embryonal rhabdomyosarcoma are from two to four.

Robert Miller, a pediatrician and cancer epidemiologist at the National Cancer Institute, obtained the death certificates for children from the entire United States for a five-year period, 1960 through 1964, and classified the types of cancer that had caused deaths in children. This is the best record available on the relative incidence of the different types because, in contrast to contagious diseases, cancer is not a reportable disease. Among children under 14, leukemia came first, then cancer of the central nervous system, lymphoma, neuroblastoma, Wilms' tumor, bone sarcoma, embryonal rhabdomyosarcoma, liver, and retinoblastoma—in that order. By contrast, in children from 15 to 19 years old, leukemia was still the leading cause of death from cancer, but lymphoma was second, bone sarcoma was up to third place, and central nervous system cancer was fourth.

Leukemia was the most frequent type of cancer in the children who were referred to Memorial Hospital in 1970, but bone cancer, embryonal rhabdomyosarcoma, and lymphoma were ahead of the abdominal tumors. (This referral pattern is also characteristic in other cancer centers such as the one at the M.D. Anderson Hospital and Tumor Institute in Houston, Texas.)

Each year more and more children with cancer are surviving for five years or longer. Recent developments in chemotherapy and in treatment that combines surgery, radiation, and chemotherapy have brought about a decided change in the prognosis for a child with cancer, even when it is disseminated at the time of diagnosis. Twenty years ago, Wilms' tumor, the most commonly occurring kidney cancer in children, was considered about 20 percent curable whereas, today, 80 percent of the children with this disease are cured. One of the reasons for this has been earlier diagnosis and the cooperative efforts of surgeons, radiation therapists, and chemotherapists. In addition, intensive nursing care and supportive nursing actions have been helpful in carrying children through extensive operations and serious illnesses. Nevertheless, all cancers in children are desperate diseases, and the treatment may have to be desperate. The complications of treatment may sometimes appear to be life-threatening but, if they are anticipated they can be treated as they occur. Getting a child through one of these illnesses is a gratifying experience for physicians and nurses as well as for the child's parents.

THE HOLISTIC APPROACH TO THE CARE OF
CHILDREN WITH CANCER

The holistic approach to the care of children with cancer is multidisciplinary and involves physicians, nurses, dietitians, child psychologists and psychiatrists, social workers, recreation specialists, teachers, clergy of all faiths, volunteers, referral agencies, and personnel from other hospital departments. The center of the team approach is the patient and his family. The goal is to reduce the trauma of hospitalization and to return the child to as full a life as possible. The family concept of treatment must be kept in mind, as well as the enormous trauma they are experiencing. To set up a nursing care plan that will meet both the patient's and the family's physical and emotional needs, the nurse must ascertain the degree of the patient's illness and its severity, and whether this is a new diagnosis or whether the child is in relapse or terminally ill. She must also seek answers to many questions. What is the family constellation? Are the parents alive, separated, or divorced? Is the patient an only child and, if not, what is his place among his siblings? Is the child adopted or fostered? Has he been previously admitted to this or another hospital? Has the patient been an outpatient? Does he know the reason for his admission and its implications? Is the family experiencing any other crises at this time? In addition to this information, a profile of the child is obtained. This includes the child's age, religion, special likes and dislikes (this is extremely important in diet and fluid management), sleep habits, favorite toys or games, special routines, and whether he speaks or understands English.

Each child and each family will react in an individual way, both physically and emotionally, to the diagnosis and proposed treatment. Either may exhibit antisocial behavior that must be recognized and understood. The nurse needs to be aware of the special problems created by the child's changed physical appearance. Weight loss, alopecia, enlarged tumors, or the presence of certain lesions may lead to rejection of the patient by the family, other children, and visitors. The child becomes angry and fearful and, subsequently, isolated if this problem is not worked through. By her acceptance of the patient, the nurse acts as a guide for others.

At Memorial Hospital, interdisciplinary conferences are held on a regularly scheduled basis and interim ones as necessary for identifying problems or crises that may occur or are current. Together, the team views these situations through the eyes of the patient and his family, and they respond accordingly. Honesty with both parents and child helps to develop a sense of trust.

Children's greatest fear is that of separation from parents. Those under the age of about six experience an intense feeling of abandonment. This is one reason why it is important that visiting rules and regulations be flexible on a child's first hospital admission, or if he is critically ill. The night nurse is often the first to observe signs of anxiety. The child may be unable to sleep and require a light left on in the room. He may use symbols in trying to communicate and the nurse must be astute to recognize what he is trying to say. For example, a child may exhibit extreme apprehension about an impending procedure and, when the nurse speaks gently to the child, she often discovers a deeper anxiety.

Patient and family teaching is one of the nurse's primary responsibilities. Careful explanation and discussion of procedures or changes in condition aid in relieving anxiety in both patient and family. To be able to participate in activities, the patient must be as comfortable as possible. Adequate pain medication and good nursing care help realize this goal. Children are special people, and when they have repeated admissions or lengthy stays in the hospital, all disciplines must work together to provide as normal an atmosphere as is feasible under the circumstances. Personnel from other departments, as well as members of the team, all make contributions toward creating such a milieu. For example, the dietary department assists in planning birthday and holiday celebrations; the clergy provide a non-denominational Sunday service on the unit, and the children derive great pleasure from their participation, from singing, and from the use of musical instruments. Volunteers help to occupy many hours of the day for them. The philosophy is to maintain an informal atmosphere that serves to familiarize the patient and family with the members of the team and personnel on the unit. The play deck, with its flowers and play houses, is utilized whenever the weather permits.

Attendance at the hospital's school for children provides a normal activity. When a child and his parents first come to the hospital, they are very apprehensive, anxious, and frightened. When they are taken on a tour of the unit and see the schoolroom, some of these feelings of strangeness are dispelled, for, to a child, school is part of his daily life — familiar ground — something he knows about. The school at Memorial Hospital is a public school conducted under the supervision of the New York City Board of Education. (About one hundred such classes are conducted in hospitals in New York City.) The teachers are well trained and qualified, and all have degrees in special education. School is in session from 9:00 A.M. to 3:00 P.M., Monday through Friday. Ambulatory children receive their instruction in the schoolroom and others are taught at the bedside. Instruction is given in small groups or individually as needed. The grade range is from one through twelve, and the teacher tries to keep the children up to their grade level. Some children miss entire blocks of learning experience because of prolonged illness or long hospital stays. Therefore, remedial work plays a very important part in the educational program. The teacher sends each child's records back to his home school so he will receive credit for instruction as well as attendance. The teacher must keep in mind the emotional, psychological, physical, and educational needs of all the children in the group, and map out a program that will meet these needs as well as the individual needs of each child.

The social worker contributes to the total care of the child through a network of tangible services that can be utilized to provide relief for the family confronted with the constant burden and awareness of a child's diagnosis of cancer. These services might include advice about nearby hotel accommodations, homemaker services, special transportation plans, or advice about how financial assistance can be secured. Some families may feel particularly uncertain and unprepared for a sophisticated treatment program. While many families manage well and independently, others may ask the social worker to help interpret a protocol that seems beyond their depth. They may need an interpreter and guide, since the words they hear, the behavior they observe, and the complex treatment system seen in the pediatric pavilion and the outpatient department may have an effect that one father described as being like a surrealistic dream. For him, and others like him, every incident in the unfamiliar environment can be a source of uncertainty. Because these are intially acutely anxious families, the social worker may use a stream of supportive techniques which, at this stage, might include efforts to improve communication between the hospital system and the family's private system, slowing down the input of newness, and bolstering the parents' sense of control and mastery by helping them live from day to day. Above all, she might communicate her willingness to anticipate their needs in a totally generous spirit, as this is the essence of providing a climate of emotional support.

The course of treatment for children with cancer may be marked by unnerving unpredictability and seemingly random periods of remission and relapse. It is a uniquely stressful course of treatment, since it compels a family to tolerate uncertainty and conflict for prolonged periods of time. For many families, the physicians, nurses, and other staff members become a treasured and trusted second family; others are particularly vulnerable and react with panic, much like people caught up in a natural catastrophe. Constant change and newness can boost the price of making decisions. Families need to know that they may be affected by the child's illness on three levels — the sensory level, the cognitive level, and the decisional level. They may sense the new situation, think it through, and finally decide on courses of action which may or may not be appropriate. The social worker can help the family to try to "re-program" themselves, since all their painfully pieced together bits of behavioral routines may not help them in solving this new medical problem. In fact, clinging rigidly to familiar behavior may even intensify the new problems, and the social worker may serve as a kind of guide who can provide them with rather special knowledge that can be helpful in reducing the seemingly unbearable level of stress created by a sequence of what appear to be unending and unmanageable problems. She must convey that her service exists to offer support to patients and that her policies and procedures are shaped by their needs.

The child psychiatrist views the pediatric cancer patient as a child first of all—regardless of his diagnosis, his pain, his suffering. From the point of view of the child, the first situation he faces in his illness is the learning of his diagnosis. The crucial question as to whether the patient should be told his diagnosis has been discussed for years. The child with cancer is unique in that his life experiences have been different from those of other children. For a child, the process of learning must be accompanied by affect. Often, in clinical practice, nurses will observe a child being taught without affect by a teacher or by his parents. He learns as a computer learns, and stores the data he collects but it has no emotional meaning for him. Cold, detached mothers have been observed explaining diagnoses and prognoses to their terminally ill children. The child who collects data that is presented without affect may later express what he has learned by broadcasting his terrifying diagnosis to staff members and other patients who, in turn, become anxious and sometimes even panicky. This is not a picture of healthfulness or acceptance on the part of the patient, but rather the result of a disturbed learning process. The anxiety it creates in nurses is not pathological; it is the consequence of being in contact with bizarre behavior. New knowledge that comes to a child must produce a pleasurable sensation in order for him to explore it further — to go ahead. It is impossible to really learn in the vital sense of the words "to learn" if those who are teaching or telling one things display no affect. When his mother, or someone who does not give him the proper affect along with the information, tells a child with cancer about his diagnosis and about the probable course of his disease, the child becomes aware of the facts but he does not know what they mean. Then he is likely to run about saying, "I'm dying" or "I'm very sick," and both patients and nursing staff are shocked at hearing a seven-year-old child say such things. The mother may remark, "See how wonderful my child is. He's only seven years old, but he knows all these big words and everything about his illness. Can you see how strong, how mature he is?" The child's behavior, however, does not represent strength, or maturity. It represents disturbed learning, and the child's behavior can be classed as disturbed behavior. Such behavior produces disturbed reactions in the staff — sometimes fear, sometimes confusion.

On the other hand, the nurse often sees children who are isolated from their fears. To staff members and physicians, such a child appears uncooperative, irritable, hostile, demanding, depressed, uncommunicative, and to have poor sleeping and eating habits. This child lacks trust, and what he exhibits is despair. He is extremely infantile, in panic and desperate, fighting for his life. Nurses often feel ambivalent, helpless, and unable to deal with this chaotic situation which deteriorates day by day. But the child can not behave in any other way. Typically, in such cases, the child's mother is isolated from the parents of other children on the ward; is demanding, intolerant, abusive, nasty, and sometimes hostile to the nurses; is inconsiderate of other patients; does not follow hospital rules regarding visiting or other privileges; is critical of everyone and especially of the hospital staff. The social history of the family reveals that the patient was always "different". He had few friends and poor relations with his siblings, was fearful at night and many times shared his mother's bed. His father was a busy, distant, uninvolved, passive but angry man who, in the hospital, is more reasonable than his wife. But he is also ineffective. This symbiotic syndrome between mother and patient existed long before the child's diagnosis was known. Often nurses who are caught up in such a situation react with helplessness, frustration, and even anger, and this is understandable.

In both of the examples described above, what is needed is the intervention of someone with warmth and compassion; someone who can infuse some affect into the concept of the child's illness. Otherwise, the child will continue to be unreachable. The intervening person may be a psychiatrist, but not necessarily. The patient has to find out that tears are healthy and fear is normal. But to learn this he has to have someone with him, and it must always be remembered that he is still a child.

The term "symbiosis" is defined as "an advantage relationship" between two abnormal people who become dependent on each other. This is the kind of relationship that exists between the mother and child in the second illustration cited earlier. The therapeutic approach in such a situation involves everyone concerned with the care of the child; individuals who try to combat this kind of syndrome alone will be destroyed. Expecting adherence to rules and regulations and taking the professional approach with firmness and honesty is the only possible therapeutic tool that the staff can use in dealing with this painful syndrome. The nurse's role should not be that of judge or jury, but rather that of an observer who has special skills and training, who consults with supervisors for psychiatric advice in order to learn the patient's whole situation, and who acts accordingly, always with the sense of being part of the whole effort.

The holistic approach to the care of the pediatric cancer patient pays high dividends. The nursing care of these children is intensive and sometimes very frustrating because small children are unable to relay their symptoms or significant feelings. However, more and more children with cancer are doing well because they are receiving early diagnosis and treatment, and because *all* of their needs are being met — not just those that are created by their disease. Briefly, a few of the encouraging outcomes observed by one nurse in the children's pavilion at Memorial Hospital include the following:

A newborn baby with a diagnosis of neuroblastoma was treated with surgery, x-ray, and chemotherapy, and has survived to the age of four months.

Another patient who had a hemipelvectomy for embryonal rhabdomyosarcoma at the age of 18 months is now a young teenager living a very active normal life.

A six-year-old boy with a diagnosis of lymphosarcoma of the neck was treated with surgery, x-ray, and chemotherapy, and has survived to the age of 16. He has no apparent symptoms of disease and he, too, is leading an active, normal life.

A child of 14 months with a diagnosis of neuroblastoma who had such severe symptoms that his prognosis was completely negative, has survived to the age of 21 with no evidence of disease or disability.

A set of identical twins in whom Wilms' tumor was diagnosed — one nine months after the other — were treated with x-ray, surgical removal of the kidney, and actinomycin D, and have received several courses of actinomycin D since. Now, after several years, they, too, are alive and leading normal lives.

EARLY DIAGNOSIS AND TREATMENT ARE VITAL

Diagnosis and early treatment at a curable stage of cancer is as important in children as it is in adults. But, since cancer in children is very rare, how can early detection be accomplished when the average pediatrician will probably encounter only one or two cases in a lifetime of practice? Cancer is not a reportable disease, and thus public health departments cannot publish statistics regarding the number of children in whom cancer is diagnosed in a given week, month, or year.

The first responsibility of the nurse who is a member of a care team that takes the holistic approach to pediatric cancer nursing is to assist in securing early diagnosis and treatment for children with cancer. Since cancer is second only to accidents in causing death in children, the professional nurse plays an important role in all efforts to reduce this statistic. She may observe children in the hospital, in schools, in well baby clinics, public health stations, or among relatives or friends. Because of her knowledge of the early signs of malignancy, she can be instrumental in directing children to the help they may need.

Ideally, however, everybody belongs on the team for improving the survival of children who will be developing cancer. Adults who are responsible for children should know the types of cancer to suspect in each age group. Children depend on adults to get them an early diagnosis. The cancer specialist is of little value in the population laboratory, where among 57 million living children only about four thousand will develop cancer each year; one of his major roles must be educational.

Infants' monthly visits to physicians' assistants should include a cancer examination. The preschool child should have a cancer examination twice yearly and, after five years of age, at least yearly with special attention to the presence of anemia, fatigue, and an unexplained lump or abdominal mass. The adolescent should have a yearly examination that includes examination of the genitalia. An estimated 500 cases of Wilms' tumor are diagnosed in the United States each year, of which 80 percent are curable. Another 500 develop neuroblastoma each year. Until cancer research comes forth with some better kinds of tests than we now have for identifying susceptibility to cancer in children, the only way it can be found early enough for cure is by searching for it in the asymptomatic child. Leukemia, the most frequent of the cancers that occur in children, may be misdiagnosed, and this results in long delays in instituting proper treatment. Because of the bone and joint symptoms of this disease, it is often erroneously diagnosed and treated as rheumatic fever, sometimes for as long as six or more months. Second come abdominal tumors which are diagnosed as subacute appendicitis or mesenteric adenitis and, a few weeks or months after the child is operated on, the true diagnosis is made, often through the discovery of a metastatic lesion. Third, a tumor is often incised under the impression that it is an abscess. Finally, a mild athletic injury may be suggested to explain bone pain which may, in fact, be a lytic and proliferative bone lesion in progress.

The diagnosis of leukemia is confirmed by bone marrow aspiration, and that of a solid tumor by histologic examination. These tests are probably best carried out by the team who will initiate the treatment. Ideally, treatment should be at a cancer center, for two reasons: 1) the accumulated cancer experience of the medical staff is greater than that of the staff of a general hospital and, since supportive therapy is often complicated, chances of cure are better; and 2) the urgency of collecting information that characterizes each type of cancer, and for searching out distinguishing features of each type is considerable. For example, in addition to the histologic study of biopsied material, an electronmicroscopic study should be made; attempts should be made to establish a tissue culture line; and studies for possible viruses and for chromosomal abnormalities of the malignant cells should be carried out. Small amounts of serum should be collected and frozen for future identification of antibodies as the science of immunology opens up new understanding of cancer. Characteristics of the normal family members should also be studied.

One such center is located at the Memorial Hospital for Cancer and Allied Diseases, in New York City where, in 1934, the first cancer ward in the world for children was established. It consisted of four beds. Now the children's pavilion at this hospital has 13 rooms and 26 beds, of which four are especially designed for postoperative patients. The pavilion includes a treatment room, an intravenous room, a children's library, classroom, recreation room, and outside porch. (The new Memorial Hospital will have 25 rooms and 40 beds for children.) Four hundred children, ranging in age from the newborn to teen-age, are admitted annually. The outpatient department and the Day Hospital handle approximately 12,000 visits a year. Separate medical and nursing staffs in addition to those who care for the children around the clock are required for these day patients. They number 65 to 85 a day and are seen by appointment between 8:00 A.M. and 5:00 P.M. five days a week. The attending staff consists of seven full-time pediatricians, a child psychologist, and a pediatric surgeon. Serving part-time are a child psychiatrist, a pediatric diagnostic radiologist, and a pediatric neurologist. In addition, all the departments, services, and research laboratories at Memorial Hospital and the Sloan-Kettering Institute for Cancer Research participate in the care, treatment, and study of the children. At all times there are eight first- or second-year pediatric interns and residents from eight pediatric training programs in New York City rotating for from four to eight weeks' intensive experience with cancer on the Children's Pavilion; they total 60 each year.

The Workup

One or all of the team members who will be giving the definitive treatment (the surgeon, the radiotherapist, and the chemotherapist) plan the workup for a child who, on preliminary examination, is likely to have a malignant tumor. The early strategy consists of determining the extent of the disease in order to delineate the anatomical areas to which treatment will be directed, and also to formulate an opinion regarding the ability of the child's normal organs and systems to tolerate the necessary treatment. Although one usually associates a bone marrow examination with a diagnosis of leukemia, the round cell sarcomas of children (neuroblastoma, embryonal rhabdomyosarcoma, and lymphosarcoma) may also invade and replace the marrow and modify the child's resistance to treatment. Therefore, a bone marrow aspiration will be done. The intravenous pyelogram (IVP) is usually associated with the diagnostic workup for Wilms' tumor or neuroblastoma of the adrenal gland. However, it is important to include an IVP in the workup of patients with newly diagnosed leukemia, since the finding of enlarged kidneys (due to infiltration by leukemic cells and decreased renal function) at the diagnosis of acute leukemia means that intensive drug treatment must be instituted cautiously because, as chemotherapy destroys the leukemic cells and causes the lymph nodes, liver, and spleen to shrink, these cell breakdown products are converted to uric acid which must be eliminated by the patient's kidneys.

The team members within the cancer center include the nurses who must reassure the child and his parents, and speed up the diagnostic workup. Detailed records concerning each child must be collected from all outside physicians, offices, and hospitals that have been involved with the child's care. The anesthesiologist and the diagnostic radiologist are also part of this team. The pathology department can be counted on to come through with a diagnosis of benign or malignant disease within a maximum of 48 hours, often within ten minutes, from the time a piece of tissue is submitted to them. Often the biopsy is not done until the patient and the surgeon are prepared to go ahead immediately with an extensive surgical procedure if the biopsy frozen section report is positive for malignancy. The radiation therapist needs to know exactly the extent of normal structures within a field that he will be asked to irradiate. Since he is included on the diagnostic team, he can give this request preoperatively to the surgeon who can then mark with tiny silver clips the margins of the kidney to be spared, or the margins of an inoperable tumor to be irradiated. The chemotherapists on the team are prepared with knowledge of results of active chemotherapeutic agents that have been used in similar cases.

Together, during the diagnostic workup, immediately preoperatively, and again postoperatively, the team members meet with a pathologist to plan the best possible treatment with a minimal sacrifice of normal structures and tissues. During the workup, the social worker, the child psychologist, and the child psychiatrist interview and test the child and the family for distinguishing characteristics that will serve as a base line for orientation to problems they might have in accepting the cancer treatment. It is important to emphasize again that parents and nurses must work closely with physicians so that children with cancer may be given the best possible chance for life and its best quality. More hope can now be given to parents than was possible in the past, because the lives of many of these children are now being comfortably prolonged and more cures are being obtained.

Most commonly, the leukemic child exhibits pallor, fatigue, adenopathy, abdominal pain, ecchymoses, or pains in the bones and joints. The child with a brain tumor may have an enlarged head, walking difficulties, early morning vomiting, headache, and behavior problems. A large abdominal mass may indicate a Wilms' tumor of the kidney, a liver malignancy, or a neuroblastoma of adrenal origin. Persistent swelling anywhere—in the muscles of the head or neck, extremities, or external genitalia—may be early signs of cancer. In older children, pain in the bones is the earliest indication of cancer, and it occurs even before a swelling is noticeable.

At present, there are more different kinds of treatment regimens being proposed than there are children with cancer to test them on. It is essential to define clearly the absolute minimum of treatment that will cure the child. If the national goal is to eradicate cancer (as defined by the President and Congress in the National Cancer Act of 1971) and, in the meantime, to diagnose and administer optimum treatment, it is imperative that we study every child with cancer and administer optimal treatment for as long as is necessary to cure him and to keep his emotional, physical, and intellectual developmental processes on schedule, and that we continue his follow-up into adulthood. On the other hand, many children referred to cancer centers do not have cancer. They may be diagnosed and referred back to their family doctors for treatment of such conditions as infectious mononucleosis, tuberculosis, toxoplasmosis, or hemangioma. A biopsy may show a benign bone or soft tissue cyst, a benign teratoma, or a benign pigmented nevus.

CHEMOTHERAPEUTIC TREATMENT

Leukemia

As late as 1947 there was no hope of palliation for acute leukemia in children. Gradually, however, eight new chemotherapeutic agents were found, all of which produce remission in this disease. When they are used one at a time to obtain a remission, the leukemic cell disappears from the bone marrow, the normal bone marrow function returns, and enlarged organs and nodes return to their normal size. When used in sequence, they will produce successive remissions. However, the 50 percent survival rate of children with acute lymphoblastic leukemia treated in this way is only about 18 months. Therefore, in the mid-1960's, a concept of treatment based on knowledge of growth rates of leukemic cells and of the mechanisms by which drugs kill cells, suggested a new strategy.

This strategy, which is still being used in the treatment of acute leukemia, is to establish the cytologic type which, in 80 percent of the children is acute lymphoblastic leukemia, and then to select a treatment protocol based on the cytologic type with the objective of restoring normal function by inducing a remission of the disease, preventing relapse after induction, and promoting consolidation of remission by vigorous drug treatment. At Memorial Hospital, the concentration presently is on the last part of the strategy—preventing relapse. Formerly, the physician would ease up on the treatment when a patient got into a remission of his disease. The present procedure is to consolidate the remission with further intensive treatment following the induction course of drugs. The remission is maintained by repeated five-day cycles of drugs alternating with five days of ᵣrest. Measures are also taken to prevent meningeal leukemia by also administering drugs periodically into the cerebrospinal fluid. Consideration is now being given to continuing the treatment for two years, but how long the treatment will be required to prevent return of leukemia is not yet known.

The L-2 protocol (at Memorial Hospital) for lymphoblastic leukemia is quite complicated. It starts with an induction series of drugs given over about four weeks to get the patient's bone marrow into a complete (or M-1) state. The induction drugs are four weekly doses of vincristine, daily prednisone, and two doses of daunorubicin (Daunomycin). The patient then has a rest period of ten to 15 days, and then the consolidation phase takes place. Cytosine arabinoside (Ara-C) is given intravenously and thioguanine orally for five days followed by five days of rest, then treatment and rest, treatment and rest; and then L-asparaginase which is very specific against leukemic cells, three times weekly for one month followed by a maintenance phase. Each maintenance phase is composed of cycles of five days of treatment, five days of rest, treatment and rest, treatment and rest, which takes a total of 50 days; then the maintenance phase is repeated over and over again. About 96 percent of children tried on this protocol have achieved complete remission. The goal is total kill of the leukemic cells. If, by calculation, there are about three trillion leukemic cells present at the time the disease is diagnosed, induction will lower this to 85 million. The strategy is to reduce the number of leukemic cells by a course of treatment; let them rest and recruit non-dividing cells into the dividing pool; let the number go up again and then give another course of consolidation with drugs which can readily kill cells synthesizing DNA just prior to mitosis, until finally all of the leukemic cells have (theoretically) been destroyed. Then the maintenance phase is carried out for years to kill any returning leukemic cells which might have been missed during the induction and consolidation.

The first 26 children who were enrolled in the L-2 protocol as their first treatment for leukemia had fewer relapses than those in another group of patients who had had some other prior therapy before they were enrolled in this protocol. The same results have been achieved in a succeeding 25 patients. In addition, meningeal leukemia is usually expected to develop in about 25 percent of the patients during the first year of their disease, in 50 percent during the second year, and 75 percent during the third year. But there have been no cases of meningeal leukemia in the patients who were enrolled in this protocol as their initial treatment, and none were given radiation therapy to avoid meningeal leukemia. The first patient enrolled in this study is now 28 months along his course.

Solid Malignant Tumors

Solid malignant tumors in children are treated with vincristine and other drugs that are classified as alkylating agents, antimetabolites, and anticancer antibiotics. In general, these agents are all active against the sarcomas of children. One drug, o,p,'DDD (discovered as a chemical contaminant of DDT), is very specific for one kind of cancer—adrenal cortical carcinoma. It can be used even in the successful management of metastatic disease, and will sometimes return the patient to a state of health. A seven-year-old girl entered Memorial Hospital in 1968 with a diagnosis of metastatic adrenal cortical carcinoma of such extent that she was having hemoptysis. She was treated with this drug and still has had no return of her widespread abdominal and pulmonary metastatic disease. An undesirable side-effect is destruction of all normal adrenal function and she must receive substitution hormone therapy as if she had had bilateral adrenalectomy. She is growing normally, however. In some cases, surgery is employed for treatment of metastatic tumors, or surgery, radiation, and chemotherapy together.

Complications Arising in Children Receiving Chemotherapy

The primary complications that arise in children under chemotherapy are infection, hemorrhage, such central nervous system diseases as leukemic meningitis, infectious meningitis, or cord compression and, sometimes, superior vena cava syndrome.

Infection is the most common non-hematologic complication in children receiving chemotherapy. It is associated with the bone marrow depression that occurs with this therapy, and/or the production of immature cells in bone marrow relapse, either of which diminishes the normal body defenses. Nursing measures and observations to be made should be included in the nursing care plan. Mouth sores may be the first indication of difficulty in the gastrointestinal tract. Therefore, the patient's mouth must be checked daily (using a flashlight) for redness, white patches, or ulcers. Frequent mouth care including sprays or oral irrigations with saline and Cepacol, is started when therapy is initiated. This routine is preventive as well as therapeutic and, when started early, helps the child to become accustomed to the procedures before sores develop. Severe mucosal breakdown is treated with half strength hydrogen peroxide for effective debridement. The physician often orders Mycostatin in suspension at this time. All mouth care must be done around the clock because, with intensive nursing care, these infections clear in approximately four to eight days. Soft toothettes are used so as not to cause bleeding of the gums, since a low platelet count may make bleeding from any source dangerous. Special precautions must be taken when handling nursing bottles and pacifiers, and their use should be limited whenever possible. Because nausea and vomiting are common side-effects of chemotherapy, and breakdown of the mucosal tissue frequently occurs, a full liquid to soft diet with protein supplements should be used.

The rectal and perineal area should be checked daily for redness, fissures, or other signs of infection. Rectal temperatures are eliminated whenever possible. Thorough cleansing is essential. Sitz baths and the use of a bedside lamp as a heat lamp are very helpful, as are the antibacterial ointments that are applied after cleansing.

Upper respiratory infections require prompt supportive care in order to prevent pneumonia. These children often do not develop the usual bacterial types of pneumonia, but are prone to fungal infections. Any change in the child's condition, even the development of a slight cough, must be reported to the physician immediately, so that prompt action can be taken. A slight cough may be the first sign of rapidly progressing pneumonia. If pneumonia should develop, routine nursing measures must be intensified. The small child will not move or turn from side to side when he is very ill. Therefore, it is essential that the nurse turn him frequently and institute deep breathing and coughing on a one- to two-hour basis. For the child who is reluctant to breathe deeply, the use of blow bottles can be helpful; often one child will challenge another and they make a game of using the bottles. Humidification in the form of cold steam, or a control tent with compressed air or oxygen will help to relieve congestion. When oxygen therapy is required, the tent is preferred because it is less frightening to a child than having a mask put over his face. A tent with thermostatic controls can be used for cooling purposes when the patient's temperature is greatly elevated, and is preferred over the cooling mattress. A child tends to curl up into the fetal position when ill and, in addition, the severe chills and petechiae that may occur when the cooling mattress is used for these particular patients, make the tent preferable. Children with large lymph nodes, or tumors in the head or neck area, must be closely observed for respiratory obstruction.

Skin infections may result from needle punctures, leukemic infiltrates, or general breakdown of tissue. Children on chemotherapy have frequent spinal taps and bone marrow aspirations, and venipuncture is frequently necessary to obtain blood for various diagnostic procedures, to maintain fluid balance, and to administer chemotherapeutic drugs, high doses of antibiotics, blood and blood products, or analgesic agents. Every venipuncture creates a potential site of infection; therefore, extra care is taken with regard to cleanliness, and all possible precautions must be taken to prevent infection. The child's skin is cleansed with alcohol before any venipuncture is performed. Continuous intravenous infusions are carefully dated as to the time they are started, and the needle site is changed every three days. All tubing used with continuous intravenous infusions is changed daily. The tendency to bleeding that results from lowered platelet counts also requires the nurse to consistently take such precautions as rotating the injection sites and applying prolonged pressure after venipuncture. Intramuscular injections cannot be given to children with decreased platelet counts. Cutdowns are almost never used because they increase the potentiality of infection and bleeding and because they destroy veins that will be needed in the future. These children require more blood studies, diagnostic procedures, intravenous infusions, and drugs than patients in any other situation. The nurse can be instrumental in keeping venipunctures to a minimum by attempting to coordinate all these procedures.

The white cell count may be low, and this makes the patient less resistant to invading organisms and also unable to form pus. Therefore, the nurse must be careful to observe, and quickly report, the appearance of any localized reddened areas. Thorough, frequent inspection and cleansing of the skin, and changing of bandages and dressings are essential. Dressings should be limited whenever possible in order to allow constant observation of the skin. Nursing responsibilities include observation for streaks, redness, swelling, or patient complaints of discomfort. Good manicures are important since small children will scratch themselves and transfer bacteria to broken skin areas. *All* skin surfaces should be observed daily for redness, swelling, tenderness, open lesions, and Pseudomonas lesions. Pseudomonas lesions are usually tiny with a black center at first. It is extremely important to notice these lesions early so that prompt treatment can be started, since progression of infection and septic shock can be extremely rapid and may not be reversible in the later stages. Just picking at a toe or the cuticle around a fingernail can break the skin sufficiently to create a portal for entry of such infections. When the lesion is caught early, the area is cleansed with Betadine Surgical Scrub and antibiotics are administered. Large, progressive lesions are covered with Adaptic gauze which does not stick, or Kerlix gauze. This reduces the possibility of contamination, makes dressing changing easier, and prevents the child and his family from seeing the lesion which might be very upsetting to them.

The patient must also be protected from infection by the organisms that cause any of the *communicable diseases*. The child with cancer may have more severe reactions and complications from such diseases than other children because of the chemotherapeutic agents he is receiving.

Any of the infections or conditions mentioned here may lead to overwhelming sepsis. Often this will occur even when all necessary care and precautions have been taken. Children with depressed bone marrow are very susceptible. Therefore, in order that prompt treatment can be initiated, the nurse must observe the patient closely and immediately report to the physician such developments as: 1) sudden change in any of the vital signs, including either an elevated or a subnormal temperature; 2) acute abdominal pain, which may indicate a ruptured abscess; 3) lethargy or confusion; 4) skin changes or lesions; and 5) decreased urinary output. It is very important for the nurse to be aware that a child who has a depressed or a recovering white blood cell count, who is not on antibiotics or running a fever, and who suddenly "spikes" a fever, is most probably septic. *Treatment must be prompt.* This usually consists of an immediate blood culture and, without waiting several days for a result, initiating high doses of broad spectrum antibiotics, sometimes adrenal steroids, and other supportive measures to maintain life. Constant monitoring of the child's condition is imperative. Children whose white blood count is below 1,000 are usually placed in room isolation for protection. Routine isolation technique is carried out for any child with a suspicious rash or lesion.

Hemorrhage is the second most important complication that must be considered in the nursing management of children with cancer, particularly leukemia. The nurse's responsibilities include the monitoring of vital signs; being alert to symptoms of shock; checking daily the skin and orifices for petechiae, ecchymoses, or bleeding; seeing that stools, urine, and vomitus are tested for guaiac; being aware of the daily blood count reports and their possible implications, such as epistaxis that may result from a low platelet count; and reporting any sharp abdominal pain or severe headache to the physician. The nurse must be skilled in handling any bleeding complication; she must know how to do nasal packings, and how to use pressure dressings or Gelfoam pads, if necessary.

Platelet transfusions can be a tremendously helpful factor in reducing the incidence of hemorrhage. A type and cross match specimen record is kept up-to-date for all children with any tendency toward bleeding. When the platelet count is low, antibiotics, analgesics, sedatives, and other necessary medications are administered orally or intravenously. The use of intramuscular injections is severely restricted as they may cause large hematomas, continuous bleeding or oozing, lack of absorption of a vital medication and, in addition, may become sites of infection. Such procedures as bone marrow aspiration or spinal tap should be scheduled after the child has had a platelet transfusion whenever this is possible; if the coagulation and bleeding time are abnormally prolonged, pressure must be applied for a much longer interval.

Central nervous system involvement is the most difficult complication to handle in children with cancer. The nurse should report immediately the following symptoms, any one of which may indicate increased intracranial pressure: headache; dizziness; nausea; vomiting; dilated pupils; cranial nerve palsies; any change in vision; increased blood pressure; slow pulse; or decreased respirations.

The physician will usually initiate treatment with a regimen of adrenal steroids and intrathecal methotrexate. He may also employ x-ray therapy. The patient is placed on convulsive precautions, and anticonvulsive drugs are administered as necessary. Bacterial invasion of the central nervous system is treated with high doses of antibiotics intrathecally as well as intravenously.

Children with solid tumors may develop metastasis to the brain or lesions of the spinal cord. The nurse must carefully observe for any of the symptoms mentioned above, as well as for indications of cord depression. These changes include any alteration in urinary or bowel habits; lack of movement, feeling, or sensation in the extremities; gait changes; and changes in muscle tone and activity. It is extremely important that these symptoms be reported promptly to the physician so a diagnosis can be made and therapy begun immediately in order to prevent the development of paralysis.

Leukemic infiltrations can occur in organs, bones, nerve roots, and the central nervous system. Fortunately, aggressive and prophylactic therapy has made these infiltrations less common now than they were in the past.

Bone marrow depression is one of the major toxic effects of cancer chemotherapy. The bone marrow might be described as a factory that constantly produces both red and white blood cells and platelets. However, it is extremely sensitive to all drugs, thus limiting the dosages of chemotherapeutic agents that can be given. A course of chemotherapy that produces bone marrow depression causes a serious reduction in the manufacture of elements the bone marrow normally produces. As a result, the patient may become anemic and susceptible to infection, and may develop bleeding tendencies due to the reduction in platelets. The chemotherapy nurse carefully records the amount of blood that is drawn each day in an effort to aid the physician in his treatment of the child with anemia which may be due either to the disease or to bone marrow depression. Blood studies are extensive in cancer patients. Hence, the nurse must report any large amounts of blood drawn from a child with a falling hemoglobin, and request a reevaluation of all blood tests ordered. Because of their small blood volume, this is especially true of pediatric patients.

The nursing problems encountered in providing good care for the child with leukemia or a solid tumor that is being managed medically, are the results of the complications of his illness and of the therapy that is required. Whatever drugs the patient is receiving, the nurse must be acutely aware of their effects and keep the patient under constant observation. She must know exactly what drugs the child is receiving, their modes of action, their toxic effects, and whether these effects will be evident immediately or later. One important nursing function is the keeping of strict intake and output records in order to monitor renal function. Cell breakdown in patients receiving chemotherapy results in high uric acid formation; therefore, the doctor usually orders electrolyte and renal function tests frequently. The nurse should encourage the patient to take fluids; record intake and output accurately; make frequent specific gravity determinations of the urine; and promptly report excessive lethargy and confusion which may indicate an elevated blood urea nitrogen or uric acid.

The Nurse's Role on the Chemotherapy Team

The great number of venipunctures required for workup and treatment of neoplastic diseases, and the obvious difficulties in carrying out this procedure in children, have made the development of a team of nurses skilled in this technique essential. These nurses perform all of the procedures that require venipuncture—starting continuous and intermittent infusions of blood, plasma, and platelets; drawing blood for routine testing and research studies; and preparing conventional and research chemotherapeutic drugs to be administered by physicians. They work in the inpatient department during the children's initial workup and treatment, and continue to work with them as they come to the outpatient department for their frequent intravenous injections and blood tests. Therefore, the chemotherapy nurses pose no new threat to the children when they begin therapy as outpatients, or at any time that re-admission to the hospital is necessary. While the responsibilities of the nurses on this team are many and serious, the rewards are very special, for it is probably only through clinical research that a cure for cancer can be found.

Anticancer drugs are given to destroy, or at least alter, the reproductive ability of malignant cells. Unfortunately, these drugs are not selective enough to act only on malignant cells; many of them are equally toxic to normal cells and, therefore, the treatment plan may have to include treating the patient for toxicity which may manifest itself before a therapeutic effect can be obtained. The chemotherapy nurse must be aware of the drugs the child is receiving, their mode of action, and how their actions will affect procedures she performs on the child. Because cancer chemotherapy can cause such dangerous toxicities as bone marrow depression which can lead to anemia, infection, and bleeding, certainly these potentialities must always be uppermost in the nurse's mind as she draws up the drug for administration by the physician. She must be certain that the dose is accurate, and no physician ever objects to having his calculations checked by a nurse. If the appropriate dose of a chemotherapeutic agent can cause such dangerous toxicities, the nurse must surely be aware of the fact that an error leading to an overdose would most certainly be catastrophic—perhaps lethal.

Chemotherapy doses are calculated according to the patient's weight and, especially in pediatrics, are based on the surface area of the body (in square meters). Both the height and weight are used in calculating the "square meter" of a child, thus accurate heights and weights are essential. Since weight loss is a frequent side-effect during courses of chemotherapy, the child is weighed every day and any needed adjustment is made in the dosage of the drug to be given. Heights are taken at least once a month. Many children who are on high doses of prednisone retain fluids and have a markedly increased appetite, and thus they become cushingoid and overweight. Therefore, the nurse should be aware that the doses of chemotherapeutic drugs for these children should be based on the actual or pre-steroid weight; that is, the weight before the steroids were begun. If the drug were to be calculated on a child's steroid weight, with no allowance being made for this weight gain, an overdose of an extremely toxic drug would occur. The importance of correct calculation of chemotherapeutic drugs is illustrated by the following incident.

A child in relapse from acute lymphoblastic leukemia was admitted to Memorial Hospital after having been treated with prednisone for over two years. Along with tapering her dose of prednisone, the physicians had treated her with adriamycin, a new antitumor antibiotic whose side-effects include mouth lesions, bone marrow depression, loss of hair, gastrointestinal disturbances, and fever. Obviously, this child could not be allowed to receive an overdose of such a potentially dangerous medicine. Because of her severe obesity and the length of time she had been on steroids, her dose of adriamycin was calculated according to the average square meter surface area of a normal six-and-a-half-year old. Had this child's dose been calculated according to her steroid weight, she would have received almost twice as much adriamycin as she should have and surely would have suffered a severe toxic reaction.

The chemotherapy nurse's responsibility does not end with drawing up what she is certain is the accurate dose of drug for the physician to administer to the child. Both conventional and research drugs have many side-effects. Anaphylactic or allergic reactions to any of these drugs is a constant danger, and the nurse must be alert to this possibility. For example, a child may develop a rash over the entire body after being given an injection of L-asparaginase, an enzyme used in the treatment of acute leukemia; he develops antibodies to this enzyme and careful observation after administration is essential.

The nurse must also be aware of the toxicities that are specific to a drug, whether it is being used in conventional or research chemotherapy. Before a research drug is used on a pediatric patient, the chemotherapy nurses study all the available background data on the compound (sometimes only preclinical studies in animals are available) so they have an indication of what acute side-effects they must anticipate in the children to whom the drug is given. They also give a summary of this information to the staff nurses prior to the first patient trial, and aid the physician by keeping daily toxicity records on children after they are started on a new drug. These records include all expected and unexpected side-effects and toxicities a child develops during a course of the new drug as the dose is being advanced each day, and help the physician to know the tolerated dose and what to expect in future patients.

Still another danger that may accompany the use of many of the chemotherapeutic drugs that are given intravenously, is that leakage from the needle or vein into the tissues may cause necrosis at the site of injection. The nurse who starts either a continuous or an intermittent infusion of such a drug must be confident that the vein is patent before she asks the physician to administer the drug. For an intermittent infusion, patency is assured by rinsing the vein with sterile saline for injection before the drug is administered. The vein is again rinsed with saline after the administration to avoid allowing even a drop of the medicine to leak out of the vein into the tissues. Antecubital veins are never used for the administration of chemotherapeutic drugs. Despite all precautions, drug infiltrates can occur, and they are far more disastrous if they occur in the region of the antecubital veins than elsewhere. Should an infiltrate occur, continuous ice packs for 24 hours, intravenous antibiotics and fibrinolysin are utilized and, possibly, debridement of the necrotic area will be necessary.

SURGICAL TREATMENT

The parents' fear of surgery and their hope for the child's recovery make it essential to carefully prepare them for what to expect postoperatively. The nurse must stress the positive aspects of the situation and help parents to realize that the surgery to be performed is necessary to save the child's life. Their fears may be related to the possibility that the child will have a permanent handicap postoperatively, and that he will have to make a tremendous adjustment. Experience has shown that, with supportive help from the nurse, the child adapts very well, and that it is the other members of the family who require the most help in accepting the situation.

Nurses who give postoperative care to children who have undergone major surgery for a malignant tumor must know the patient's diagnosis and the special procedures that were performed. The nursing objective is to return the child to normal activities as soon as possible. To help prevent complications, the nurse must be fully aware of all therapies that the child may be receiving concurrently. Including preoperative teaching in the nursing care plan will help her identify what the child's physical and emotional needs are preoperatively and what they will probably be postoperatively.

In pediatric surgical nursing, all routine post-surgical measures (such as coughing and deep breathing) are carried out. In addition, when the child patient has undergone a major procedure, the nurse must have a sophisticated awareness of what complications may arise due to the patient's age, body size, and the anatomical proportions of his organs, or that may be the result of the child's response to surgery, previous operations, or other therapies he may have received—radiation therapy or chemotherapy, for instance.

Specialized Postoperative Care

The pediatric surgical nurse must know and understand how the vital signs and the anatomy of children differ from those of adults. The normal pulse rate for a child under two is over 100. A child who weighs 4 kilos will have a normal pulse rate of 130, whereas his blood pressure will be lower than that of an adult—78/50. A child who weighs 15 kilos normally has a pulse rate closer to that of an adult—95—and a blood pressure of 100/70. The tracheal lumen in a baby that weighs only 4 kilos measures 4 millimeters, and this must be kept in mind when the need for resuscitation measures arises. The normal tidal volume of an infant or baby weighing 4 kilos is 18 cc's for total lung expansion. Thus, if resuscitation is undertaken in any child under two years of age, extreme caution must be used, since the common cause of pneumothorax in these cases is excessive volume. As little as 15 cc's of water pressure will rupture an infant's pleura; thus, only two fingers pressure should be used when applying an Ambu bag.

The most important immediate responsibility of the nurse who cares for the postoperative pediatric patient is monitoring of the airway. A well-equipped emergency cart should be closely available. After intubation, the respiratory tract in all patients will be irritated and the bronchial secretions increase. The smaller the child, the more difficult the problem. If an endotracheal tube is used for more than four hours, a child may develop laryngeal edema. Decadron may be given to the child while he is still in the operating room in order to reduce the amount of spasm, which can increase dangerously without warning. Postoperative sedation should be limited; a crying child is the best indication of full lung expansion, and sedation is one of the most common causes of lung collapse in young children. The best indication of airway obstruction is a slowing of the pulse rate which will occur even before cyanosis, noisy respirations, and color change.

If the child has a tracheostomy, an x-ray should be done immediately to determine the position of the tube and the absence of pneumothorax. Silastic tubes are preferred, since mucus does not cake along the inside of the lumen. Even a small mucus plug can be fatal; therefore, frequent suctioning and excellent tracheostomy care are required. Since the trachea dries out very quickly, humidity is essential to prevent the development of a condition called *tracheitis sicca* in which the mucosa sloughs off. Antibiotics are not effective in treatment of this condition which is almost always fatal to children. The first sign of *tracheitis sicca* may be a small amount of bleeding when the child is suctioned. Infants who have this complication must be provided with 100 percent humidity for a minimum of 30 minutes of each hour.

Fluid replacement following surgery is of prime importance, and because this is based on the child's weight, correct postoperative weights are essential, particularly if a large tumor mass has been removed, or if the child has an amputation. If the child is in the zero to 10 kilogram weight range, his minimum 24-hour requirement will be 100 cc's per kilogram (e.g., weight = 8.5 kg; requirement = 850 cc's); if he is in the 10 to 20 kilogram range he will require 100 cc's for the first 10 kilos plus 50 cc's for each kilo over 10 (e.g., weight = 12 kilos; requirement = 1000 cc's for the first 10 kilos plus 100 cc's for the 2 kilos over 10, or total of 1100 cc's); if he weighs over 20 kilos he will require 20 cc's for each kilo over 20 (e.g., weight = 22 kilos; requirement = 1000 cc's for the first 10 kilos, 500 cc's for the next ten kilos and 40 kilos for the 2 kilos over 20, or a total of 1540 cc's).

As to electrolyte replacement, the sodium requirement is 40 mEq per 1,000 cc's of fluid, and 30 mEq of potassium per 1,000 cc's.

In addition to normal fluid losses during major surgery, there is a third space loss of fluid which is a hidden loss caused by fluids moving into the space previously occupied by the organs or nodes that were removed. These areas fill with fluid and serum which is composed of isotonic saline and plasma protein. Children generally require a plasma replacement equal to one-fourth of their blood volume for the first two or three postoperative days. Monitoring of third space loss is primarily a nursing responsibility. Since this is a hidden loss, the nurse must be aware of signs that she can use in monitoring the patient for this loss: 1) increase in pulse rate; 2) decrease in blood pressure; 3) a falling central venous pressure (CVP); and, 4) a falling urinary output. The CVP is a measure of the blood volume that passes through the heart and is accomplished by means of a catheter that is placed in the superior vena cava during the operation. The normal CVP in a child ranges from 6 to 12. A rising CVP means that the heart is overloaded, while a falling CVP indicates hypovolemia. Urinary output falls off after any surgery but should return to normal, unassisted, within 24 hours. The kidneys are very sensitive to blood volume changes, therefore, urinary output should be measured hourly. Output per day should measure two-thirds of the total fluid intake. The specific gravity of urine also provides a guideline and this, too, should be determined every one or two hours.

Fluid loss may also occur as a result of swelling of the bowel that is caused by ileus, which most children develop in some degree after surgery. To maintain circulation, the body replaces this loss by pulling fluid out of the tissues, thus causing dehydration. Insensible loss through lungs and skin must also be taken into consideration.

Postoperative fluid balance must be achieved, but not necessarily on a day to day basis. Because of the various fluid losses and the rentention of fluids, diuresis normally occurs on the third or fourth postoperative day when bowel function returns and fluids are again absorbed from it. Urinary output will rise markedly for a period of two or three days and, at the end of that time, intake and output should achieve balance. When strict monitoring of a small child's intake and output is required, it may be necessary to insert a Foley catheter.

The nurse who is responsible for the fluid and electrolyte management of the pediatric patient must be knowledgeable about the purposes of the various tubes and the methods that are used to convey different types of drainage to the exterior. The nasogastric tube drains gastric contents and, because this material is acid in reaction, alkalosis may occur and the child will require acid replacement. The loss of potassium is minimal, but chloride loss can be excessive and should be replaced with half strength normal saline, volume for volume, approximately every eight hours. The Anderson tube is frequently used for gastric suction and this requires the use of such an appliance as the Emerson pump. A gastrostomy tube is frequently used instead of the nasogastric tube for infants, because the larynx in these patients is small and the trachea can easily be blocked by a nasogastric tube. The management of a patient with a gastrostomy tube is the same as for one with a nasogastric tube. A tube that is placed in the ileum will drain normal saline which is alkaline. The fluid loss may cause the patient to become acidotic and to require replacement which is generally normal saline with bicarbonate as needed. Not much fluid is lost through a colostomy because the drainage becomes solid very quickly. Food intake should be resumed as soon as possible, since recovery progresses much more rapidly once the child is receiving his required daily caloric intake.

Fever, which may reach 103° the night following surgery, is most commonly caused by atelectasis or pneumonia. Fever that develops during the first two or three postoperative days is usually caused by an upper respiratory infection, although it may also be due to a urinary tract infection. The child who "spikes" a fever on the fourth or fifth day after the operation most likely has a wound infection or, possibly, an internal abscess. If he is receiving radiation therapy, the wound edges must be carefully checked frequently, since breakdown of tissue may occur. Temperature regulation is not the same in children as in adults. For example, a child may develop an infection but have little or no fever, or his temperature may be subnormal. Infection may also be hidden if the child is receiving, concurrently, therapy that causes immune suppression. The only indications of infection in a child may be weakness, lethargy, or lack of crying. On the other hand, an older child may have a significant rise in temperature when only a slight infection is present. Because infants have no means of regulating their body temperature, extra precautions should be taken for all children under the age of two. For example, warm "preps" should be used in the operating room, the child should be placed in a warming blanket, and waterproof Steridrapes should be used. The child should be kept very warm postoperatively; the infant should be placed in an Isolette.

Children have a tremendous ability to tolerate and recover from major surgery. They have excellent pulmonary, cardiovascular, and kidney functions. However, the first 48 postoperative hours are critical. Good nursing management can ensure a safe transition. The pediatric surgical nurse is rewarded by the fact that her patients recover quickly and by the knowledge that she has helped relieve some of the parents' and child's anxiety and fear through her teaching and supportive activities.

DAY HOSPITAL CARE

The pediatric day hospital is a specialized unit of Memorial Hospital that provides outpatient care and management for children with leukemia and other malignant diseases. Although this is a relatively new concept in cancer care, the increase in the number of patient visits during the year 1971 was over 2,000. The philosophy behind day hospital care for children is that the best place for any child is with his family and his friends, and at home if at all possible. The day hospital makes feasible the administration— on an outpatient basis—of intensive daily treatment that previously could only be carried out for a hospitalized child.

The day center is open daily from 8:00 A.M. to 5:00 P.M., and arrangements are made for weekend, evening, and night coverage should this be needed. The nursing staff includes a head nurse, three staff nurses, one nurses' aide and a clerk receptionist. In addition, a nurse is rotated monthly from the inpatient area for two reasons: first, the child is happy to see a nurse he knows from his previous hospital stay and second, the nurse benefits from seeing that children who had been very ill are now well enough to live at home and come to the day center for their treatments. One permanent staff member, the liaison nurse, has the special assignment of screening all incoming calls regarding new patients, makes the first appointments, interviews the parents, and obtains contagious disease and immunization histories. She is usually the first nurse contact that the patient and his parents have, and it is she who sets the tone for future child-parent-nurse relationships. Since the children are under treatment for prolonged periods of time, it is important that this relationship get off to a good start. Other staff members include a team of chemotherapy nurses, three hematology technicians, a record librarian, and a specially trained nurse and her assistant who collect data for statistical purposes.

Physically, the day hospital consists of six treatment rooms that are fully equipped for carrying out procedures ranging from physical examination to minor surgical operations that sometimes require anesthesia. Two bed-holding rooms contain six beds. Laboratory space is set aside for the use of the chemotherapy research nurses, and a small but complete hematology laboratory accommodates three technicians. Games, toys, and books are available in the waiting room where children can play until the time for their examination and treatment. Volunteers, called Bluebells by the children, help a great deal in keeping them occupied until time for their appointment. A large conference room, a record library, and a work area complete the unit.

All patients' parents are given a medication sheet so they can keep a record of anticancer drugs that the child is given by mouth, as well as any other medication that may be ordered, such as an antibiotic. They are asked to be extremely careful about recording accurately the medications, the time they are given, and whether the child has retained it or vomited it. They bring this record whenever they come to the day hospital with the child and it becomes a part of the permanent record.

The new patient is usually hospitalized for a battery of diagnostic tests, induction of therapy, and sometimes surgery. After only a few weeks of chemotherapy, a young child with acute leukemia may reach a stage of remission and be discharged to the day hospital for continued treatment. Often, both the child and his parents are apprehensive about future treatment. The parents, particularly, may be frightened or even angry at the ramifications of the diagnosis. The mother may feel inadequate and unable to meet the new needs of her child. The outpatient nurse must be aware of the emotional and physical ordeal that parent and child are experiencing, and realize that it is normal for these parents to be bitter, hostile, bewildered, frightened, and depressed. But, with patience and understanding, she can win their confidence. She explains all the points the doctor has made about the treatment, the medications that must be given, and how to keep the medication record. The mother is given all the information she needs and is instructed to watch for signs of toxicity and for any other sign that may indicate the child is not doing as well as he might. She is assured that help is close at hand and that she is free to call the doctor or the hospital at any hour of the day or night. If a call comes in from a parent after the day hospital is closed, it is put through to the pediatric service where a physician is available to answer any queries. To provide even more assurance, she is given a printed list of all the attending physicians' and pediatric residents' home telephone numbers, so she need never feel alone with her problem. Gradually, the mother's confidence in her ability to care for the child is rebuilt.

Each outpatient visit routinely begins with the child having a "finger-stick" for hemoglobin, white cell count, and platelet count. He is then weighed and his temperature and blood pressure are checked. The nurse questions the child and his parents on his eating habits and tries to find out whether he is able to take an adequate amount of fluids. She asks if there has been any change in the character of the stools or urine, whether there has been any nausea or vomiting, and whether the child has complained about abdominal pain. After the nurse has obtained all of this information, she reports it to the physician who then completes the examination. Usually, by this time all blood factors have been obtained and a decision is made about the dosages of the child's medications, or his need for blood replacement.

Because of the rotating residency program at Memorial Hospital, the outpatient nurse is the one constant, familiar, and always present person that parent and child both come to rely on. When the nurse is able to achieve good rapport with the patient, many procedures which may be frightening and uncomfortable can be done with a minimum of trauma to the child. Sometimes a child is subjected to lumbar puncture twice a week, venipuncture for the administration of chemotherapeutic drugs daily, multiple "finger-sticks," and bone marrow aspiration every six weeks. Understandably, many children become so apprehensive about these procedures that they cannot cooperate and, in such instances, a sedative or even light anesthesia may be used.

Children are considered day-hospital patients if they spend three to eight hours there at each visit. These are children who receive intravenous cyclo-phosphamide, amphotericin B, and intrathecal methotrexate. Those who need transfusions, or intravenous fluids because of dehydration are kept for longer periods. Also, when children are first given such drugs as L-asparaginase they, too, must remain long enough to determine whether they are going to have any untoward reactions.

Children who are on a protocol that requires just one intravenous injec-tion can be seen during a 15- or 20-minute visit. Then they can be off to school, play, or home. These children are still monitored closely, however. One complete physical examination is done weekly. The patient who must come in daily will have blood counts done three times a week. If the white count is too low, therapy may be discontinued for a short time to allow for bone marrow recovery. Low hemoglobins and low platelet counts may show the need for replacement by transfusion.

The outpatient nurse must be just as alert as the nurse on the inpatient unit to the earliest signs of anaphylactic shock, infiltration, chills, and high temperature that may follow the administration of chemotherapeutic drugs. Side-effects such as any unpleasant sensation or burning at the site of the IV needle, nausea, vomiting, and rash must be watched for. Individual re-actions can be anticipated when the nurse knows her patient well. She can anticipate the occurrence of nausea and vomiting, perhaps, and give the child an antiemetic before the symptoms arise. Other children, she knows, will develop a rash if not given a dose of Benadryl before the chemo-therapeutic drug is given. One unfortunate side-effect of chemotherapy is alopecia which, in a teenage patient, can be quite devastating. The patient needs to be reassured that the hair will grow back in, sometimes with the bonus of having it grow in curly or of a different color. In the meantime, the nurse can help to see that the patient is fitted with an attractive wig.

QUESTIONS AND ANSWERS

Q. To what extent is the patient's family encouraged to participate in the care of the pediatric cancer patient?

A. Actually, they are encouraged to participate a great deal in giving care to the child. When they learn to do the different things that must be done for the patient, the whole family becomes involved, directly or vicariously, in the child's care. This increases the child's sense of security.

Q. How does the care team deal with parents who never request a diagnosis or ask about their child's progression or regression?

A. Parents who react to their child's illness in this way are either completely denying what is happening, or are in a tremendous panic about it. They do not want to hear anything. So how are they going to hear their son or their daughter? If they do not want to listen to the physician, how are they going to listen to the voice of a little seven-year-old, in panic, feeling dreadfully sick—sicker by the day? Perhaps some of these parents should be talked to by a qualified team member who can convince them that they should start opening up and being receptive to information about their child.

Q. How long has L-asparaginase been in use, and has it fulfilled the early expectations for it?

A. This drug was first used at Memorial Hospital in 1967. L-asparaginase works very fast. It gives remission within a week or ten days. Alone, it gives very short remissions so it is usually followed with other agents and, as indicated by the L-2 protocol, it is now combined with a number of other agents in the attempt to reduce the leukemic cell population very early in the course of treatment.

Q. How is abdominal tumor in a five-day-old baby recognized?

A. An abdominal tumor in a very young infant is extremely difficult to recognize. The physician has to rely on the probabilities and, in the end, the child comes to laparotomy.
Various tests can be used. The commonest tumors in the newborn are Wilms' tumor and neuroblastoma, so an intravenous pyelogram, inferior vena cavagram, lymphangiogram, and arteriogram should all be done. In about half of the cases, the diagnosis is not known until an exploratory laparotomy is done.

Q. Are external or internal sources responsible for the infections that flare up in patients with leukemia?

A. Surgical wound infections are practically always caused by patients' own bacterial flora. If the source is below the navel, the causative agent is usually a Gram-negative organism from the stool or urine; if the causative organism is from the upper part of the body it is usually a staphylococcus.

Q. What treatment is given to the patient with a diagnosis of Hodgkin's disease if he has not been treated elsewhere?

A. In a newly diagnosed case of Hodgkin's disease, the abdomen is explored surgically, the spleen is removed, the lymph nodes are biopsied and, in little girls, the ovaries are moved out to the iliac crest so that if the child subsequently gets radiation therapy, the ovaries are protected from radiation and the child—hopefully, cured of Hodgkin's disease—will be fertile. A liver biopsy is taken and this is very useful in finding out whether there is disease below the diaphragm. This kind of surgery can only be done if there is a backup team and a great deal of intensive nursing care available.

Q. What are the important problems that come up in the rehabilitation of a child who has had an amputation?

A. The child who is going to have an amputation must be prepared ahead of time, and honestly. Usually the surgeon gets to know the child during the workup and, the night before surgery tells him exactly what will be done, that he may have a prosthesis applied in the operating room, and that he will be able to walk within two or three days.
For rehabilitation to succeed, the team needs to have the confidence of the child, and support from the parents, social service, and the nursing staff. If the team has the complete confidence of the child, he will do remarkably well and rehabilitation presents no problems.

Q. What is the present mortality rate for children being treated for cancer at Memorial Hospital?

A. At the moment, it is very low. Only two deaths occurred between January 1 and March 30, 1972. This was attributed to the more aggressive and effective therapy being employed.

Q. If the family knows that the patient is terminally ill and the patient asks the nurse, "Am I going to die?" how does she answer this question?

A. Many of the children in the teenage group certainly have an awareness of the seriousness of their illness. Perhaps they don't actually admit that they know definitely they are going to die, but often the nurse can tell that they are aware of the probability by the things they say and the questions they ask.
When a patient asks outright, the nurse can sometimes turn the question around and explore his thinking by saying, "Why do you think this?" or "What are you feeling that makes you ask this?"
Frequent team conferences are held during which different children are discussed, and the question as to whether or not they should be told often comes up.

The nurse does not proceed on her own initiative to tell the patient that he is terminally ill. However, some of the children do know their diagnoses from the start and they also know that they are going to die from their illness.

Q. What approach can be used in answering the child who asks what his diagnosis is and how long he is going to live?

A. Who knows how long an illness will last? No one really, because each illness and each child is different.

Prognosis is an even more difficult aspect of medicine than diagnosis. In some siutations, when the child is terribly ill and obviously in the later stages of his illness, the physician may presume that death is imminent.

The answer to this question, as far as the nurse is concerned, depends on the child's stage of development, how intelligent he is, and how well adjusted he is emotionally. A fairly intelligent 11-year-old who knows his diagnosis may go to a library to find out about his disease and he will know exactly what to expect. Then, when he approaches his mother with the question, "What do I have?" and the mother says, "Anemia," the child may become very angry. He will express his anger through temper tantrums, and by being very antagonistic to his mother and toward the staff. The child knows, the mother knows, and neither wants to talk to the other about it.

What the child should be told depends on all the facts in the situation. Sometimes he should be given a direct, truthful answer but, again, his question should be answered in a way that will not destroy his feeling of hope.

Q. What recreational activity or therapy helps the child most in dealing with his thoughts of death?

A. Anything that helps the child express himself creatively is helpful when he is occupied with thoughts of death, because when he does something creative he is totally alive and feeling alive. This is the most important thing to him.

SUGGESTED READINGS

Books

Bishop, H., et al. "Solid Tumors in Childhood" in *Current Perspectives in Cancer Therapy*. New York: Harper & Row, 1966.

Carter, R. "Palliation of Childhood Cancer" in *Palliative Care of the Cancer Patient*. Boston: Little, Brown, 1967.

Dargeon, H. *Tumors of Childhood*. New York: Hoeber, 1960.

Marlow, Dorothy R. (Ed.). *Textbook of Pediatric Nursing*. Philadelphia: Saunders, 1969.

Marsden, H. B., and J. K. Steward (Eds.). *Tumors in Children*. New York: Springer Verlag, 1968.

Matson, D. *Neurosurgery of Infancy and Childhood*, 2nd ed. Springfield, Ill.: Charles C Thomas, 1969.

Murphy, M. L. "Chemotherapy of Neoplastic Diseases," in *Pediatric Therapy*, H. Shirkey, (Ed.). St. Louis: Mosby, 1972.

Nelson, W., Y. Vaughan and R. J. McKay (Eds.). *Textbook of Pediatrics*. Philadelphia: Saunders, 1969.

Pack, G., and P. Ariel. *Cancer and Allied Diseases of Childhood*. Boston: Little, Brown 1960.

Shirkey, H. (Ed.). *Pediatric Therapy*. St. Louis: Mosby, 1972.

Willis, Rupert A. *The Pathology of the Tumors of Children*. Springfield Ill.: Charles C Thomas, 1962.

Periodicals

Adamek, M. "Some Observations on Death and a Family," *Nursing Science, 3*:258, August, 1965.

Armstrong, D., L. S. Young, R. Meyer, and A. Blevins. "Infectious Complications of Neoplastic Disease," *The Medical Clinics of North America, 55*:729-745, May, 1971.

Beattie, E. (Ed.). "Problems of Surgical Oncology," *The Surgical Clinics of North America, 49*:213-216, April, 1969.

Blackburn, E. K. "Acute Leukemia," *Nursing Times, 67*:509-11, April, 1971.

Bonnie, G. "Student's Reaction to Children's Deaths," *American Journal of Nursing, 67*:1439, July, 1967.

Bozeman, M., et al. "Psychological Impact of Cancer and Its Treatment: II. Adaptations of Mothers to the Threatened Loss of Their Children Through Leukemia: Part I and II" *Cancer, 8*:1-33, January/February, 1955.

Clarkson, R., and J. Fried. "Changing Concepts of Treatment in Acute Leukemia," *Medical Clinics of North America, 55*:561-600, May, 1971.

Cragg, C. E. "The Child With Leukemia," *Canadian Nurse, 65*:30, October, 1969.

Dittman, L. "A Child's Sense of Trust," *American Journal of Nursing, 66*:94, January, 1966.

Engel, George L. "Grief and Grieving," *American Journal of Nursing, 64*:93-98, September, 1964.

Ericson, F. "Helping the Sick Child Maintain Behavioral Control," *Nursing Clinics of North America*, 2:695, December, 1967.

Exelby, P. R. "Malignant Abdominal Tumors in Children," *Cancer*, 20:342-351, November/December, 1970.

Exelby, P. R. "Methods of Evaluating Children with Hodgkin's Disease," *Cancer*, 21:95-101, March/April, 1971.

Exelby, P. R., and E. Frazell. "Carcinoma of the Thyroid in Children," *Surgical Clinics of North America*, 49:249, April, 1969.

Exelby, P. R., et al. "Primary Malignant Tumors of the Liver in Children," Paper presented before the Surgical Section of the American Academy of Pediatrics, San Francisco, California, October 17-19, 1970.

Exelby, P. R., M. L. Murphy, D. Armstrong, P. P. Rosen, C. M. Ramos, G. Rosen, and B. Fish. "Pneumocystis Carinii," *Clinical Bulletin (MSKCC)*, 1:23-28, 1971.

Exelby, P. R., J. K. Sidhu, G. Rosen, W. H. Knapper, A. G. Huvos, and J. H. Dietz, Jr., "Fibrosarcoma in Children," *Clinical Bulletin* (MSKCC), 1:97-101, 1971.

Fraumeni, J. "Stature and Malignant Tumors of Bone in Childhood and Adolescence," *Cancer.* 20:967, June, 1967.

Geis, D. "Mothers Perceptions of Nursing Care Given Their Dying Children," *American Journal of Nursing*, 65:105, February, 1965.

Goldfogel. "Working with the Parents of a Dying Child," *American Journal of Nursing*, 70:1675, August, 1970.

Graham, P. J., et al. "Leukemia in Childhood," *Nursing Mirror*, 133:18-20, July, 1971.

Green, A. P. "Meeting the Needs of a Child in Hospital," *Nursing Times, 66:* 210-2, February, 1970.

Gutowski, F. "Nursing the Leukemic Child with Central Nervous System Involvement," *American Journal of Nursing*, 63:87-88, April, 1963.

Helson, L. et al. "Urinary Cystathionine, Catecholamine and Metabolites in Patients with Disseminated Neuroblastoma," *Clinical Chemistry* 18:613-615, 1972.

Heyn, R. M. et al. "Vincristine in the Treatment of Acute Leukemia in Children," *Pediatrics, 38*:82-91, July, 1966.

Hope, J., et al. "Radiologic Diagnosis of Primary and Metastatic Cancer in Infants and Children," *Radiation Clinics of North America*, 3:353-374, December, 1965.

Holland, P., et al. "Prevention and Management of Acute Hyperuricemia in Childhood Leukemia," *Journal of Pediatrics*, 73:358, March, 1968.

Holton, C., et al. "Chronic Myelocytic Leukemia in Infant Siblings," *Journal of Pediatrics*, 72:377, March 1968.

Howard, J. "Response of Acute Leukemia in Children to Repeated Courses of Vincristine," *Cancer Chemotherapy Reports, 51*:7, December, 1967.

Iriarte, P., et al. "CNS Leukemia and Solid Tumors of Childhood: Treatment with BCNU," *Cancer, 19:* 1187, September, 1966.

Krakoff, I., et al. "Hyperuricemia in Neoplastic Disease in Children: Prevention with Allopurinol, A Xanthine Oxidase Inhibitor," *Pediatrics, 41*:52, January, 1968.

Krivit, W., et al. "Induction of Remission in Acute Leukemia of Childhood by Combination of Prednisone and Either 6MP or MTX," *American Journal of Nursing, 68*:965-968, June, 1966.

Knapper, W. H. (Ed.). "Hemangioma of the Tongue in an Infant," *Clinical Bulletin* (MSKCC), *1*:143-146, 1971.

Leikin, S. L. "Varying Prednisone Dosage in Remission Induction of Previously Untreated Childhood Leukemia," *Cancer, 21*:346, March, 1968.

McKenna, R., et al. "Osteogenic Sarcoma in Children," *California Medicine, 103*:67-170, September, 1965.

McMillan, C. W. "Coagulation Defects and Metastatic Neuroblastoma," *Journal of Pediatrics, 75*:347, March, 1968.

Meighan, S. "Leukemia in Children," *Cancer, 16*:656-664, May, 1963.

Mulelly, K. A. "A Child with a Nasopharyngeal Sarcoma," *Nursing Times, 67*:348-51, March, 1971.

Omer, Burget, E., et al. "Chemotherapy of Malignant Lesions Unique in Children," *Cancer:* American Cancer Society. January/February, 1967, pp. 15-20.

Pacyna. "Response to a Dying Child," *"Nursing Clinics of North America, 5*:421, September, 1970.

Patton, J. et al. "Ministering to Parent Groups in a Pediatric Hospital," *American Journal of Nursing, 68*:1290, June, 1968.

Phillips, R. et al. "The Curability of Ewing's Endothelioma of Bone in Children," *Journal of Pediatrics, 70*:391-397, March, 1967.

Pinkel, D. "Chicken Pox and Leukemia," *Journal of Pediatrics,* May, 1961, p. 729.

Porter, L. S. "The Impact of Malignancy as a Chronic Illness Upon the Ill Child and His Family," *Philippine Journal of Nursing, 39*:63, April/June, 1970.

Preston, K. O. "Nursing Children with Cancer," *Nursing Times, 67*:467-9, April, 1971.

Reilly, D. et al. "Cure of Three Patients Who Had Skeletal Metastasis in Disseminated Neuroblastoma," *Pediatrics, 41*:474, January, 1968.

Schneider, K., et al. "Neonatal Neuroblastoma," *Pediatrics, 36*:359, September 1965.

Skor, J. T., et al. "Malignant Melanoma in Children," *Cancer, 19*:620, May, 1966.

Smith, Evelyn. "Pseudomonas, the Ever-Present Menace," RN, *35*:63-70, February, 1972.

Tan, C. et al. "Chediak-Higashi Syndrome in a Child with Hodgkin's Disease," *American Journal of Diseases of Children, 121*:135-139, February, 1971.

Vernick, J., et al. "Milieu Design for Adolescents with Leukemia," *American Journal of Nursing, 67*:559, March, 1967.

Wesseling, E. "The Adolescent Facing Amputation," *American Journal of Nursing, 65*:91-94, January, 1965.

Whitmore, W. J. "Wilm's Tumor and Neuroblastoma, Medical Considerations," *American Journal of Nursing, 68*:527, March, 1968.

Wiener, J. M. "Attitudes of Pediatricians Toward the Care of Fatally Ill Children," *Journal of Pediatrics, 76*:700-5, May, 1970.

Patients with Head and Neck Tumors

Regional Medical Program — Oncology Nursing Seminar

on

NURSING MANAGEMENT OF PATIENTS WITH
HEAD AND NECK TUMORS

Seminar Leader

Elliott W. Strong, M.D.

Seminar Participants

Daniel Catlin, M.D., Assistant Coordinator, Department of Surgery, Memorial Hospital Regional Medical Program and Associate Attending Surgeon, Head and Neck Service

Alice Costello, R.N., Head Nurse

Nancy Frankel, R.N., Public Health Nurse; Team Leader, Central Harlem Visiting Nurse Service

James B. Lepley, D.D.S., Chief, Dental Service

John E. McClear, Chief, Post-laryngectomy Clinical Service, Speech Rehabilitation Institute

Blanche Scheib, M.S.W., Social Worker

Elliott W. Strong, M.D., Chief, Head and Neck Service

Alice Tanona, R.N., Treatment Room Staff Nurse

Judy Wilcox, R.N., Head Nurse

The designation, head and neck cancer, includes tumors that occur in multiple sites, but all of which lie above the clavicle. It includes neoplasms that originate in the skin, soft tissues, mucous membrane, salivary glands, thyroid gland, and various other specialized tissues. It even includes bone tumors. Tumors of the brain or spinal cord, even though they may lie within the head or neck area, are not considered in this category because their treatment falls within the province of the neurosurgeon; nor are tumors of the axial skeleton or vertebral bodies, because their treatment is ordinarily the responsibility of the orthopedic surgeon. Increasingly, the treatment of head and neck tumors involves representatives from many professional disciplines including general surgeons, plastic surgeons, otolaryngologists, radiotherapists, chemotherapists, dentists, prosthodontists, speech therapists and, of course, nurses.

To place the incidence of head and neck cancer in perspective, one needs to remember that, in men, skin cancer comprises 22 percent of the total cases of cancer, lung cancer 17 percent, and prostatic cancer 11 percent. In women, 24 percent of the cancers arise in the breast, 14 percent in the uterus, and 13 percent in the skin. In one of its publications, the American Cancer Society estimated that in 1970 a total of 625,000 new cancers would be diagnosed in this country; that 14,000 of these would be oral cancers and 7,000 laryngeal cancers; and that 50 percent of patients who developed cancer of the mouth or larynx would die of the disease. The same source also estimated that in 1970 approximately 1,050 patients would die of cancer of the thyroid gland and its ramifications. Thus, it can be seen that head and neck cancer comprise only a relatively small part of the cancer spectrum. However, it is one of the most devastating forms of the disease, not only to the patient but also to his family and friends, by virtue of the cosmetic and functional effects that so frequently occur as a result of the disease and its treatment. What is more vital to one's self-esteem than the integrity of his face? And what is more important to one's daily life than the ability to take his food normally and to communicate normally?

The most common site of head and neck cancer is the skin. In fact, skin tumors are the most common neoplasms that occur in man and, since a significant percentage of them arise on exposed areas of the skin, there is an obvious implication of a relationship between them and exposure to the sun's rays. The next most common site is the tongue. (These statistics are from the files at Memorial Hospital and may not be representative of the country as a whole.) Third in order of incidence is cancer of the vocal cords, followed closely by tumors that arise in the larynx in locations other than the vocal cords. Then follow tumors of the thyroid, mouth, tonsil, gums, lips, buccal mucosa, major salivary glands, nose and sinuses, nasopharynx, palate and pharynx—in that order. The great bulk of head and neck tumors arise from the oral mucous membrane and are epidermoid squamous cancers. Ninety percent or more of oral cancers occur in people over the age of forty-five. It is primarily a disease of men, but whereas in the past the ratio was four males to one female afflicted with this disease, the ratio now more nearly approaches two males to one female. The reason for this striking relative increase in the incidence of head and neck cancer in the female is not known.

The survival rates for patients with cancer of the head and neck vary greatly. For example, the tumor registry at Memorial Hospital demonstrates these variations: The survival rate for patients with cancer of the thyroid gland varies from 13 percent for anaplastic tumors of thyroid origin to 94 percent for certain other thyroid tumors. The five-year survival rate for patients with localized intraoral cancer is 70 percent; but once it has metastasized to the regional node-bearing areas, the survival rate drops to 24 percent. Only 34 percent of oral cancers that are less than 22 mm in diameter metastasize to the cervical area. Of those that are from 22 to 35 mm in diameter, 58 percent have cervical metastasis, and of those greater than 35 mm in diameter, 80 percent have such metastasis. Thus, once again, the importance of early diagnosis is stressed as a factor of importance in increasing the patient's chances of survival. In one series, patients with cancer of the tongue who never developed a cancer of the lymph nodes, had an anticipated survival rate of 67 percent but when they developed cancer of the lymph nodes in the neck subsequent to their initial tumor, the survival rate fell to 31 percent.

A patient whose disease is so advanced on admission to the hospital that he presents with evidence of regional lymph node metastasis, has only a 16 percent chance of survival. In spite of the fact that the head and neck are anatomic areas easily examined with relatively inexpensive diagnostic equipment, many patients present with advanced cancer of these parts. It appears obvious that both patients and physicians often delay overlong in seeking diagnoses of pathological conditions in the head and neck.

ETIOLOGY

Probably no single factor is responsible for head and neck cancer, but rather multiple interacting factors. Whether leukoplakia, a white patch that forms in the mouth and does not scrape or rub off, is a true precursor of cancer is debatable. Various studies have demonstrated its coexistence with oral cancer in percentages ranging all the way from 14 to 60 percent of the patients studied. In some studies it has appeared that leukoplakia was the antecedent of oral cancer in from 1.4 to 36 percent of the subjects—an extremely wide range. The word leukoplakia means white patch, and is often used as a descriptive term for a condition that may or may not be precancerous. Cancer in situ may also appear as a white patch but this is recognizable as cancer on biopsy and should not be referred to as leukoplakia. Leukoplakia is a descriptive term only and may actually refer to several varied histologic entities from lichen planus to squamous carcinoma.

Viruses have been implicated, but the only tumor in which there is reasonable assurance of a viral etiology is Burkitt's tumor which occurs in children largely in a specific geographic area of Africa. It is interesting, however, that in a high precentage of patients with carcinoma of the nasopharynx, antibodies against a virus that is similar to, or even identical with the one found in Burkitt's tumor, have been found.

There is certainly a positive relationship between the use of tobacco and mouth cancer. The mortality rate from oral cancer is 4.2 percent greater in cigarette smokers than in non-smokers. Oral cancer has the highest mortality rate of all diseases in people who smoke cigars or pipes. A very interesting study was done in Louisville, Kentucky, in which a group of patients who had been cured of a first oral cancer were followed for six years. Of the 65 patients who continued to smoke after their cure, 21 or approximately one-third, developed a second oral cancer. In the control series of 37 patients who stopped smoking after their cure, only two, or 5 percent, developed a second oral cancer. Of 636 patients with oral cancer seen at the University of California Medical Center in San Francisco, 90 percent of the males and 67 percent of the females were smokers.

The ingestion of alcohol and the coexistence of cirrhosis of the liver appear to be positive etiological agents of oral cancer. Studies have shown that a high percentage of patients with this disease not only drink but that they drink excessively. In a study carried out some years ago, it was found that more than one-third of a group of 540 male patients with mouth cancer consumed more than seven ounces of whiskey daily. In a control group of patients without mouth cancer, only 12 percent admitted to consuming this much alcohol. Frequently the heavy consumption of alcohol parallels the heavy use of tobacco. As far as the etiology of mouth cancer is concerned, there may be a synergistic relationship between the two.

In India and some other parts of Asia where many people have a habit of chewing betel nuts, cancer of the buccal mucosa has a high incidence rate. Actually what these people chew is a wad composed of tobacco, slaked lime, betel nut, and various other agents. They keep this wad in their mouths around the clock and usually in the same place. The buccal mucosa is subjected to an intense inflammatory response and cancer often develops in the area immediately adjacent to the place they carry the wad of material. In another area of the world, the Philippines, some people have the habit of smoking cigarettes in reverse; that is, they put the lighted end in the mouth. These people often develop cancers on the top of the tongue and on the hard palate, presumably as a secondary effect of the exposure to the heat of the lighted cigarette.

Several other etiological agents have been suggested, and sometimes implicated, in cancer of the head and neck including vitamin deficiencies—particularly A and the B complex—a history of radiation, poor oral hygiene, and syphilis. Sharp teeth and ill fitting dentures have been cited as possible causes of oral cancer and it is a fact that frequently a malignant tumor will be found adjacent to a poorly fitted denture or a clasp.

DIAGNOSIS

As in most forms of cancer, the diagnosis of head and neck cancer rests on the histological examination of a specimen. In these cases, however, the physician may be guided by an asymmetrical enlargement of the lymph nodes in the neck. Whenever this occurs in an adult, metastatic cancer should be suspected. About two-thirds of such patients will be found to have a primary cancer in the head and neck area. A thorough search for the primary cancer should be carried out with biopsy of the enlarged cervical lymph node as the last step in this examination, being prepared to proceed with the appropriate treatment at once. Unfortunately, patients often pay no attention to early signs and do not seek medical advice until the intraoral lesion has advanced to the stage that it can only be treated by radical means.

TREATMENT

At Memorial Hospital the treatment for head and neck cancer is primarily surgical. A radical neck dissection, or removal of the regional node-bearing areas in the neck is often included. This procedure is carried out whenever a) there is clinical evidence of regional node metastasis; b) the surgical removal of the primary tumor necessitates entry into the neck in order to remove it; or, c) the clinical or actual history of the case illustrates the real probability that the patient will develop regional node metastasis. Many years ago, a review of the head and neck cancers treated at this hospital showed that cancer of the lip was the most common tumor seen, and that of these cases only 8 percent ever developed regional node metastases. In our more recent experience, only 8 percent of patients with cancer of the true vocal cords have developed regional node metastases. Therefore, in the absence of clinically involved lymph nodes, there appears to be no justification for the use of radical neck dissection in the routine treatment of lip or vocal cord cancer.

On the other hand, it has been demonstrated that when cancer of the larynx arises above the vocal cord, 65 percent of patients will ultimately develop regional node metastases. This undoubtedly accounts for the relatively standard practice of subjecting patients with this kind of laryngeal cancer to radical neck dissection at the time their primary disease is treated. It should also be stated that a significant number of patients with clinically negative neck nodes will be found to have positive nodes at the time of surgery; therefore, it would seem that the error should be on the side of doing rather than not doing the neck dissection.

If bone adjacent to the tumor is involved, especially the maxilla or mandible, it should be removed at the time of the primary surgery. This should also be done when the tumor approximates the bone so closely that to preserve it would not provide an adequate surgical margin. The surgeon is dealing with a malignant disease that will recur if it is incompletely excised. Therefore, he is compelled to look at the overall situation when considering the sacrifice of two or three millimeters of bone. When oral cancer destroys some of the alveolar ridge, the operative and postoperative problems that are created are very difficult to handle. Unfortunately, there is no way of determining absolutely whether or not the underlying bone is involved. Therefore, of necessity, adequate surgical therapy demands removal of the bone in question. Radiotherapy can sterilize tumor in bone but it does so at the expense of necrosis of the bone, so that the ultimate result may be the same, whether the patient has a clean surgical excision or is allowed to slough out the radio-necrotic bone.

Tracheostomy is indicated whenever there is actual or anticipated laryngeal or pharyngeal obstruction. Such instances include a) patients who have had a partial laryngectomy; b) those who have had a segmental or complete resection of the mandible; c) those who have a history of therapeutic radiation to the neck; d) those who have a second or simultaneous bilateral neck dissection. It is far easier to do this procedure under controlled circumstances in the operating room than in the middle of the night under uncontrolled emergency circumstances.

A nasal feeding tube is also put in place in the operating room whenever the patient has—or it is anticipated that he may have—difficulty in swallowing. Also, it is thought that intraoral wounds heal more satisfactorily when they are not subject to contamination by food.

Basal cell carcinoma is probably the most common type of tumor of the head and neck area. It has a high cure rate by surgery or radiation therapy. However, when it exists in proximity to the eye or eye socket, removal of the eye may be necessary to obtain adequate margins on the tumor to prevent local recurrence. So the consensus is that in the presence of normal vision in the other eye, sacrificing the eye in order to eradicate the tumor completely is justified.

Melanoma, particularly of the scalp, is very aggressive and its behavior differs according to its location on the scalp or neck. The treatment is surgical and demands wide excision. Whenever feasible, the operation includes radical neck dissection, depending on the location and the depth of invasion of the tumor.

Cancer of the lip is fairly common and potentially highly curable; in fact, cure rates of 80 to 90 percent have been reported for lip cancer that is uncomplicated by neck node metastasis. Cancer of the lower lip is ten times more common than cancer of the upper lip. It also behaves in a much less aggressive fashion except when it is neglected, as sometimes happens with older people who may be inclined to delay treatment. Lower lip cancer calls for complete surgical excision, often with radical neck dissection when indicated on the involved side. Lip cancer seldom metastasizes to regional lymph nodes, but when it does it becomes more aggressive and the survival rate falls. When the lesion is in proximity to the midline, a significant percentage of patients will have bilateral lymph node metastasis because the lymphatics actually cross the midline. Fortunately, this is a relatively rare development.

Cancers of the floor of the mouth also tend to be highly aggressive. These lesions are likely to metastasize bilaterally, and adequate surgical excision results in a high incidence of severe cosmetic and functional disturbance. The tongue is brought down to the buccal mucosa; therefore, the patient initially has difficulty talking and swallowing until retraining can be begun. His cosmetic appearance has also been affected. Newer methods of reconstruction have made it possible to remedy some of these problems. The patient with an exophytic, polypoid lesion enjoys a better prognosis by virtue of the fact that rather than infiltrating and rapidly invading adjacent lymphatics, this type of tumor tends to grow outward and is somewhat less aggressive.

Buccal mucosal cancer is often moderately bulky in size and infiltrative, and metastasizes to regional lymph nodes in a significant number of patients, so that complete removal results in extensive deformity. Surgery is usually employed if the lesion is large, although radiation sometimes gives equally satisfactory results. As a general rule, the earlier the lesion is diagnosed the more likely the surgeon or radiotherapist is to be enthusiastic about its treatment. Overall, the results of treatment are not impressive, but surgery seems to be somewhat more effective for the larger lesions than radiation.

Cancer of the salivary glands may arise in the major glands—the parotid, the submandibular, and the sublingual—but a significant number arise in areas of the mouth, oropharynx, pharynx and larynx where there are innumerable salivary glands. The histologic and clinical behavior are similar in all of these tumors. They are characterized by a much longer clinical course than their counterparts that arise in the mucous membrane, that is, the epidermoid carcinomata, and are highly likely to recur locally because of clinically occult dissemination peripherally, which is difficult at times to evaluate. In a significant number of patients, they metastasize to the lungs where they may remain asymptomatic for five to ten years or more.

In some patients large parotid tumors exist for many years without producing any symptoms or without affecting the facial nerve. When there is no pain and no interference with the function of the facial nerve, a tumor in this location may be benign. Both benign and malignant tumors of the parotid gland may grow slowly so the patient often procrastinates in seeking medical advice. Finally, pain may develop and facial paralysis soon follows.

The clinical history of an insidious onset of a mass in and about the angle of the mandible, accompanied at first by a rather dull and indefinite but progressive pain and facial nerve paralysis, is diagnostic of primary cancer in a high percentage of patients.

The treatment for cancer of the parotid gland is complete excision of the gland and affected area. This is sometimes difficult to achieve without removing the facial nerve which would cause facial paralysis on the affected side. When excision is not feasible, radiation therapy may be employed for palliative purposes and may effect a diminution in the size of the tumor.

Parotid tumors often recur unless completely excised, and each recurrence is progressively more invasive. Postoperative radiation to the entire operative area may be beneficial in such patients.

Tongue cancer is localized to the lateral border of that organ and involves the anterior two-thirds of it in a very high percentage of cases. This is the portion of the tongue that is mobile and which lies anterior to the circumvallate papillae. Cancers of the dorsum of the tongue are distinctly uncommon; they comprise less than 5 percent of all cancers of the tongue and, when they do exist, are commonly associated with the preexisting changes that are consistent with leukoplakia or carcinoma in situ. Again, in view of the location of the lesion, it is apparent that there may well be some relationship between dental trauma and the generation of cancer. Surgical treatment of cancer of the tongue may involve, in addition to removal of the primary lesion, sometimes with wide excision of part of the tongue, a radical neck dissection, and partial or complete mandibulectomy.

Cancer of the thyroid occurs in individuals of all ages. Some patients who develop this disease in later life have a history of radiation to the neck early in life for treatment of a skin condition or for an enlarged thymus gland. The relationship between neck radiation and thyroid cancer now appears to be substantiated by the reports of the Atomic Energy Commission following studies of data from Hiroshima and Nagasaki which show a definite statistical increase of thyroid cancer among the survivors of the atomic bomb explosions. The anticipated survival rates of those patients with well differentiated thyroid cancer are similar to those in comparable age groups of the population as a whole without thyroid cancer. While thyroid cancer may be fatal, it is often a very prolonged and protracted disease.

The diagnosis of thyroid cancer rests on the histologic examination of the specimen, but patients who are suspected of having such a tumor are given a radioiodine uptake test, and if the scan demonstrates that the suspected area of the thyroid does not pick up the radioiodine, this may well be the site of cancer in from 10 to 40 percent of such nodules. The usual treatment is removal of the offending area. Papillary cancer of the thyroid grows slowly and the patient may survive for several years without symptoms. It may metastasize to the adjacent lymph nodes. Hence the usual policy is to do a complete lobectomy on the side of involvement with adjacent lymph nodes, reserving neck dissection for those patients with positive nodes. The giant cell type of thyroid cancer may be the most malignant of all the malignant tumors. It has a survival rate of less than 2 percent. Many of these patients have a previous history of a long-time thyroid mass. Whether or not such tumors develop from benign growths, the policy of removing all suspicious masses found in the thyroid appears to be the best one to follow.

Cancer of the larynx includes that of the vocal cords and of the supraglottic and subglottic areas. The importance of this differentiation of cancer of the larynx rests on the clinical behavior of the disease in the three parts of this organ. Early true vocal cord cancer, when adequately treated, can be expected to have a survival rate of 80 to 90 percent. Cancer of the vocal cord may be confined to that area for a long period of time during which the patient may present symptoms but the disease still remains localized. In these cases, a partial laryngectomy or radiation therapy may be performed with an equal degree of success. However, if the tumor has infiltrated the vocal cord extensively and fixation of the cord has occurred, a partial laryngectomy(a voice-saving procedure) for the most part is impossible and a total laryngectomy is advisable to ensure complete removal of the cancer.

Cancers of the supraglottic area have a survival rate of about 30 to 50 percent. Those of the subglottic area are more subtle in their clinical presentation and may remain silent for a long time before they reach considerable size and produce symptoms. They then become aggressive and often metastasize to the regional lymph nodes thus reducing the survival rate considerably.

COMPREHENSIVE NURSING CARE

The nursing care plan that evolves for the patient who has extensive head and neck surgery is not only complex but often difficult to execute. Team work is essential if the patient is to receive skilled pre- and postoperative care. The nurse must not only be able to give the nursing care required, but she must also be adept in teaching patients self care. To accomplish these activities, she needs to have a positive attitude toward the patient's disease and the kind of surgery involved, as well as a complete understanding of the patient's attitude toward his illness.

Careful physical and mental preparation of the patient is necessary if extensive head and neck surgery is to be at all successful. The surgeon has the responsibility of discussing the operative procedure with the patient and a responsible member of the family. However, the nurse should be aware of how much and what information the patient and/or his family have been given so that she can provide the additional reenforcement necessary, and clarify any misconceptions the patient or his family may have. She can play an important part in helping to instill confidence in the patient by explaining to him the reasons for the various preoperative tests and procedures. This preparation includes x-rays, biopsies, and a complete medical evaluation that includes biochemistry screening and liver profile studies. A thorough physical evaluation may reveal the need for improving the patient's general physical status preoperatively. He may be in a state of malnutrition because it has been painful or difficult for him to swallow, or because of the presence of fistulae or chronic infection. The deficiency may involve depletion of total blood volume, extracellular fluids, electrolytes, or vitamins. Vigorous replacement therapy carried out before surgery will not only provide for greater safety during the operative procedure but will result in a smoother postoperative course.

To prepare the patient emotionally for the postoperative period the nurse must be aware of the fears and anxieties he may be experiencing, especially the fear of mutilation which is particularly strong in a person awaiting head and neck surgery. She should encourage the patient to express his concerns so that he can be helped to view them realistically. Depending on the planned surgical procedure and the patient's level of understanding, simple explanations are given regarding aspects of his postoperative care such as the purpose of the tracheostomy and the nasal feeding tube. In addition he should be told that he will be provided with an effective means of communicating with others during the postoperative period when he may have a temporary or permanent loss of speech.

Preparation for Surgery

The immediate preoperative preparation includes a bath (or shower) and shampoo using a bacteriocidal soap the night before surgery and again on the day of surgery. The areas of skin to be prepared will depend on the kind and extent of surgery to be done and will be ordered by the surgeon. Male patients are instructed to shave on the morning of surgery. A sedative is ordered to ensure a restful night's sleep and fluids are omitted after midnight.

After the patient's departure for the operating room, his unit is prepared for his return. A suction apparatus is provided as well as a nasal feeding tray, magic writing slate, mirror, and disposable tracheostomy cleaning set. The patient often remains in the recovery room overnight following surgery because of the necessity for constant observation and intensive nursing care.

Postoperative Care

Upon reaching the recovery room, the patient is immediately placed in semi-Fowler's position to facilitate drainage and promote adequate respiration. He will probably be on Hemovac suction and this apparatus will be immediately connected to wall suction. The purpose of the Hemovac is to provide continuous evacuation of wound secretions and thereby promote rapid healing. For this reason, it is absolutely necessary that the Hemovac remain compressed and in proper working order.

If the patient has a tracheostomy he will have a cuffed tracheostomy tube in place when he leaves the operating room. The reasons for using the cuffed tube are 1) to prevent aspiration and 2) to permit ventilatory assistance. As soon as the patient arrives in the recovery room the nurse checks to see if the cuff is inflated. Routinely, the tracheostomy cuff is kept deflated unless otherwise ordered. If it is to remain inflated, it will be deflated periodically, according to the doctor's written order. Prior to deflating the cuff, the oropharynx must be suctioned thoroughly to prevent aspiration of the secretions that have collected above the cuff. For this same reason, the trachea must be suctioned at the time the cuff is deflated. It is essential that the nurse understand the reasons for using the cuffed tube and the possible complications that may develop from its improper use.

Suctioning is done, under aseptic conditions, as often as necessary to remove secretions, prevent airway obstruction, and to prevent atelectasis. Humidified oxygen is administered by means of a plastic disposable tracheostomy collar. A high degree of humidity is required during the immediate postoperative period.

The patient is constantly observed for adequate respirations, the occurrence of swelling, excessive bleeding or drainage, level of consciousness, and any change in vital signs. Extreme restlessness may be due to respiratory distress, anxiety, pain, or reaction to anesthesia. If the restless patient has a history of heavy alcohol intake, a solution of 5 percent alcohol and 5 percent glucose in water may be ordered. Inasmuch as sedation after surgery tends to decrease the cough reflex, the use of narcotics and sedatives is usually kept to a minimum. Aspirin will usually control the pain but, on occasion, codeine may be required.

Although he may have had excellent preoperative psychological preparation, the patient is almost invariably anxious and depressed when he awakes from anesthesia and finds that he can neither speak nor breathe in the normal manner. The nurse can do much to counteract his anxiety by anticipating his needs. In addition, he is given a magic writing slate as soon as he is reactive and this helps to minimize his frustration when he finds that he cannot speak.

Close nursing observation continues after the patient is returned to his unit where the nursing care plan is directed toward maintaining an adequate airway, providing adequate nutrition and hydration, preventing complications, and teaching the patient the elements of self care and rehabilitation. Providing for adequate suctioning is probably the most important factor in early postoperative management. A number 14 or 16 whistle-tip catheter is used for tracheal suctioning. For mouth suctioning a plastic suction tip is used. These two catheters are kept at the bedside in a solution of 1:750 aqueous zephiran chloride. The tracheostomy tube must be aspirated as often as secretions are present. Clean (rather than sterile) suctioning technique is used once the patient returns to his nursing unit. The patient is encouraged to cough frequently and especially prior to suctioning, so the mucus can be reached with the catheter. In the early postoperative period secretions are often blood-tinged. Later on they are mucoid in character and whitish or colorless. A purulent secretion indicates infection, and requires more frequent tracheal suctioning.

The tracheostomy tube must be kept patent and in the proper position. The tube is secured by tape ties which are inserted through openings in the outer cannula and tied at the back of the neck. In the early postoperative period the outer tube is never removed or changed except by the doctor. The inner tube is removed by the nurse for cleaning as often as necessary. It is cleaned under cold running water using a test tube brush. The outer tube is suctioned prior to reinsertion of the inner tube to remove any secretions that may have accumulated.

A tracheostomy dressing is placed under the tube next to the skin and is changed as often as required.

To filter and moisten the air a wet compress of one thickness of gauze is worn over the opening and is held in place by tape ties.

The obturator, which would be used to reinsert the outer cannula should it become accidentally dislodged, is always kept at the patient's bedside.

If the patient has a bulky dressing, the inner tube is extended so that the airway does not become occluded by the dressing.

The tube may become occluded by a crust or mucous plug with resulting signs of respiratory embarrassment such as restlessness, dyspnea, cyanosis, and possibly substernal retraction. Close observation, proper suctioning, frequent cleaning of the inner cannula, the use of a humidifier, and keeping a moistened 4 x 4 gauze dressing over the tracheal airway can do much to prevent such occurrences.

The length of time the patient has the tracheostomy tube depends on the reason for its insertion. When surgery has been extensive, the tube may be left in place for some time. As soon as the patient returns to his nursing unit, he is taught to do his own suctioning and, as he gains strength, he is encouraged to assume increasing responsibility for his own care. He learns to clean the inner cannula, and to change the tracheostomy dressing. If the teaching is done before a mirror, the patient will learn more readily. Providing him with strong assurance of his ability to care for his own tracheostomy will give him a feeling of independence and security. Patients with a temporary tracheostomy may be taught to speak by holding a finger over the tracheal opening thus diverting air through the larynx and making speech possible. Prior to the actual removal of the tube by the doctor, a cork is placed in the tube opening, sealing off the airway. For greater safety, this is best done in the morning. For the remainder of the day, the patient is observed for signs of labored breathing, cyanosis, stridor, and retraction. Corking of the tracheostomy tube is often a gradual process because the cork must be removed at frequent intervals during the day and night for suctioning purposes. A successful corking off period of 24 hours usually guarantees removal of the tube without subsequent difficulties.

If the tracheostomy opening is to be permanent, as happens following a laryngectomy, it is called a tracheal stoma. A patient with such a stoma can no longer inhale or exhale through the nose or mouth since the esophagus is the only remaining connection with those areas.

If the patient has had a total laryngectomy, both patient and the family member responsible will be instructed in the insertion, removal, and care of the laryngectomy tube prior to the patient's discharge. Because there is so much for the patient to learn and accept, teaching must begin early if he is to learn all the facets and entirely understand the various aspects of his care. Several days after surgery, the laryngectomy tube will be removed for a few hours during the day and replaced at night. As the stoma heals, the tube will no longer be needed. The patient is taught to suction himself, clean the inner cannula, and apply the moistened gauze. The tracheal stoma is kept clean by gently removing any crusts with a gauze moistened with hydrogen peroxide or water. Even the most intelligent and cooperative patient may need a great deal of instruction, supervision, and time to practice before he becomes competent and confident enough to give himself the care he needs.

Nutrition is maintained by tube feeding from the first postoperative day whenever there is an intraoral suture line, edema, pain, or inability to swallow. A number 16 French catheter is used as a nasal feeding tube, to which a rubber nasal stopper flange and a rubber band are attached and anchored to the nose so that the tube will not slip too far into the esophagus. The patient is started on water only, and gradually progresses to a full-strength feeding formula. He receives a daily total of 2,000 cc's of formula —400 cc's at four-hour intervals five times a day. This feeding regimen may be adjusted to conform to any special dietary requirement. Coffee, tea, and even carbonated drinks will give some measure of satisfaction and help raise the patient's morale even though he cannot taste in the literal sense of the word. Additional liquids are encouraged with the intent of improving hydration, thus preventing tenacious secretions from developing in the trachea. Medications are given through the feeding tube; pills are either crushed or dissolved in water, and whenever possible, liquid preparations are used. If the patient was accustomed to taking alcoholic beverages preoperatively, these may also be given through the tube at feeding time, according to the doctor's order. To prevent regurgitation, it is advisable to suction the patient prior to feeding and to place him in a comfortable sitting position.

Starting with the first liquid meal, the nurse should encourage the patient to feed himself. The use of the feeding holder will help him to manipulate the funnel and reduce his apprehension about spilling the formula. As soon as he begins to swallow, he is started gradually on oral feeding, but the feeding tube may be left in place for supplementary feedings until he is taking sufficient calories by mouth. For oral feedings, semi-soft food and heavy liquids are often handled better than clear liquids. The nurse should plan to spend some time with the patient during his meals to provide any assistance, encouragement, and support he may need. He will feel a great sense of satisfaction and accomplishment when he can finally manage the technique of eating again.

If it is necessary to continue tube feedings after the intraoral suture line is healed, the patient is taught to pass the catheter himself whenever possible. This is especially important if he is going to need tube feeding over a long period of time—not only is he more comfortable, but he feels less conspicuous if the tube is in place only during the actual feeding. For greater ease in passing the catheter, the patient is instructed to sit upright in a comfortable position. The tube is lubricated with water-soluble jelly and held in one hand while with the other hand the patient raises the edge of the nostril. He inserts the tube directly backwards along the horizontal plane until it reaches the back of the throat. Then the patient is instructed to swallow repeatedly until the tube is advanced into the esophagus. The nurse may check the position of the tube by oral examination using a flashlight and tongue depressor. If the tube is to one side of the midline it is probably in the esophagus, but if it is in the midline it is probably in the trachea and should be reinserted. Even if the tube appears to be in the proper position, a further check may be made by injecting a few drops of Dakin's solution into the tube. If it is in the trachea the patient will cough immediately and there will be no further injury. Should this occur, the tube is removed and reinserted. When the proper position has been established, the feeding tube is corked and fastened securely to the nose. The patient sits in front of a mirror so he can watch the nurse insert the tube. At the next feeding, the patient does the insertion under supervision. Instruction and supervision continue until he demonstrates skill in the procedure. Some patients are handicapped by impaired eyesight, hearing, or inability to manipulate the catheter. In such a case, a relative or friend is taught the procedure. Some patients want to be dependent and prefer to have a relative or someone else care for them. Others, having been taught the procedure while in the hospital, lose their courage when at home and require supervision and demonstration by a visiting nurse.

All patients who have intraoral surgery at Memorial Hospital are taken every morning to the treatment room where they see the doctor and the treatment room nurse and where a program of oral hygiene and daily wound care is carried out. Good oral hygiene helps to promote healing, prevent infection, and control unpleasant odors.

The use of a power spray and suction apparatus is an effective means of cleaning the oral cavity or the defect that results when a patient has an orbital exenteration or maxillectomy. Throughout the patient's hospitalization, he is given an oral spray treatment once or twice every day, the solution usually being half strength hydrogen peroxide followed by normal saline. In addition to the power sprays, irrigations are given at the bedside, beginning 24 or 48 hours postoperatively. The solution used is a quart of warm water containing one teaspoon each of salt and sodium bicarbonate. This is a simple procedure but an extremely important one. Irrigations are usually done after meals and before bedtime throughout the patient's hospitalization. This not only serves to convey their importance but also helps to establish a habit pattern that the patient will continue after he goes home.

Patients who have oral prostheses to cover defects in the palate and to aid in speaking and eating are taught to remove and clean the prosthesis before irrigating and to continue this process at home.

Operative wounds or defects are sprayed and packed in the treatment room in accordance with the doctor's instructions. Gauze packing soaked in Dakin's or acriflavin solution is commonly used. Dressings are adapted to the type of wound or defect the patient may have. Because these dressings need frequent changing, gauze rolls or 4 x 8 compresses folded lengthwise are used to secure dressings applied to the neck area, thus reducing the need to apply tape to skin surfaces.

Unfortunately, complications do occur after extensive head and neck surgery despite the best of care. If hemorrhage from one of the main arteries appears at all likely, precautions are instituted. Emergency equipment is placed in readiness and blood is held in reserve. If a "blowout" occurs, the nurse applies pressure over the bleeding point until the medical team can ligate the vessel involved. The split-second timing and teamwork inherent in comprehensive care of these patients has saved many lives. The hazard of acute hemorrhage following the rupture of an artery can be handled quickly and efficiently if all members of the team follow the prescribed rules and procedures set up for this emergency.

Prostheses

Maxillofacial prosthetics is an important aspect of the postoperative care of the patient who has had face and neck surgery. Many of these people need a maxillofacial prosthesis to restore missing parts for either functional or cosmetic purposes. Functionally, prostheses are often essential for restoring the patient's ability to speak, eat, and swallow. A cosmetic restoration is often necessary, of course, simply because a person cannot function very well in society after losing an eye, his nose, or some other part of his face.

Prior to surgery or radiation therapy, the prosthodontist joins the care team. After surgery he usually does not see the patient until the sixth or seventh day at which time the construction of an obturator is begun. This temporary prosthesis allows for speech and the removal of the feeding tube which was used for passage of liquid meals. Then later, after three months or so, the prosthodontist provides a more definitive, permanent prosthesis which is more sophisticated, lighter in weight, less bulky, and more comfortable to wear.

The basis of most prostheses is the obturator, which is simply defined as a "cork" to plug a hole or seal off an opening. The obturator fits into the defect created by the surgery thus making many natural functions of the parts possible and also helping to build out the face cosmetically when parts of the mandible or maxilla have been removed. Some patients have defects of both hard and soft palate and their situation is much like that of a child born with a cleft palate. For these people, the prosthodontist makes a "speech bulb" obturator that fits into the oropharynx and permits the patient to eat and to speak clearly.

Recent figures indicate that approximately 65 percent of head and neck cancer patients require some form of dental care. Of these, about 50 percent require some form of prosthetic restoration to attempt to restore function, cosmetic appearance, or a combination of both.

Fifty-four percent of patients receive a prosthesis known as an obturator which closes, or obturates, the defects created by removal of portions of the maxilla and soft palate, or both. Prosthetic closure of the defects is preferred over reconstructive surgery since frequent observation of the defect area is necessary to ensure the patient's being free of disease. Obturators may be constructed prior to surgery, adapted in the operating room, and inserted into the defect at the time of surgery. However, at Memorial Hospital, obturators are usually constructed and inserted on the sixth or seventh postoperative day. These early obturators are regarded as immediate postoperative care. Upon insertion of the prosthesis, the patient recovers his functions of speech and feeding by mouth.

Eighteen precent of patients need a mandibular repositioning prosthesis following a segmental resection of the mandible. This prosthesis guides the mandibular teeth into contact or occlusion with the maxillary teeth and enables the patient to regain chewing function. Prostheses that restore this function usually are either a guiding plane prosthesis which fits on the maxillary teeth and palate and provides an inclined plane on which the mandibular teeth slide into contact with the maxillary teeth or a guiding flange prosthesis which fits upon the mandiblular teeth and has an upright flange which glides upon the buccal surfaces of the maxillary teeth when the mandible is elevated and the teeth are brought into occlusion. Both of these prostheses function on the unoperated side of the mandible.

If replacement of the mandible is indicated, it may be done by bone grafting procedures, or by use of a metallic mesh implant which is firmly screwed into the mandibular fragments.

Approximately 10 percent of patients receive prosthetic replacement of missing parts of the face such as the nose, eye, ear, or combinations of these. Also in this category are patients who require either temporary or permanent closure of pharyngostomies, tracheostomies, esophagostomies, or laryngostomies. These prostheses are made by sculpting the missing or defect areas in clay or wax on casts of the defect. Molds are then constructed and the prostheses fabricated of a flexible plastic which may be a polyurethane resin, a polyvinyl resin, or silicone. These prostheses are tinted to match patients' skin, and patients are often supplied with several prostheses tinted to match skin color variations at different seasons.

Personal hygiene habits become of utmost importance whether the patient wears an intraoral or facial prosthesis. Usual skin cleansing habits plus the careful removal of adhesive which retains a facial prosthesis is basic for the patient wearing an extraoral or facial prosthesis. Strict and scrupulous oral hygiene becomes a daily requirement for the patient wearing an intraoral prosthesis. For the dentulous patient thorough, proper tooth-brushing technique, the use of a fluoride dentifrice after each meal, and the daily correct use of dental floss will usually contribute to an excellent state of oral health. For the denture patient, proper denture cleaning, tongue brushing, and oral irrigation will provide a feeling of oral well-being.

For patients receiving radiation therapy, the above described oral hygiene regimen is of paramount importance. In addition, these patients receive flexible polyethylene molds which fit exactly over their teeth. These molds are used to carry a concentrated fluoride gel to cover the teeth and to bathe them thoroughly. This procedure is very helpful in preventing radiation damage to the teeth, the unnecessary loss of teeth, and the possibility of osteoradionecrosis of the jaw.

Prosthodontic dental rehabilitation is often very successful. For example, one Memorial Hospital patient who had very extensive head and neck surgery became rehabilitated sufficiently to function as the Worthy Matron of the Eastern Star—an office that involves considerable public speaking. Many others have been able to return to their various positions in the community and to function as effectively as they did before their surgery.

A common problem of the patient who has a maxillectomy is that the operative procedure often includes the removal of the contents of the orbit, sometimes including even the eyelids. Thus the defect extends upward from the teeth to the top of the orbit. The prosthesis utilized in these cases consists of a silicone rubber plug that serves as a maxillary obturator and to which an artificial eye is attached. This device can be made so that it is not noticeable if the patient wears eyeglasses.

When the nose or part of it is removed, an artificial nose can be made of silicone rubber and tinted to match the patient's skin. These prosetheses are often very satisfactory. The nose can be made according to the patient's liking and often is a copy of someone else's nose of which a cast is taken. The prosthesis is first made in wax and fitted to the patient and then a cast is made which can be used at any time to make a duplicate if this becomes necessary. Sometimes polyvinyl is used for nose prostheses, but the silicone rubber takes color better.

Sometimes the ear or part of its removed during radical surgery, and this too can be replaced with a silicone rubber prosthesis that can be attached by adhesive tape. Usually the patient can arrange his hair to cover the device so that it cannot be seen.

FOLLOW-UP AND REHABILITATION

Even though the patient and his family have been capably instructed in all procedures pertinent to his care prior to discharge, he may panic after leaving the secure hospital atmosphere and forget all or part of what he has learned. For this reason, a return visit to the dressing room is scheduled for one to three days following his discharge.

Should the patient live a distance from the hospital, a visiting nurse referral is initiated before he goes home. The visiting nurse will evaluate the home situation and make recommendations helpful to those who are planning his future management. The visiting nurse can play a vital role giving the patient the nursing care he requires, plus encouragement, reassurance, and reenforcement of the teaching that he and his family received while in the hospital. Knowing ahead of time that the visiting nurse will see him at home the day following discharge can do much to lessen a patient's fear of leaving the hospital. Therefore, it is important that the referral be made as soon as the patient's discharge date is known.

When a person has had extensive head and neck surgery, many problems arise during the recovery period. Depending on his needs, he may be seen at the clinic two or three times a week, or even every day. The nurse makes every attempt to establish good rapport with both the patient and his family. Although self-care is stressed, a member of the family is usually included in the teaching from the very beginning in order that he may assist the patient when necessary. Sometimes this person will try to do everything for the patient and this should be discouraged but, at the same time, the follow-up team should try to instill in the family a sense of responsibility for participating in the patient's treatment and rehabilitation.

The cleansing of the oral cavity with the power spray and the oral irrigations that were done while the patient was hospitalized are continued in the outpatient department. Any dressings the patient has must be constructed so that he can manage them himself. If he has a pharyngostome, a pharyngeal fistula from which saliva drains, the use of a surgical mask lined with 4 X 8's, placed over the drainage area and tied on top of his head, is a simple and effective method of holding the dressings in place.

Outpatients who are receiving radiation therapy come to the clinic after each treatment, for an oral and nasal spray. Dilute Dobell's solution, followed by normal saline, is used. Dobell's solution is preferable to hydrogen peroxide because it is less irritating to irradiated tissue and is very effective in cutting thick mucus. Initially, the patient receiving radiation develops an oral mucositis which is followed after a period of time by annoying dryness. The therapeutic effects of frequent irrigation, both in the outpatient department and at home, help to alleviate both conditions. In addition, patients are advised to avoid highly spiced foods or those with a high acid content while undergoing radiation therapy. The patient is instructed not to use soap because it is irritating to irradiated skin. As a substitute, he may gently cleanse the skin with mineral oil. If erythema develops, he may apply A & D ointment; and for severe weeping reactions there is nothing more soothing than boric acid patches applied every two hours.

If the patient has had a radical neck dissection, he is taught a series of special shoulder exercises. The nerve and muscle resection necessitated by the operative procedure results in shoulder drop and a forward curvature, and this may eventually result in a "frozen" shoulder if not corrected early. The clinic nurse demonstrates the exercises emphasizing the importance of relaxation, and evaluates the patient's learning through return demonstration. On subsequent visits to the clinic, his progress is observed and, if necessary, he receives reenforcement of the instruction.

After oral surgery, continued mouth care is very important for these patients because many of them wear some sort of prosthesis. Wound contracture following a partial or radical maxillectomy is very rapid in the early stages of recovery. For this reason, the patient is cautioned against removing the obturator for prolonged periods of time. He is instructed to wear it even at night, and to remove it only for oral irrigations and for cleansing. It is important that the patient understand the real function of the obturator, which is to allow him to eat, speak, and swallow. If the patient is receiving speech therapy, the clinic nurse emphasizes the virtues of patience and relaxation while learning this new skill and always should spend a few minutes with him, listening to him speak and applauding his progress.

Tracheitis sicca is a frequent development in patients who have had a total laryngectomy. This is the result of prolonged inhalation of cold, dry air. Respiratory obstruction occurs as a result of the accumulation of dried mucous plugs, crusts, and blood clots. The patient may help forestall this by always wearing a moistened "bib" over the stoma. He is also advised to turn off the heat in his bedroom at night, to keep a steam vaporizer going at his bedside, or to keep a basin of water on the windowsill or radiator. Should sicca develop, a small amount of 5 percent sodium bicarbonate solution may be sprayed directly into the stoma to help dissolve the crust, and intensive cold steam inhalation therapy is instituted. The physician may order 2 cc's of Mucomyst inserted directly into the stoma. To allow the patient to receive the full benefit of this medication, and to prevent his coughing it out, he is instructed to take a deep breath and to hold it while the medication is being instilled, and then to exhale slowly—if possible, to the count of ten. In severe sicca, it is sometimes necessary for the physician to do a bronchoscopy and remove the plugs manually. It may even be necessary to re-admit him to the hospital or to have him return daily to the dressing room until all the problems have been resolved.

Patients who must continue on tube feedings after they leave the hospital often go on a "blender" diet. With the exception that the food is put through a blender, the patient partakes of the same menu as the rest of the family. Most people prefer this regular diet. The patient's wife finds it less trouble to prepare than the MSKCC (Memorial-Sloan Kettering Cancer Center) nutritional liquid meal, and the patient feels that he is beginning to return to a normal way of life. To be told that he may eliminate the fifth feeding if he is able to absorb the total prescribed amount in four meals is a good morale builder.

Esophageal Speech Therapy

Patients who have had a total laryngectomy are referred to a speech school once the stoma is healed. The teaching of esophageal speech usually begins about seven to ten days postoperatively and after the feeding tube has been removed. Actually, instruction involves voice therapy rather than speech therapy, since it is the production of sound that the patient must learn. At first, he is simply given tips on how to produce voice and is carried along gradually until he is ambulatory and can come to the speech school. Then he becomes a member of a formal class in speech that meets for about an hour and a half three times a week. It takes the average person from one week to three months to complete the course. The prime requisite for speech rehabilitation of the laryngectomee is motivation, and this is borne out by the fact that those who learn esophageal voice quickly are those who expect to succeed—those who can apply their ambition and their previously successful experiences to their new situation. People who have a problem in adjusting to their post-laryngectomy situation are those who continue to compare their esophageal voice to their preoperative one and, therefore, can never feel successful. On the other hand, many patients conceive of their postoperative situation as life versus no life, and voice versus no voice, and these are the fortunate ones, because they can learn to produce voice again.

The Social Worker's Contribution to the Patient's Rehabilitation

For everyone, the face is a primary means of communicating attitudes and feelings. Through it we convey our personalities by the expression in our eyes, by our smile, and by subtle nuances of speech—media that are often denied to the person who has had head and neck surgery. This patient often finds that life presents some particularly devastating circumstances for him, once he begins to try to resume his normal life in the community. His physical appearance is usually unsightly, and it is there for everyone to see. His image of himself is so diminished that he sometimes sees himself as worthless and burdensome to everyone. At the same time, he is called upon to make major adaptations so as to carry on the functions of living—speaking, eating, and swallowing, for example. Frequently, the patient had formerly kept to a life style characterized by limited personal ties and excessive drinking. Because of his marginal social adjustment and tenuous financial situation, members of his family are inevitably caught up with the patient in the crisis of his illness. Within such a constellation, a social worker can provide services that support the patient's ego and help ease some of the environmental stresses.

While all team members have a concern with the total patient, the primary concern of the social worker is to provide a sustaining relationship in which counseling and the creative use of community resources take priority. The social worker is involved in all phases of comprehensive patient care, even to the planning of his hospital admission when he is burdened by personal attitudes or family problems that hinder his full participation in the treatment needed. During his hospitalization, and afterwards, the social worker's skills are available to both the patient and his family when they need help in adapting to the dramatic physical and social changes that accompany malignant illness and radical surgery. A special period of anxiety occurs when the patient and his family must plan for his return to the community, sometimes when he is still on tube feeding and tracheal suctioning. Another period of anxiety is when the patient and his family are exhausted by the demands of the patient whose illness has become progressive but when plans must still be made for his care at home or in an outside setting. One example will illustrate some of the ways in which the social worker functions when working with patients who have had extensive head and neck surgery.

Mr. W., 58 years old, had surgery for the resection of his tongue, cheek, gum, and tonsils, plus a radical neck dissection. He was in the hospital for many months for reconstructive surgery. He had lived in a dreary, substandard room over a tavern, had been a heavy drinker for many years, was separated from his wife, and had only a fragile relationship with his daughter who reluctantly responded when she was contacted by his friends during his alcoholic crises.

During the first weeks of his hospitalization, he was apparently accepting of his situation but, as time went on, he missed increasingly the freedom of the out-of-doors and his employment in the commissary of a military academy. This restlessness, compounded by anxiety, made him so dejected that he felt his life was of no value and that he was a burden to himself and everyone else.

These feelings were intensified when the patient's younger brother died of lung cancer. Then his daughter's child was still-born, thus thwarting his long anticipated joy in grandfatherhood. In addition, he said people on the bus stared at him when he went home on a weekend pass, as though he had leprosy, when they observed his feeding tube, the gauze between his lips to absorb saliva, and the dressing that covered the open area on the side of his face.

The social worker acknowledged the realities of Mr. W.'s experience and worked toward restoring his self-esteem by emphasizing his basic worth as a human being. She shared his pleasure when he succeeded in learning the procedures involved in self-care and encouraged him to hold to the goal of ultimate reconstruction and return to his former employment. She also let his daughter know that she realized what hardships she had experienced through the years in her relationship with her father, and at the same time encouraged her to continue as a daughter to him through correspondence and telephone calls, using the social worker as an intermediary. The kindness of the patient's landlord was also acknowledged, for in spite of some revulsion, these compassionate people—the tavern-keeper and his wife—always had a furnished room ready for the patient when he came home for weekends.

The social worker also kept the hospital nurses and the medical staff informed all through the weeks of the patient's treatment so that the efforts of everyone on the team could be coordinated. When the time came for the patient to go home, a more comfortable and secure transition was provided by the supervision and concern of the visiting nurse to whom the patient was referred.

QUESTIONS AND ANSWERS

Q. Should all moles or nevi on the head and neck area be removed?

A. Moles that are of substantial size, or that increase in size, change in color, bleed, become ulcerated, or are subject to constant irritation should be removed and, of course, subjected to histologic examination.

Q. Should vocal cord polyps always be removed?

A. No. Usually true vocal cord polyps result from irritation and, if they are not of major size, will go away when the source of the irritation is removed. Sometimes they need to be removed because they cause a deterioration of the voice. They rarely, if ever, are malignant.

Q. What measures can be taken to prevent the development of oral cancer?

A. Most of the dental schools in the country have elaborate programs in clinical cancer training so that students of dentistry are now receiving instruction in cancer detection and management. Since 1948, the federal government has sponsored these programs which have made considerable impact on dental practice and early detection of oral cancer.

Q. Do many patients have psychotic reactions after radical, disfiguring procedures, and are they seen by psychiatrists?

A. Frank psychotic reactions are extremely rare; there is much less trauma associated with these procedures than one would imagine. However, many of the head and neck cancer patients have a history of alcoholism and may develop delirium tremens, a serious complication that may well threaten the patient's life. In these cases, the patient may be given tranquilizers or sedatives, but probably giving them alcohol at specific intervals accomplishes control of the complications with greater ease.

Q. How is mouth infection managed after head and neck surgery?

A. Mouth infection seldom occurs. Most patients who have an intraoral wound are placed on antibiotics preoperatively, intraoperatively, and postoperatively. When infection does occur it is usually of saprophytic origin and is treated by opening the wound and providing for drainage, doing a mechanical debridement with a power spray, and then using such oxidizing agents as hydrogen peroxide or, better yet, zinc peroxide —the most effective agent available for the treatment of anaerobic oral infections. If these infections are not properly treated, massive destruction of tissue and tremendous defects result.

Q. Is there any problem with aspiration during the oral spraying procedure used in oral hygiene?

A. Not really. The patient is instructed to lower his head, almost putting his chin on his chest, and to keep his mouth open to prevent the solution from trickling down the back of the throat.

Q. Why is the inner tracheostomy tube cleaned with water rather than hydrogen peroxide?

A. Hydrogen peroxide mottles the tube. Along with the plain water, the nurse may use a little abrasive action with a small tracheostomy brush. If tracheostomy care is given as frequently as it should be, plain water will suffice.

Q. How much air should be put into the tracheostomy cuff; and what happens if the cuff is not deflated periodically?

A. The amount of air used is variable depending on the size of the patient's trachea. Normally, 10 cc's of air are drawn up into a syringe. When inflating the cuff, place your hand over the patient's mouth or nose and begin injecting the air. When you no longer feel the patient's breath, the cuff is properly inflated. The number of cc's injected should be noted and recorded. When deflating the cuff you should know the amount of air in it initially. If 10 cc's or more are required to inflate the cuff, there may be a slow leak and the cuff must be changed.
If the cuff is not deflated periodically, the continued pressure on the tracheal wall will lead to inflammation, necrosis, and possibly stricture.

Q. How can the nurse help the patient who is frightened by the prospect of going home with a tracheostomy tube in place?

A. Sufficient time must be allowed to plan for his discharge. The patient must be given opportunity to learn how to care for his tracheostomy tube and the technique of suctioning. This is started early in the postoperative period and the teaching is intensified as the day for his discharge approaches. The family should be included in the teaching because many of the patients not only have the tracheostomy tube but a nasogastric feeding tube as well and, in addition, may have an open area in the head and neck that is covered with a dressing that needs to be changed often. Often, the patient cannot manage all of these things without help. Reassurance that many others have been able to learn self-care is helpful. Arrangements are made for the patient to return to the dressing room within three days after he goes home, even if he lives out of town. Also, referrals are made to the Visiting Nurse Association so that a nurse from that organization can visit the patient in his home and continue with the instruction and reassurance.

Q. What are some of the problems associated with self-care for the laryngectomee?

A. After surgery, the patient is taught self-care. This includes care of his laryngeal tube and his tracheal stoma. To communicate he uses a magic slate on which to write until he eventually learns esophageal speech or another effective method.

Q. To what extent are physiotherapists involved in caring for the patient while he is hospitalized?

A. This varies from patient to patient. Many patients do not require physiotherapy. If the patient does require it, however, it is not begun in the postoperative period in the hospital but in the clinic or outpatient department where he goes for follow-up care. It is instituted if he is not using the affected shoulder and there is danger of its becoming "frozen." At the first visit he is instructed how often to do the exercises between visits. Then on each visit the nurse checks to see that he is doing them properly and notes his progress or corrects anything he is doing wrong.

Q. What percentage of laryngectomee patients can be taught effective esophageal speech, and is there any alternative?

A. About 80 percent of laryngectomees learn esophageal speech. The voice that is developed may be excellent, good, bad, or indifferent. For the other 20 percent there are various mechanical devices that are more or less satisfactory, including the electrolarynx.

Q. Is one more susceptible to colds and sore throats after laryngectomy?

A. Not necessarily. It depends upon one's activities and general health, and the amount of exposure one may have to people who may have such infections.

Q. Will an oral prosthesis last the lifetime of the patient?

A. All prostheses require constant surveillance and periodic adjustment, just as normal dentures require periodic adjustment.

Q. Is every patient who has head and neck surgery at Memorial Hospital provided with a prosthesis, or only those who can pay for them?

A. A prosthesis is provided for every patient who needs one, whether they can pay for it themselves or not.

Q. Why is the patient under radiation therapy advised to avoid spiced and acidic foods?

A. The simple reason is that they burn the mucous membranes of the mouth. Instead, patients are advised to use bland foods and liquids such as apricot or apple juice which are soothing to the membranes.

Q. Why is sterile suctioning not used after the patient returns to his nursing unit?

A. Clean suctioning is used because sterile suctioning is really impractical, since the first thing the patient is taught is to suction himself. Although patients do sometimes develop tracheitis, they seldom have clinical evidence of infection, and the tracheitis is usually resolved after the tracheostomy tube is removed.

Q. Why is the Water Pik not used to facilitate oral care?

A. The Water Pik would probably be more efficient than irrigation with the regular setup but it is not used for two reasons. It is more expensive than the regular irrigating outfit; and it has a water-pressure regulating device on it that produces a pulsating jet stream that may literally force food into the tissues and result in the formation of an abscess.

SUGGESTED READINGS

Books

A Cancer Source Book for Nurses. American Cancer Society, Inc., 1968.

Beland, Irene. *Clinical Nursing, Pathophysiological and Psychosocial Approaches,* 2nd ed., London: MacMillan, 1970.

Bouchard, Rosemary. *Nursing Care of the Cancer Patient.* St. Louis: Mosby, 1967.

Brown, Martha and Grace Fowler. *Psychodynamic Nursing, A Biosocial Orientation.* Philadelphia: Saunders, 1971.

Cancer Management. A Special Graduate Course on Cancer Sponsored by the American Cancer Society, Inc. Philadelphia: Lippincott, 1968.

Fletcher, Gilbert and Bao-Shan Jing. *The Head and Neck.* Chicago: Yearbook Medical Publishers, Inc., 1968.

Healey, John (Ed.). *Ecology of the Cancer Patient.* Proceedings of Three Interdisciplinary Conferences on Rehabilitation of the Patient with Cancer. Washington: The Interdisciplinary Communication Associates, Inc., 1970.

Lauder, Edmund. *Self-Help for the Laryngectomee.* 2nd ed. San Antonio: Lauder, 1968-1969.

Martin, Hayes. *Surgery of Head and Neck Tumors.* New York: Hoeber, 1957.

Murphy, Walter. *Radiation Therapy.* Philadelphia: Saunders, 1967.

Nealon, T. F., Jr. *Management of the Patient with Cancer.* Philadelphia: Saunders, 1961.

Rand, Robert and Arthur Rinfret. *Cryosurgery.* Springfield, Illinois: Charles C Thomas, 1968.

Thoma, Kurt. *Oral Surgery.* Vol. I, II. St. Louis: Mosby, 1969.

Travelbee, Joyce. *Interpersonal Aspects of Nursing.* Philadelphia: Davis, 1971.

Periodicals

Beattie, Edward and Steven Economou. "The Current Status of Radical Laryngectomy," *Nursing Clinics of North America, 3*:515-18, September, 1968.

Binder, S.C., B. Cady, and D. Catlin. "Epidermoid Carcinoma of the Skin of the Nose," *The American Journal of Surgery, 116*:506-12, October, 1968.

Cady, Blake and Daniel Catlin. "Epidermoid Carcinoma of the Gum," *Cancer, 23*:551-69, March, 1969.

Catlin, Daniel, and Elliot Strong. "Preoperative Irradiation for Neck Dissection," *Surgical Clinics of North America, 47*:1131-37, October, 1967.

Francis, Gloria. "Cancer : The Emotional Component," *American Journal of Nursing, 69*:1677-81, August, 1969.

Frazell, Edgar. "Management of Cancer of the Thyroid," *American Journal of Surgery, 112*:473-75, October, 1966.

Frazell, Edgar L., Elliot Strong and Barbara Newcombe. "Tumors of the Parotid," *American Journal of Nursing, 66*:2702-08, December, 1966.

Garde, Sister Mariana. "Cancer of the Thyroid," *American Journal of Nursing, 65*:98-102, November, 1965.

Moore, Condict and Daniel Catlin. "Anatomic Origins and Locations of Oral Cancer," *The American Journal of Surgery, 113*:510-13, 1967.

Murphy, Eleanor R. "Intensive Nursing Care in a Respiratory Unit," *Nursing Clinics of North America, 3*:423-36, September, 1968.

Newcombe, Barbara. "Care of the Patient with Head and Neck Cancer," *Nursing Clinics of North America, 2*:599-607, December, 1967.

O'Brien, Paul and Daniel Catlin. "Cancer of the Cheek (Mucosa)," *Cancer, 18*:1392-98, November, 1965.

O'Dell, Ardis J. "Objectives and Standards in the Care of the Patient with a Radical Neck Dissection," *The Nursing Clinics of North America, 8*:159-64, March, 1973.

Rosillo, Ronald, Mary Jane Welty and William Graham III. "The Patient with Maxillofacial Cancer, Psychological Aspects," *The Nursing Clinics of North America, 8*:152-58, March, 1973.

Sandler, Henry. "Oral Cytology," *Ca; Cancer Journal for Clinicians, 16*:97-101, 1966.

Sovie, Margaret and Jacob Israel. "Use of the Cuffed Tracheostomy Tube," *American Journal of Nursing, 67*:1854-56, September, 1967.

Sykes, Eleanor. "No Time for Silence," *American Journal of Nursing,* 66:1040-41, May, 1966.

Totman, Lawrence and Roger Lehman. "Tracheostomy Care," *American Journal of Nursing,* 64:96-99, March, 1964.

Tyler, Martha and Norwin Synnestvedt. "Artificial Airways," *Nursing '73,* 22-39, February, 1973.

Welty, Jane, William Graham III and Ronald Rosillo. "The Patient with Maxillofacial Cancer, Surgical Treatment and Nursing Care," *The Nursing Clinics of North America,* 8:137-51, March, 1973.

Wolf, Edith. "Where Hope Comes First," *Nursing Outlook,* 12:52-54, April, 1964.

Zavertnik, J. J. "Emotional Support of Patients with Head and Neck Surgery," *Nursing Clinics of North America,* 2:503-10, September 1967. pp. 503-510.

Patients with Lung Cancer

Regional Medical Program — Oncology Nursing Seminar

on

NURSING MANAGEMENT OF PATIENTS WITH
LUNG CANCER

Seminar Leader

Edward J. Beattie, Jr., M.D.

Seminar Participants

Edward J. Beattie, Jr., M.D., Chief Medical Officer and Chief of
   Thoracic Service

Karamat Choudhry, M.D., Thoracic Service

Bennie Davis, R.N., B.S.N., Professional Nurse Practitioner

Paul L. Goldiner, M.D., Associate Attending Anesthesiologist

Patricia Mazzola, R.N., B.S.N., Clinical Nursing Instructor

Dulce Twist, B.S., R.P.T., Physical Therapist

Cancer of the lung is the commonest killing cancer among men. Some 60,000 American men get it every year and less than 10 percent of them are cured. Of all deaths from cancer in men, 48 percent are due to cancer of the lungs, colon, prostate, and bladder, with cancer of the lung accounting for 18 percent of this figure. Women do not seem to be as susceptible as men to this form of tumor; four to five times more men than women develop cancer of the lung. Assuming a life span of 70 years and a continuation of the present incidence rate, 4.2 million males living in the United States today will get lung cancer in the next 70 years and 90 percent of them will die of it. The situation is even worse in Scotland where the incidence rate is 75 per 100,000 men—50 percent higher than in the United States with its rate of 50 per 100,000; in fact, Scotland has the highest rate in the world. Scottish women too have a higher incidence rate than American women. However, lung cancer is on the rise among women in the United States and this seems to be directly related to the fact that the number of American women who smoke is increasing every year.

All cancers of the lung have a high degree of malignancy. The oat cell carcinoma, which causes only about 5 percent of lung cancers, is probably the most malignant type. Most patients who develop this die within a few months; some who are treated with chemotherapy and radiotherapy survive somewhat longer. Terminal bronchiolar carcinoma, or the alveolar cell carcinoma, has about a 40 to 50 percent cure rate, more women being cured than men; when distant metastasis is present at the time treatment is started, the usual survival time is three years. The well keratinized lung cancers that grow to be big bulky tumors without lymph node metastases are very curable.

ETIOLOGY

It has been difficult in the past to obtain accurate statistics on the relationship between air pollution and the incidence of lung cancer. Reliable investigators have now studied this problem, however, and have found that there is a definite link between the pollution of the air, either by cigarette smoke or industrial pollutants, and the incidence of cancer of the lung.

Epidermoid cancer, the commonest type of lung cancer, is unquestionably linked to smoking. It is generally believed that if everyone who now smokes would stop, there would be a remarkable decline in the number of people who get lung cancer.

Among the studies that have been done on the effects of air pollution on carcinogenesis, that of Dr. Ernest Wynder, carried out in New York, Detroit, and Los Angeles showed that, in experimental animals, the pollution from cigarette smoke was 50 times more likely to cause skin cancer than the polluted air from any one of these three cities. This and other reports have led to the general observation that industrial pollutants have been overrated as a cause of cancer as compared to pollution from cigarettes.

It was once thought that arsenic miners were particularly susceptible to lung cancer until a definitive study showed that the incidence rate was high among those miners who smoked but that among the non-smokers it was no higher than in the general population. Uranium miners too have been thought to be particularly susceptible to lung cancer but, again, a study of radioactive mines has shown that people who work in them and do not smoke do not get cancer any more frequently than non-smokers in the general population. One kind of mining, however, does expose miners to carcinogenic material—that is, asbestos mining. It causes malignant tumors of the pleura that are usually non-curable. Asbestos may also be an air pollutant, a fact that became publicized during the building of the World Trade Center in New York City. Asbestos powder, a fireproofing material, was sprayed on the steel beams used in the construction of this 100-story building. An alert public health officer found that the percentage of asbestos dust being thrown off into the air constituted a serious health hazard to the entire city and was able to secure a cease and desist order against this procedure.

It is often thought that patients who have chronic bronchitis or chronic emphysema are quite likely to develop lung cancer. Some of them do, of course. But the real cause is not the bronchitis or the emphysema, but smoking. Both of these diseases are caused by smoking, and many smokers get cancer of the lung, so undoubtedly people with either of these diseases often also get cancer.

Alcohol is another agent that is often suspected of causing lung cancer, but this does not appear to be a fact.

The question often arises as to whether lung cancer may be hereditary. The consensus among physicians is that lung cancer is not hereditary in the sense of genes being passed from parents to children. It does appear, however, that certain types of cancer tend to occur more often in some families than in others. The general belief is that the reasons for this are environmental. For example, children whose parents both smoke usually also become smokers and thus their chances of developing lung cancer are enhanced. Oncologists who entertain the theory that some cancers are caused by a virus hold that when cancer occurs frequently in certain families, it is caused by exposure to the same virus, rather than being hereditary.

PREVENTION

Everyone who smokes heavily should have a semiannual chest x-ray examination and, after the age of 40, a sputum test twice a year as well. (A heavy smoker is defined as one who smokes over a pack of cigarettes a day and has done so for a period of at least 20 years.) These tests could be staggered; for example, the chest x-ray could be done in March and September and the sputum test in June and December, thus increasing the likelihood of discovering cancer earlier than usually happens at present.

Because it is very difficult to break the habit once it is established, it is essential that children be educated as to the deleterious effects of smoking, in the hope that this will keep them from ever starting to smoke. A number of studies have shown that the majority of children whose parents smoke also develop the habit, and that children of non-smokers are less likely to become smokers. The American Cancer Society has presented a series of television commercials aimed at teaching children the possible ill effects of smoking, and has sponsored several anti-smoking programs in schools. Many public schools have a good ACS-sponsored anti-smoking program which often includes two excellent films—"The Huffless Puffless Dragon," a film geared to elementary grade children, and "I'll Take the High Road" for junior high-school students. The aim, of course, is to teach children the advantages of never starting to smoke.

It is very difficult to motivate smokers to give up the habit. Some of the "stop smoking" clinics have been quite successful, but not many of the clinic members who stopped have remained non-smokers.

If one cannot stop smoking, he should switch to filter cigarettes with a low tar and nicotine content and then smoke only part of the cigarette; it is the last part that is most harmful. This should reduce one's chances of getting lung cancer by about four or five times. Dr. Ernest Wynder has shown that if a person switches to filter cigarettes, even though he does not cut down on the number he smokes per day, he reduces the risk of getting cancer by 50 percent. However, it will take that person 14 years to reduce his risk to that enjoyed by the non-smoker.

DIAGNOSIS AND PROGNOSIS

Lung cancer is a fairly slow growing type of cancer. Ordinarily, about 20 months elapse between the time the lesion becomes visible on x-ray and the appearance of symptoms. The first symptom is usually a change in the character or severity of a chronic cough the patient may have, especially if he is a smoker. Consequently, he often waits two or three months before seeing a doctor, and tries various cough syrups and other self-treatment measures. Even after he goes to a physician there is more delay— often as much as four months during which the patient is treated first with one antibiotic and then another and, by this time, 27 months will have passed since the lesion became visible on x-ray. Unfortunately, in many cases the lesion has grown and metastasis has taken place to the extent that cure is no longer possible. After all this delay, the patient is in poor condition and this, coupled with the fact that many of these patients are in their 50's and 60's, are heavy smokers, and may also have a heart condition, increases the surgical risk.

In one-third of the patients with lung cancer, the tumor has become inoperable by the time a diagnosis is made, and nothing can be done to save their lives. These patients live, on the average, seven months. Thus, two-thirds of the patients who are diagnosed as having lung cancer go to surgery for removal of the tumor and, at operation, one-half of them are found to have tumors that are technically non-removable, and these patients, too, have a survival of about seven months. Only one-third of the patients who have their cancers removed are alive five years later and free of disease. These depressing statistics show why the cure rate for cancer of the lung is only about 10 percent.

The two most important tests utilized in diagnosing lung cancer are 1) an x-ray of the chest, which is the more common, and 2) a cytological examination of the sputum. In about 20 percent of cases, a definitive diagnosis can be made only at the time of operation and thus thoracotomy becomes a diagnostic maneuver.

There is no way of telling how long a cancer lesion seen on x-ray has been growing, because the lesion has to be four or five millimeters in diameter before it is visible on film. Millions of cancer cells can be found in an area the size of the head of a pin, so that the number in a lesion with a four-millimeter diameter can be very great. Obviously, cancer can be easily missed on routine x-rays. If a lesion is found on the films of a person who has an annual chest x-ray, the chances are that no objective symptoms will yet be present because of the 20-month interval between the time the lesion is visible on x-ray and the appearance of symptoms.

Even though a cancer lesion in the lung may not be large enough to be recognized on x-ray examination, the person who has such a lesion constantly throws off cancer cells in his sputum, so a cytological sputum examination is an important diagnostic procedure. A positive sputum test may be followed by more sophisticated x-rays or a bronchogram to locate the lesion and then, if the tumor is removed, the patient has a 60 percent chance for cure as compared with the national cure rate for cancers treated after the lesion is visible on x-ray. A lesion that can be seen on x-rays when the patient still has no symptoms is described as a "coin lesion." It may be as small as a British farthing or as large as an American silver dollar. Surgical removal of such lesions results in a 30 to 60 percent cure rate.

The person who does not have annual chest x-rays and who does not see a doctor until he is symptomatic may present with a condition resembling pneumonia or some other disease because asymptomatic lung cancer can, and does, mimic almost any number of other disease conditions of the chest. It can cause hemoptysis, shortness of breath if the diaphragm is paralyzed or if the chest is full of fluid, hoarseness if the vocal cords are paralyzed, pain if the cancer has invaded the chest wall or the nerve fibers. Cough is the most consistent symptom, however, and the fact that it may be a sign of cancer is apt to be overlooked because all smokers cough. The person who notices a change in his cough—perhaps it is more annoying, more difficult to control, or more productive—naturally tries to take care of himself for a while. He changes his brand of cigarettes, switches to filters, or asks the local pharmacist for a good cough medicine. He may even stop smoking for a while. What finally takes him to the doctor is the recognition that none of the things he has tried has done him any good. And by this time his chances for a cure have been substantially reduced.

Two major diagnostic procedures that are usually carried out when the patient is suspected of having cancer of the lung are bronchoscopy and bronchography. Even though x-ray reports and physical signs and symptoms are positive for cancer of the lung, proof of the presence of the disease requires a demonstration of tumor cells.

Bronchoscopy, performed by passing an endoscope into the trachea and bronchi, allows the physician to visualize these structures and to biopsy any visible lesions. The procedure should be fully explained to the patient. He should be told that he will not be allowed to take anything by mouth after midnight of the day before the bronchoscopy; that he will be given a medication that will permit him to be more relaxed during the procedure and will decrease the amount of his secretions; that he will be awake and somewhat alert during the test; but that an anesthetic will be sprayed along the path of the bronchoscope. Most importantly, he should be assured that he will be able to breathe through his nose. If he has a denture or removable bridge, this is removed before the examination.

The idea of visualizing the tracheobronchial tree is not new. Philipp Bozzini of Frankfurt first attempted to visualize the esophagus by means of an endoscope (1807), but with little success. In 1889, Adolf Kussmaul, also a German physician, performed the first successful esophagoscopy and demonstrated carcinoma of the gastric esophagus. Gustav Michaelis first examined the stomach endoscopically in 1831. In 1890, Chevalier Jackson, an American laryngologist, removed two foreign bodies from the esophagus. Gustav Killian of Freiberg, Germany, was called the father of bronchoscopy; he demonstrated in 1897 that rigid tubes could be passed into the bronchi and he removed a foreign body, a bone, from the right bronchus. In 1902, Max Einhorn, a Russian in the United States, devised a tube with distal illumination. In the following year, Chevalier Jackson, who was at that time in Pittsburgh, combined the lighting principles of Einhorn's tube with the Killian tube to make a bronchoscope to which he later added aspirating tubes.

The indications for bronchoscopy are diagnostic and therapeutic. Even if there is a positive sputum cytology and the diagnosis is known, it is essential to know the status of the airway, whether the vocal cords are moving, whether the trachea is clear, and whether there is an obstruction in a bronchus. Any patient who has an unexplained cough needs a cytological examination and thus may be scheduled for bronchoscopy; specimens for examination may be obtained through a bronchoscope by washing with saline. A second indication is the need to determine the extent of all visible lesions in the endotracheal tree, and to obtain specimens for biopsy. A third indication is the need to evaluate, before the operation, the extent of the lung resection that is required. In addition, when a patient has unexplained hemoptysis, bronchoscopy makes it possible to locate the source of the bleeding—the site, the lobe, and even the segment of the lobe that it is coming from. Patients with wheezing, especially if it is localized to one part of the lung; patients with persistent, unexplained cough; and patients whose x-rays show atelectasis are also candidates for bronchoscopy. Although sputum cytology is more accurate as a diagnostic test than examination of bronchial washings, bronchoscopy is useful in providing information about the size, location, and extent of lesions to be biopsied.

The therapeutic indications for bronchoscopy are: 1) the need for drainage in cases of lung abscess; 2) to dilate any stricture in the tracheobronchial tree; 3) to aspirate secretions when there is an obstructed lobe, or segment of a lobe of the lung; and, 4) to apply electrocoagulation to small bleeding points at the time bronchoscopy is done.

Bronchoscopy is often thought of as an extremely uncomfortable procedure, but it need not be if the endoscopist and the anesthesiologist are skillful and the patient has been properly medicated with a tranquilizer or a sedative. Strict aseptic technique is employed. The anesthesia usually consists of 1) a block of the superior laryngeal nerve on both sides of the neck as it travels between the hyoid bone and the thyroid cartilage (to desensitize the posterior part of the tongue, pharynx, and part of the vocal cords); and, 2) a topical anesthetic spray directed into the larynx and down the trachea. The patient becomes relaxed but is very cooperative, responsive to instructions, and remains awake although he will not remember much of the procedure afterwards.

The patient's head is draped with towels and his eyes covered with a piece of vaseline gauze to protect them, and sponges are provided to protect the patient's upper gums and teeth. Included in the setup are a biopsy forcep; a basin containing formalin to place the specimen in, and a series of test tubes of different colors that are used for collecting the cytology specimens from each bronchus and the trachea; a suction apparatus; additional anesthetic if needed for the farther reaches of the tracheobronchial tree; the bronchoscope, and fiberoptic telescopes that can be introduced through the bronchoscope to visualize the lobe orifices and segmental openings. There is a trap in the bronchoscope through which sterile saline solution can be instilled; the patient is instructed to cough it back up and this provides a bronchial washing.

The telescopes have a flexible tip with a remote control that makes it possible for the endoscopist to steer the tip so that he can visualize the area from which washings are desired. The first thing one sees is the bifurcation of the trachea, the carina. The right stem bronchus goes almost straight down; one can see the orifices into the three lobes of the lung and can take biopsies or washings from the different areas for bacteriologic or cytologic examination. Then the tube is brought up as far as the carina and lowered into the left bronchus which is at somewhat more of an acute angle, and the performance is repeated for the two lobes of the left lung. Some patients have cancer cells on one side and not the other, and thus the bronchial washings are valuable in actually localizing both the side and the lobe affected.

The nurse assists with the instillation of sterile saline solution through the aspiration line that goes into the bronchoscope. Because of the irritation caused by the instrument, the patient will cough thoroughly. This produces the most valuable specimen for cytology.

Only about 20 percent of lung cancers are detectable by bronchoscopy, and these occur in patients who cannot cough up any secretions. Peripheral coin lesions will not be detected. Hence the reliance on sputum cytology for accurate diagnosis.

Bronchoscopy is also sometimes used to help clear out secretions postoperatively when the patient will not cough. In this case, it is more uncomfortable because the procedure is performed without much anesthesia.

Because of the danger of aspiration, the patient is not permitted to eat after having a bronchoscopic examination until the gag reflex has returned. This may be determined by touching the back of the pharynx with a cotton swab. Usually it takes four hours for sensation to return. Throat and mouth soreness, which may persist for several days, may be relieved by gargles and lozenges. Frequently, during the first 24 postoperative hours after the examination, all sputum specimens from the bronchi are saved for the cytologist. The patient should be told that his sputum may be blood-streaked for a day or so, but that this is a normal occurrence and he should not be alarmed about it.

Bronchography is a visualization of the bronchial tree after the insertion of a radiopaque dye into the trachea. The physician tries to make this procedure as painless as possible. Often, he simply numbs the neck, inserts a fair-sized needle directly into the trachea, passes a fine catheter through the needle into the trachea, and injects the contrast medium. The patient is tilted in various positions to distribute the dye into his lungs and throughout the tracheobronchial tree, and then the lungs are x-rayed. The dye is sometimes injected through a bronchoscope, and then the care includes all measures employed in a bronchoscopy.

Scalene node biopsy is another preoperative test that may be done. Although complications following this kind of biopsy are rare, there may be bleeding or the formation of a hematoma that will require evacuation; pneumothorax; wound emphysema; wound infection; or lymph fistulae.

Pulmonary function tests are done preoperatively for three reasons: 1) to determine whether surgery is feasible and, if so, what kind of surgery can be done when the patient's pulmonary function is already compromised by concomitant obstructive disease; 2) to find out if there is any possibility of improving the patient's pulmonary function before the operation takes place; and, 3) to establish base lines for his postoperative care. Fully 90 to 95 percent of the patients who come to the hospital for treatment of cancer of the lung are long-time smokers. Because the cancer is the culmination of cigarette smoking and breathing polluted air over the years, most of these patients have a concomitant obstructive pulmonary disease which, in some, is quite severe. The older the patient and the more extensive the cancer, the more extensive the concomitant pulmonary disease. Consequently, what the surgeon can do for the patient often depends on factors other than the cancer.

Pulmonary function tests are a simple and painless method of finding out whether the patient will be left with sufficient lung function after the contemplated surgery. The usual tests are basically studies of the capacity of the patient's lungs to move gas. Vital capacity, tidal volume, and residual volume are all measured. Vital capacity and tidal volume are both lower than normal in patients with lung cancer. This is due to the chronic obstructive disease, possibly an emphysematous condition, and the overlying tumor. On the other hand, the residual volume, that is, the amount of air that remains trapped in the lungs, is increased. Functional volumes indicate the patient's ability to get air out of the lungs within a certain time. The normal individual gets out between 95 and 100 percent of his tidal air in 3 seconds, but patients with lung cancer can get out only between 50 and 60 percent in that time. These patients can probably be helped considerably by preoperative instruction in deep breathing and coughing, inhalation therapy, IPPB treatments, and bronchodilator drugs, all of which aid in reducing the obstruction and thus diminish postoperative complications.

The patient does not need any special preparation for these tests. He should be told, however, that they are time-consuming and that they will include blood gas determinations as well as tests of his breathing ability.

Blood gas studies include determination of the pH, the partial pressure of oxygen (PO_2) and the partial pressure of carbon dioxide (PCO_2). Because most of the patients with cancer of the lung also have chronic pulmonary disease, their blood pH is somewhat lower than in normal individuals in whom the range is from 7.35 to 7.45. In other words, the average lung cancer patient has a basic respiratory acidosis. The normal partial pressure of carbon dioxide is between 35 and 45 mm Hg, but almost all patients with significant emphysema have a preoperative PCO_2 of above 45. This indicates that they are retaining more than the normal amount of CO_2 and thus their capacity for diffusion and ventilation are diminished, resulting in a lowered or acidotic pH. The PO_2 range in normal individuals is between 90 and 100 mm Hg, but in lung cancer patients it is usually between 70 and 80. Occasionally, in severely compromised patients, it is as low as 55 to 60.

It is important for the physician to know the patient's preoperative PO_2 so as not to over-oxygenate him by mask or cannula postoperatively. Much of the patient's respiratory drive is based on lack of oxygen, and if the PO_2 is brought to too high a level postoperatively, the patient may have severe respiratory difficulties and possibly respiratory arrest. More patients have a near normal PCO_2 preoperatively because it is easier to get rid of the excess CO_2 than it is to take in enough oxygen to bring the PO_2 up to a normal level.

TREATMENT

As with other forms of cancer, the earlier lung cancer is detected the better the chance for cure. When the patient is in good general health and the tumor is confined to one lung, and if it can be resected adequately without leaving the patient a cripple, he has a 30 to 40 percent chance of having at least a five-year survival. X-ray therapy alone produces five-year survival in less than 1 percent of patients. Implantation of such radioactive materials as radon or radioactive iodine seeds, which requires a surgical procedure, results in a cure rate of 8 to 16 percent. Chemotherapy is useful as an adjunctive treatment but, to date, there are no statistics to show that chemotherapy, by itself, effects a cure. Immunotherapy is still in its infancy; how effective it might become in the future is still not known. Surgery, then, appears to be the only effective treatment for lung cancer.

If lung cancer is diagnosed early—that is, before the lesion is visible on x-ray, there is a 60 percent chance that surgery will effect a cure; if diagnosed during the "coin lesion" stage, but the patient is still asymptomatic, the chance that surgery will effect a cure is 30 to 60 percent if the tumor is resected thoroughly; and if diagnosed after symptoms are present, the chance for cure through surgery is 30 percent if excision is possible.

If the tumor has spread to the other lung, or if it has invaded the pleura, it is already incurable and no longer treatable by surgery, but cobalt therapy and chemotherapy may be used as palliative measures. Patients who have a curable lesion and who elect to try cobalt therapy stand a 90 percent chance of dying within a year, a 99 percent chance of dying within two years, and only one in 500 of these patients will be alive five years later. However, when a patient has a large lesion in the lung and is short of breath because of compression by the tumor mass, cobalt radiation can reduce the size of the mass enough to allow the patient to breathe adequately for carrying on his life activities.

In certain types of cancer, the preoperative or postoperative use of radiation gives better results than surgery alone. A tumor that is located at the top of the lung, the superior sulcus, will respond to surgery with a cure rate of about 20 percent; to implantation with radiation with a rate of about 16 percent; and to radiation plus surgery with a rate of about 30 percent. At the present time, treatment of these tumors with preoperative radiation, surgery, and then implantation of residuals is resulting in a two-year cure rate for 50 percent of patients. In a national study of patients who had irradiation followed by surgery, the results were no better than those for surgery alone, and the morbidity was higher. Consequently, preoperative irradiation is not used routinely for patients having surgery for lung cancer.

Implantation of radioisotopes is sometimes used for treating nonresectable cancer lesions of no more than 6 or 7 centimeters in diameter, and experience has shown that when radon seeds are used, about an 8 percent cure rate can be achieved. Whether iodine-125 will give a better cure rate remains to be seen; it is being used because it is less strong, it is readily available, and the effects last longer—actually, about a year (half life = 60 days).

For advanced cancer, chemotherapy may be of value in the treatment of extended metastasis and, in these cases, palliation is achieved in 5 to 10 percent of cases, although it may not be effective in reducing the size of the mass.

The surgical risk in diagnostic thoracotomy should be less than 1 percent; the risk in patients with extended resection is from 5 to 10 percent. Pneumonectomy is avoided whenever possible, particularly when the right lung is involved, for this lung is responsible for 55 percent of total lung capacity. In the 50- to 60-year age group, pneumonectomy has an operative mortality of 20 percent. The present cure rate after radical lobectomy, taking out as many of the lymph nodes as possible, is about 45 percent.

Preparation for Surgery

The amount of time that goes into preparing the lung cancer patient for surgery will have a directly proportional effect on the success of the treatment. These patients require exceptionally intelligent preoperative care. During the period before the operation, the nurse's first responsibility is to establish rapport with the patient, since it is she who works closest with him and functions as interpreter and teacher as well as nurse. She must assess his physical and mental capabilities and his fears and understandings in order to determine his physical, psychological, and spiritual needs. Her accurate observations and reports are important to the patient, the physican, and other responsible personnel.

The patient usually comes to the hospital knowing he will have certain tests, x-ray examinations, and blood studies, but he often has many misconceptions about them. Therefore, it is important for the nurse to explain the reasons for the tests, how they are done, what is expected of him, and what he will experience during them. He should be assured that these routine but time-consuming procedures are very important in establishing a diagnosis, prescribing treatment, and determining the type of surgery that may be done. For example, if the complete blood count shows that the patient should receive blood, packed cells, or plasma, he must be told why this is necessary and approximately when the transfusion will be started.

The analysis of blood gases will reflect the patient's ventilation efficiency, the ability of the hemoglobin to carry oxygen and carbon dioxide, the rate of cellular metabolism, and the state of the buffer system. The patient should be told that the blood samples will be taken from his radial or femoral artery and that afterwards direct, steady pressure will be exerted over the site for five minutes to prevent hematomas and hemorrhage.

Obtaining good sputum specimens for cytology is another important nursing procedure because this is the most useful type of specimen for cytologic diagnosis of lung cancer. The best specimens are obtained in the early morning when the patient usually coughs easily and more productively than later in the day, and when there is less chance that the sputum will contain food particles. The nurse must explain carefully, the night before the specimen is to be collected, that saliva and mucus from the back of the throat are of no diagnostic value, and that the patient must cough very deeply and expectorate into the specimen jar that contains 50 percent alcohol which acts as a fixative. The jar is left at the bedside so that it will be at hand the first thing in the morning. The patient may drink water or tea without milk to assist in producing the specimen. Frequently, three specimens are taken on different days for comparison and to increase the likelihood of finding and identifying cancer cells. If the patient is unable to cough deeply enough to produce a good specimen, a sputogenic machine may be used to assist him; this must be ordered by the physician.

A routine urinalysis is done preoperatively to determine whether the patient is spilling sugar or acetone and, if he is, therapy will be instituted.

An electrocardiogram is also done and, again, the patient is told that this is a routine test of heart action, and the procedure is briefly explained if it is the first time the patient has had an EKG.

After the routine and specific diagnostic tests have been done and the surgeon has decided to operate, the patient must be prepared psychologically as well as physically for the surgery. The surgeon, sometimes accompanied by the nurse and selected members of the care team, visit the patient at a time when his family is there, if possible, and explain what is going to be done and why. Thus, when he signs the operative informed consent form he really knows what to expect from the surgery and in the postoperative period. The nurse can help to build up the patient's morale by assuring him of the competency of the surgical team and instructing him as to the how, why, where, and when of various postoperative procedures. This will help to minimize his fear postoperatively, and having this knowledge ahead of time will enable him to be more cooperative in the period immediately after surgery when his attention span is short because of the pain and the medications he is receiving.

The thoracotomy patient should be told that he will be taken to the recovery room before returning to his nursing unit, that he will be receiving intravenous fluids, that he may have thoracotomy tubes to drain fluid and air from his lungs and help reexpand them, that he will have pain for which he will be given medication, that a nurse will check his vital signs frequently, that x-rays will be taken and probably blood samples also. The patient should know that he will be encouraged—almost forced—to cough, breathe deeply, turn frequently, perform leg exercises, and to ambulate early. He will be more cooperative if he understands why he is expected to be so active after surgery. He should understand especially that good coughing is extremely important, since it is one of the most effective means of removing excess secretions that accumulate as a result of the trauma from the surgery and anesthesia. In addition, he should be told enough about positive pressure to understand that coughing increases the positive pressure in the pleural cavity and this forces the air and fluid out through the thoracotomy tube. The nurse and the physical therapist instruct the patient in the techniques of deep breathing and coughing.

Deep breathing and coughing instruction should begin at least two days prior to the patient's operation. After surgery he is anxious and in pain, and it is impossible for him to relax sufficiently to listen to instructions. The nurse or the physical therapist, or both, explain carefully the facts about drainage, cupping, and clapping. The most difficult technique to teach the patient is how to use his diaphragm in breathing.

Before starting the breathing exercises, place the patient in high Fowler's position. Sometimes just the activity of moving around makes the patient cough. Tell him to put his hand on his belly. (Every patient will know what his belly is although some may not know what the word abdomen means.) Tell him that you want him to feel his breathing. He must be relaxed in order to breathe abdominally, so the nurse may need to talk to him quietly, put a pillow under his elbows to make sure he is not pressing down on the bed with them, and change his position somewhat. After he is fully relaxed he will discover that he does have some movement in his abdomen when he breathes; ask him to concentrate on how it expands when he breathes in and flattens when he breathes out. Ask him to try to exaggerate each breath a little, and to take deeper and deeper breaths so as to expand his abdomen more, until he is expanding it as much as he can. This will put him well on the way to abdominal breathing but he probably will still not be breathing as deeply as he could.

The next step is to teach him how to breathe out long enough to get rid of all his reserve air. To do this he blows out all the air he possibly can through pursed lips and with his hand on his abdomen so that he can feel what happens as he does this . (Pursed-lip breathing causes a back pressure that gives abdominal muscles a resistance to work against.) The patient will be able to feel these muscles working and will get the idea of using them in his coughing and while breathing. Also, exhaling this way helps move mucus upward. It also gives the patient an indication of how much air he is expiring so he can try to expire more with each successive breath. The emphysema patient needs to learn to breathe in this way in order to blow off his excess carbon dioxide. The patient's reaction to this will be to take a deep breath. After two, three, or even five minutes of this kind of breathing, he will be able to take deep breaths and can be taught coughing.

The first step in coughing is called huffing. This consists of taking a deep inspiration and filling the lungs as full as possible but, instead of blowing the air out in the usual way, letting it out against one's hand, as though steaming one's eyeglasses. This causes the abdominal muscles to contract when the abdomen is drawn in. When the patient is able to feel his abdominal muscles contract when he exhales this way, have him breathe out in short, sharp puffs or pants. If his abdominal muscles are weak, he may not be able to do this and the nurse will have to work with him for some time to help him strengthen his muscles. This is an important exercise because the abdominals are girdle muscles, and when they contract the abdominal contents are pushed up against the diaphragm and this helps to force the air up and out of the lungs, and any excess mucus along with it. The reason for "steaming the eyeglasses" is to make sure the patient has an open airway and does not constrict his throat. Have the patient build up from small huffs to one strong huff, and cough as he expires this air.

If the patient's abdominal muscles are so weak that he cannot use them to assist in coughing, try to get him to breathe as basely as possible because the base of the lung is so much larger than the apex. This kind of breathing will result in lateral costal expansion. First, have the patient hug himself by reaching one arm over the opposite side as far as he can without twisting his torso, and breathe in while squeezing himself lightly so that he can feel the hug. He should breathe quietly through his nose and try to expand the chest as much as possible on that side. As the chest expands he should press hard with his hand. The lungs expand along with the chest and therefore a space is created in the lungs and the air rushes in. If the patient has a large flabby abdomen, the nurse may try supporting it when he coughs; if this is not successful, she may apply a tight abdominal binder to give him support. This may make it difficult for him to inspire deeply but it will help him to accomplish lateral costal breathing followed by coughing.

If there are secretions at the base of the lung that the patient has difficulty in coughing up, have him lie on the side opposite to where the ronchi are heard, and cough. Then he should lie on the other side and cough. Have him hug his chest with the under arm, and with the other arm reach as high as he can. This will expand the side of the chest that is uppermost and which is probably the side with the atelectasis or collection of mucus (he is probably lying on his sound side). He cannot breathe as deeply with the sound side because he is lying on it, so he is forced to expand the affected side. He will not be able to do this immediately following surgery; he must work into it gradually. If he cannot do this at all, it is important to change his position frequently.

One important point about coughing the patient is that the incision must always be supported. The thoracotomy patient can be taught to support himself by reaching around as far as he can with the arm opposite to the side with surgery. The nurse should place her hand on the back near the spine at the same time. Another way to splint the patient while coughing is to roll down the top of the bedclothes and use this to support the thoracotomy, or a rolled up towel or pillow can be used. Whatever method is used, it is vital that the patient be supported or "splinted" while coughing.

COMPREHENSIVE POSTOPERATIVE
NURSING CARE

The two procedures of first importance after surgical intervention via thoracotomy are the maintenance of a patent airway and the reestablishment of negative intrapleural pressure. Measures most frequently used to maintain a patent airway include deep breathing, coughing, suctioning, humidification, frequent turning, and keeping the patient in semi-Fowler's position and well up toward the head of the bed to prevent slumping and compression of the rib cage and diaphragm.

Tracheobronchial secretions always increase following anesthesia. Their normal thin, mucoid consistency changes to one that is thick and tenacious. Ciliary action in the air passages is impaired and coughing may be ineffective because of pain and limitation of motion. Measures to maintain a clear airway and prevent accumulation of secretions to the point of atelectasis represent a principle postoperative nursing function. Atelectasis is the actual collapse of a portion of a lung or an entire lung. It may be caused

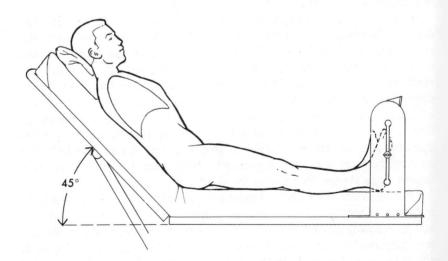

Figure 1. Patient in semi-Fowler's position

by a plugged bronchus, reduced tone of the respiratory muscles or, most commonly, by excessive mucus which can lead to emphysema or spontaneous pneumothorax and may cause death from asphyxia.

Coughing is one of the most effective ways of keeping the tracheobronchial tree free of secretions, and the nurse should continue to instruct the patient to breathe deeply and cough as he was taught to do preoperatively. Frequent turning and humidification help to loosen secretions. Keeping the patient's body in proper alignment in addition to placing him in semi- or low Fowler's position allows for better alignment of the lungs. The knee gatch should not be used because it not only tends to promote stasis in the lower extremities, but also tends to cause the abdominal viscera to be pushed up against the diaphragm and thus interfere with the downward movement of that organ.

An analgesic will be needed to make it possible for the patient to turn, cough, and deep breathe without too much discomfort. The analgesic chosen should not depress the patient's respirations or level of consciousness. The drug of choice in Memorial Hospital recovery room is Numorphan, I mg IM. Numorphan is said to have an effect equivalent to 10 mg of morphine, but does not have the same respiratory depressant effect. After the patient returns to the regular nursing unit, smaller doses of narcotics are given at more frequent intervals. Pain is a subjective experience and differs from one

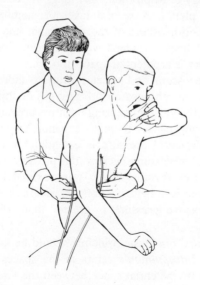

Figure 2. Supporting incision while patient coughs

person to another. Constant reassurance from the doctor and nurse often does wonders toward relieving pain. In any case, pain must be relieved, otherwise the patient will not cough.

Nasotracheal suction may be necessary if the patient is unable to cough productively. Sterile technique is always employed. The placement of the catheter is usually accomplished by gentle probing via the nasal passage with a sterile moistened catheter while a piece of gauze is used to grasp the tongue and pull it forward to lift the epiglottis from the larynx. After the catheter has entered the trachea, secretions are evacuated, using 5- to 7-second periods of nasotracheal suction, followed by intervals of oxygen administration at a rate of 10 to 15 liters per minute. During these pauses for oxygen, the suction catheter is left in place but sharply kinked or disconnected to prevent it from continuing to suck endotracheal air and suffocating the patient. After a few such sessions, the patient will make a great effort to cough well.

The Principles of Closed Chest Drainage

The reestablishment of negative intrapleural pressure is obtained primarily by closed chest drainage. To understand the principles and mechanics of closed chest drainage, the nurse must first clearly understand the basic anatomy and physiology of respiration. The lungs are covered with a membrane called visceral pleura. A second layer of membrane, the parietal pleura, covers the superior aspect of the diaphragm and the structures in the mediastinum, and lines the chest wall. Between these two layers of pleural membrane there is a potential space into which enough serous fluid is secreted to allow the visceral and parietal pleura to slide over one another without friction. These membranes absorb any gas or fluid that enters the space and create a partial vacuum causing negative pressure which, in turn, "pulls" on the lungs and causes them to expand. The maintenance of a constant negative interpleural pressure is essential for normal breathing. The term "negative" is misleading because the pressure is negative only in reference to atmospheric pressure, which is approximately 760 millimeters of mercury. In other words, a negative pressure is less than 760 millimeters of mercury and a positive pressure is greater than 760 millimeters of mercury.

Certain definitions and one basic principle should be kept in mind when referring to pressure. *Intrapulmonic* refers to the spaces within the lung. *Intrathoracic* refers to the potential space between the visceral and parietal pleura. The basic principle to remember is that all gases, including air, move

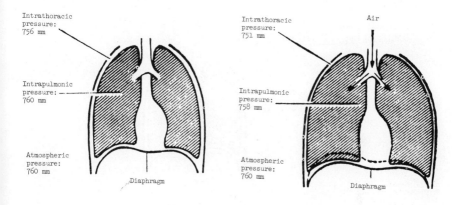

Figure 3. Chest at rest   Figure 4. Chest on inspiration

from a place of greater pressure into a place of lower pressure. (This is the principle that makes respiration and water seal drainage possible.)

Figure 3 shows the chest at rest; that is, the moment between respirations. The chest and contents maintain their normal size and position. Note that the pressure within the lungs and the atmospheric pressure are the same (760 mm Hg), but the pressure in the pleural space is slightly less (756 mm Hg) and therefore exerts a suctioning force which holds the lungs close to the rib cage. Because pressure within the lungs equals the atmospheric pressure, there is no movement of air. (Note: intrathoracic pressure is less than atmospheric pressure.)

Figure 4 shows the chest on inspiration. The diaphragm is now contracted, and is pulling downward. This has enlarged the chest cavity vertically. At the same time, the intercostal and accessory chest muscles are pulling the sternum and ribs up and out. (On taking a deep breath, one can feel these changes.) As the cavity has increased in size, the pressure within the pleural space has dropped. Thus a stronger suctioning force is being exerted and is pulling the lungs closer to the enlarged rib cage. This has resulted in enlargement of the intrapulmonic space and a decrease in the intrapulmonic pressure (758 mm Hg). According to the principle stated earlier, the greater atmospheric pressure (760 mm Hg) now causes air to move into the lungs and the person inhales.

On expiration (Figure 5), the respiratory muscles, especially the diaphragm, relax causing the chest cavity to grow smaller and, as it does so, the intrathoracic pressure rises. It is still negative, however, and continues to exert a suctioning force on the lungs, pulling them close to the rib cage and

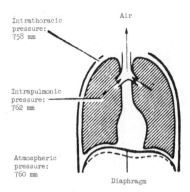

Figure 5. Chest on expiration

preventing them from collapsing. The rise in pressure within the intra-pleural space, coupled with the shrinking of the chest cavity squeezes the lungs and leads to a decrease in the intrapulmonic space, thus causing the pressure within the lungs to rise and the air within the lung rushes out in an exhalation. During surgery when the surgeon opens one side of the chest cavity, air at atmospheric pressure rushes into the pleural space equalizing the pressure. This causes a release of the lung from the usual suctioning exerted by negative pressure and the lung collapses. To help expand the collapsed lung or, in some cases, to prevent the danger of further collapse, the surgeon inserts a chest tube into the pleural space. The chest tube is connected to a closed chest drainage system with an underwater seal. The underwater seal allows air and fluid to drain out at the same time that it prevents air and fluid from returning to the pleural space.

Closed Chest Drainage Systems

The purpose of closed chest drainage is to remove blood, fluid, and air from the pleural space in an attempt to reestablish negative pressure which will promote and support the reexpansion of the lung. Proper drainage also prevents infection from developing in the pleural space and prevents compression of the trachea and mediastinum toward the unaffected side.

All equipment must be sterile in a closed drainage system, including the water or saline used, and all connections should be airtight and sealed with waterproof adhesive. Closed chest drainage systems operate on a one-bottle, two-bottle, and three-bottle gravity plus suction system.

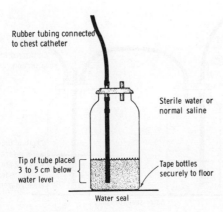

Rubber tubing connected
to chest catheter

Sterile water or
normal saline

Tip of tube placed
3 to 5 cm below
water level

Tape bottles
securely to floor

Water seal

Figure 6. Apparatus for one-bottle system of closed chest drainage

In the one-bottle system, the drainage is affected only by gravity. There-fore, the bottle and the connecting tubing are always kept lower than the chest. The tubing extending from the chest catheter is connected to a long tube the end of which is submerged in water to obtain an underwater seal. Before the patient is attached to the system, sufficient water is put in the bottle to ensure a water seal and the water level is marked so that the drainage from the patient's chest can be measured accurately. Any amount over the water seal mark is the actual drainage. Another, shorter tube pro-vides an air vent and this tube must never be obstructed. If the system is tight and functioning adequately, water will oscillate in the underwater tube and air will bubble from the tube when the patient breathes if there is air in the pleural space. On inspiration, water rises in the long tube and on expiration the water level drops below the water level in the bottle. Bubbles of air and drainage will pass out into the water if they are present in the pleural space. If, early in the postoperative period, water does not oscillate in the water seal tube, the nurse "milks" the tube from the pa-tient's chest down into the drainage bottle to dislodge clots and fibrin that may be occluding the tube. If this does not restore patency to the tube, the physician must be notified.

The two-bottle system is used when gravity drainage is insufficient to cause the lungs to reexpand. Suction is applied from a wall outlet or by an electric pump. To make sure that only the desired amount of suction will be obtained, a suction control bottle is added to the system. When suction is applied, bubbles should be observed in this control bottle. If bubbles are not seen, the suction from the suction outlet should be increased. Bottle 1

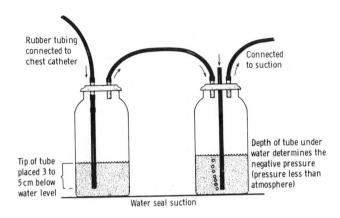

Figure 7. Apparatus for two-bottle system of closed chest drainage

provides the underwater seal and also serves as a drainage bottle. Fluid collects in bottle 1 and air travels from bottle 1 to bottle 2 (the suction control bottle) where it bubbles out. The depth of submersion of the long tube in the suction control bottle (2) determines the amount of negative pressure in the pleural cavity. The upper end of the long tube is open to the air and should never be obstructed.

In the three-bottle system with suction, a separate bottle is added for collecting drainage thus making it easier to measure and observe the nature of the drainage. Bottle 1 is the collection bottle; it is connected with rubber tubing to the patient's chest catheter at one end and at the other end to the

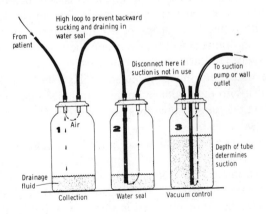

Figure 8. Apparatus for three-bottle system of closed chest drainage

long tube of bottle 2 (the water seal bottle). Bottle 3 is the suction control bottle. Again, the depth of the long tube in the water in the suction control bottle (3) determines the amount of negative pressure that reaches the patient's chest. And, again, this tube is open to the air and serves as an air vent that must not be obstructed. There will be bubbling in bottle 3 when it is connected to a suction source.

A Pleur-evac is a sterile, disposable plastic unit that provides underwater seal drainage of the pleural cavity. In principle, the Pleur-evac duplicates the three-bottle system by incorporating in a single package three separate chambers for collection of drainage, for providing a water seal, and for providing suction. It is more compact and easier for the nurse and the patient to handle than the three bottles.

Before connecting the patient's chest catheter to the Pleur-evac drainage system, the physician fills the water seal chamber to the level of 1 to 2 centimeters (not cc's) of water. (Note that this is centimeters and that to get 1 centimeter of water one must add approximately 70 cc's of water.)

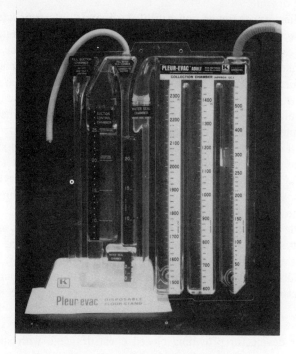

Figure 9. Adult Pleur-evac unit

Sterile water is added to the water seal chamber through a short rubber tubing that extends from the top of the chamber. A float valve situated high in the small arm of the water seal chamber allows the patient to develop as much negativity as he needs without the danger of the water contents in the water seal chamber being aspirated over into the collection chamber.

The suction control chamber is graduated from 5 to 30 centimeters. The height of the water added to this column will determine the amount of negative pressure exerted on the pleural space; usually 10 to 25 centimeters of pressure are ordered. An atmospheric opening at the top of the suction control chamber is used to fill the chamber to the desired level with sterile water and also provides the vent to the atmosphere. This opening should never be obstructed. For the patient to receive the desired negative pressure, the system must be connected by an additional piece of tubing to a suction source or outlet, the suction is started and then increased until bubbling occurs in the large arm of the suction chamber. Since the water in this chamber evaporates, the nurse is responsible for maintaining the suction at the desired level by adding water to the suction chamber through the atmospheric opening.

The collection chamber consists of 3 separate interconnected sections. The first section is calibrated for infant use in 2 cc increments up to 260 cc. Over 260 cc, the calibrations are in 5 cc increments. When the first section becomes filled, the drainage fluid cascades into the second section and then into the third section to provide a total capacity of approximately 2600 cc. The writing surface on each section of the collection chamber allows notations of fluid level, date, and time to be made directly on the calibration scale. Connecting tubing extends from the top of the chamber to the patient's chest catheter. Two self-sealing rubber diaphragms are located on the back of the collection chamber through which small amounts (1-10 cc) of drainage for bacteriological specimens may be aspirated. Aseptic technique must be observed and a 15-gauge needle attached to a syringe is used to aspirate the drainage from the chamber.

When the collection chamber is filled to capacity a new unit must be used since emptying of any large amount of fluid content through the diaphragms may increase negativity in the chambers to unacceptable levels.

The Pleur-evac has its own tip-proof stand and at the top there are hooks for connecting it to the patient's bed or to a stretcher if the patient is in transport.

Another device for providing closed chest drainage with suction is the Emerson pump. It is possible to obtain a greater amount of negative

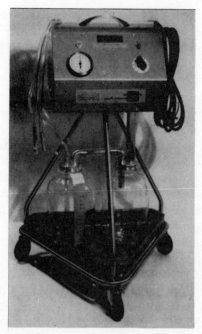

Figure 10. Emerson pump

pressure with this electrical suction pump than with the Pleur-evac. The Emerson pump duplicates the two-bottle system. The bottle on the right serves both as the water seal and the drainage bottle. Before connecting the chest catheter to the pump, 500 or 1000 cc of sterile water is added to the bottle to ensure the underwater seal. The level of the water is marked on the bottle. The patient is connected to the pump and this pump has provision for one or two chest catheters to be connected separately. After plugging in the pump, the physician turns it on to the continuous suction setting. He then turns the rheostat to the desired amount of suction which will be shown on a manometer. Tape should be put over the rheostat as a precaution against accidental changing of the setting. The second bottle is a vacuum bottle. Both bottles are kept in a mobile stand, thus making ambulation and transportation of the patient easier. When the patient is being transported, the suction may be turned off since the system will provide for gravity drainage. After the system is set up by the doctor, the nurse is responsible for its correct operation. Regardless of the system used, it is important that the nurse understand the design and operation of the unit because she has the final responsibility for the following duties:

1. Explaining the purpose of the treatment to the patient and members of his family and cautioning them not to tamper with any part of the equipment. After the dials are properly set they are taped to prevent inadvertent movement which may change the settings.

2. Observing the operation of the unit to see that the chest drainage system is functioning properly.

3. Checking all connections to be sure they are airtight and securely taped with waterproof adhesive.

4. Observing the character and amount of the drainage.

5. Preventing undue tension on the chest tube; it should be secured in a coiled fashion to the bottom bed sheet. The tubing should not be permitted to drag on the floor where it can be tripped over or caught by moveable furniture and possibly dislodged, but at the same time the patient should have enough leeway for moving about in bed.

6. Keeping all equipment below the level of the chest to prevent reflux of drainage into the pleural cavity.

7. Noting whether bubbling occurs in the drainage bottle. At first this may be due to a large amount of air being expelled from the intrapleural space but if it continues or if it suddenly increases, it may indicate the presence of a bronchopleural fistula, a tear in the lung, or a leak at the wound site.

8. Noting whether fluctuation occurs, since this will happen as long as the lung is not completely expanded.

9. Notifying the physician when the drainage bottle or Pleur-evac needs changing. The nurse assists the physician but does not change the bottles or the Pleur-evac herself.

10. Encouraging the patient to cough and breathe deeply periodically in order to enhance lung expansion and prevent bronchopneumonia.

11. Observing the dressing and reporting any evidence of bleeding to the physician.

12. Encouraging the patient to ambulate early. Most patients are up and sitting in a chair within 24 hours after surgery. When there is no evidence of air or fluid being evacuated in the chest tube, the doctor usually orders x-rays to verify the effectiveness of the treatment and, depending on the outcome, the tube is withdrawn while the patient exhales, the wound is closed with vaseline gauze, and a snug dressing is applied.

13. Checking the wound site every few hours after the chest tube is removed for evidence of air leakage.

14. Watching for symptoms of respiratory embarrassment which would indicate loss of negative pressure.

Accidents involving chest drainage systems can be fatal if not handled properly. Two dangerous accidents are a disconnected tube permitting a "sucking wound" of the chest, or an obstructed tube with an air leak from the lung producing a "tension pneumothorax." For some unexplained reason, some nurses have been taught to clamp the chest tube if anything goes wrong. One who understands the principles of chest drainage also understands the possible lethal complications of such an action. If a chest bottle that is being used for a patient with a persistent air leak is inadvertently broken, the tube should not be clamped. It should be momentarily kinked and the end placed under water in any available container—even the patient's water glass if nothing else is at hand—while the chest bottle is rapidly replaced. If a Pleur-evac should tip over and the water seal is lost, the water seal compartment should be refilled immediately.

The chest tube bubbling off air should not be clamped, for if it is, there could be a rapid buildup of positive pressure in the pleural space. This would not only collapse the lung on the same side but would cause a shift of the mediastinal structures and a tension pneumothorax to the contralateral lung. Death will result if such a situation is not corrected immediately. If the chest tubes are fluctuating and not bubbling, they may be clamped during transportation or ambulation. This is short-term clamping and the chances of the lung collapsing on short-term clamping are negligible. The danger arises when the clamps are left in place and forgotten. Over several hours, the patient develops a pneumothorax, often under tension, so many chest surgeons now recommend that chest tubes never be clamped, even when moving patients from stretchers to their beds. However, there is one exception to this rule. The chest tube inserted at the time of pneumonectomy remains clamped. A label should be placed on this clamp so that it is not inadvertently removed.

Inhalation Therapy

The main objective in giving inhalation therapy after thoracic surgery is to deliver humidified air to the patient without endangering him by exposing him to organisms that may be the source of a concurrent infection, particularly the patient who is going to receive chemotherapy or radiotherapy and whose lung cancer makes him especially prone to infections—pseudomonas infections in particular. It helps him to deep breathe, cough, and get up secretions.

The proper equipment must be selected for each patient. All inhalation therapy equipment should be gas sterilizable with disposable lines and manifolds, and should have final filters. The greatest hazard in the use of inhalation therapy is that the equipment may be dirty. Many hospital studies have demonstrated that equipment in use was delivering not only oxygen and humidity but also organisms that could cause a fatal condition in patients who have had thoracic surgery.

The least complicated and most common piece of equipment used in recovery rooms to supply humidity is simply a nebulizer which is connected to a tank or wall source of oxygen, a humidifying jar, a flow meter, and tubing that is attached to a face mask. All of its parts are either completely sterilized or disposable.

In the past, the so-called steam nebulizer was often used to humidify a room. This was plugged into a wall outlet, became contaminated by one patient and was then used immediately for another patient, was impossible to clean, and was found in various studies to be responsible for distributing many common hospital bacteria along with the humidity. Most of these nebulizers have been phased out and replaced by the high output nebulizer (Micromist) that is not electrically powered but is attached to a pressure source. It is completely sterilizable with ethylene oxide after use, and has a disposable mask. Some of the models are capable of humidifying an entire tent or room.

Ultrasonic nebulizers are also available. These devices produce supersaturated atmosphere that is adequate for most patents' needs. The humidity is delivered through a face mask or directed into a tent or croupette. The equipment is gas sterilizable and has disposable tubing. This type of nebulizer is particularly helpful when secretions are very tenacious and the patient cannot get them up by coughing. Its use should be followed by deep breathing and coughing.

Today, when IPPB treatments are ordered, the most commonly used machines are the Bennett AP 5 and the Bird respirator. Both are equipped with disposable tubing and mouthpieces, and the manifolds and nebulizers are gas sterilizable. A final filter prevents any backflow into the machine so that the danger of cross infection between patients is avoided.

The Bennett MA 1 volume-cycled respirator is preferred over the Bird respirator in the event of respiratory failure and when long-term respirator therapy is required. The patient is moved to the special care unit for this therapy. The nurse who cares for him must have a working knowledge of the machine and be able to recognize any malfunctioning. The Bennett machine has a heated nebulizer so that the temperature of the inspired gas the patient receives is warmed approximately to body temperature, thus preventing the buildup of tenacious secretions. It is possible to set the pressure limits the physician desires, and oxygen settings allow the patient to receive anywhere from 21 to 100 percent oxygen. The respirator also has a built-in sigh mechanism so that the patient can be sighed as many as 15 times an hour. This is an extremely important procedure. Sighing is just taking an extra-deep breath. When the patient is on a respirator and receiving a constant volume of gas, the lungs are not being completely expanded. If not contraindicated, the sigh volume is usually set at approximately twice the normal tidal volume with the hope of preventing atelectasis.

Tracheostomy Care

Following a thoracotomy, the patient may require a tracheostomy in order to: 1) provide an access for the aspiration of tracheobronchial secretions; 2) reduce dead space in the airway when the tidal volume and the vital capacity are critically impaired; 3) provide prolonged respiratory assistance for the patient in cardiac failure or acute respiratory failure; and 4) provide mechanical assistance for the patient with a flail chest.

All tracheostomy tubes are cuffed when inserted. Cuffed tubes are needed when it is necessary for the patient to be on a positive pressure or volume-cycled ventilator. The cuff provides a closed system so that the desired volume of gas may be delivered, and prevents aspiration. Good nursing care is essential. This includes periodically deflating the cuff to prevent tracheal necrosis and consequent stenosis caused by the constant pressure on the tracheal walls by the cuff. Before the cuff is deflated, the oral pharyngeal airway and the trachea should be suctioned thoroughly. Otherwise, secretions that have built up above the cuff could be overwhelming and cause respiratory embarrassment. The amount of air to be inserted into the cuff depends upon the relationship between the size of the tracheostomy, the size of the patient's trachea, and the size of the cuff. Only enough air should be inserted to seal off any air leaks. This can be tested easily by placing one's hand over the patient's nose and mouth. If there is no exchange of air, the cuff is inflated enough. The cuff must not be over-inflated since tracheal damage may result. As soon as the patient can tolerate it, the cuff should be left deflated.

Because the incidence of iatrogenic infection is high, sterile technique must be employed when suctioning or giving tracheostomy care. The patient is never suctioned for more than 10 seconds at a time since any longer period could cause further respiratory embarrassment. Immediately after the tracheostomy has been created, secretions are often copious and the patient must be suctioned every five to ten minutes in order to keep the airway clear.

Other Nursing Measures

Positioning the patient so that he rests on his operative side every two hours promotes drainage and gives the unaffected lung more room for expansion, thus improving respiration since the rib cage is not compressed by the weight of the patient's body. The pneumonectomy patient is positioned with his good side up as much as possible so that the lung can expand fully. To prevent pain or pull on the catheter, the nurse must be careful whenever moving or positioning the patient so there is no drag on the catheter. While the patient is in bed, the catheter should be shaped into a coil and fastened to the bottom sheet with a safety pin, being sure there is enough leeway for the patient to turn in bed. One small pillow under the patient's head and neck is preferable to one large one which would also be under his shoulders and would thus push the chest forward and out of line.

The Ace bandages that were applied to the patient's legs preoperatively to aid in the prevention of venous stasis should be changed at least once during every tour of duty.

Sometimes when the postoperative patient lifts his arms or inspires deeply, he will feel pain in the lungs. This may happen because he has not been breathing deeply since the surgery. He should be encouraged to breathe each time to the point of pain and, if he does this repeatedly, the pain will eventually subside if it is due to the thoracotomy itself. In most cases, the pain is in the chest wall and is due to the surgery, and if the patient will persist in the deep breathing, his pain on breathing will subside much more quickly than if he does not practice deep breathing.

Sometimes an older male patient, especially if he has had some prostate difficulty will have trouble voiding after thoracic surgery. Most surgeons think it wise to insert an indwelling catheter while the patient is still in the operating room and leave it in until the patient can stand for voiding. This will usually be one or two days.

Usually, intravenous fluids are given postoperatively. If the patient has a thoracotomy without complications, he will probably be taking adequate fluids by mouth and be on a liquid diet within 24 hours after the operation and then the intravenous fluids are discontinued.

Special Problems of the Pneumonectomy Patient

Mediastinal shift is the main problem that arises after pneumonectomy. No air leak is expected and the hemithorax is expected to fill in with sero-sanguineous pleural fluid. The chest tube that was inserted in surgery and has been kept clamped, may be released periodically by the doctor to prevent excessive build-up of pressure within the hemithorax. If the chest tube were left unclamped while submerged in pleural fluid, a siphon effect could result in a sudden, major pressure drop in the hemithorax and a rapid shift of the heart and other mediastinal structures.

Mediastinal shift is characterized by sudden dyspnea, tachypnea, restlessness accompanied by an anxious expression, cyanosis, rapid and irregular pulse, cardiac failure, pulmonary edema, and death. If a chest tube is not inserted at the time of surgery, it may be necessary to do repeated chest taps to equalize the pressure between the right and left pleural cavities. Pneumothorax readings may be taken and air may be added or subtracted accordingly.

Air in the mediastinum is seldom a postoperative complication but one that can be fatal. A paradoxical pulse develops if the pressure in the mediastinum becomes dangerously high and can be detected by an observant nurse while taking frequent blood pressure readings. (Paradoxical pulse is defined as "an exaggeration of the normal variation in the pulse volume with respiration, becoming weaker with inspiration and stronger with expiration . . . so called because these changes are independent of changes in pulse rate." *Stedman's Medical Dictionary.*) Paradoxical pulse occurs when venous return is obstructed by increased pressure around the heart. A significant respiration-related variation in *systolic* pressure is an important sign of increased mediastinal or pericardial pressure. The amount of variation is a good measurement of the degree of cardiac embarrassment. The technique of measuring a paradoxical pulse is as follows: A quick blood pressure reading is taken to get the approximate level of systolic pressure, and recorded. Then a repeat pressure is taken and a very accurate reading made, while deflating the cuff very slowly. By auscultation it is possible to note the maximum cuff pressure at which any systolic beat is heard. The rest of the beats at this cuff pressure during a complete respiratory cycle of inspiration and expiration will not be heard, but will be seen as vibrations on the mercury column. A slow lowering of the cuff pressure will permit more and more variable beats to be heard, until the level is reached at which all beats can be heard. This reading is also recorded. The difference between the initial and the final systolic readings is the amount of the paradox. A paradox of 10 millimeters is usually a sign of intrathoracic or mediastinal pressure or, more often, of cardiac tamponade.

Subcutaneous emphysema is not an uncommon development in pneumonectomy patients postoperatively. In all cases of subcutaneous emphysema, there is a one-way air leak into tissues. This one-way valve action at the leak results in accumulation of air in the tissues, the tissues swell, and there is crepitus on palpation. Massive subcutaneous emphysema usually originates from a torn bronchus or trachea and could be fatal; thus, the physician should be notified immediately of any marked increase in subcutaneous emphysema. When a postoperative patient with a moderate air leak develops subcutaneous emphysema during the night, the nurse can safely assume that either the tubes have been allowed to hang in fluid-filled dependent loops, or that the patient has rolled onto the tube and blocked the drainage. This could cause a tension pneumothorax and should be corrected immediately.

Hemorrhage is indicated when there is a sudden increase in drainage accompanied by a sudden drop in blood pressure or rise in pulse rate. The chest tubes will be warm to the touch due to the drainage of fresh blood. The hematocrit should be checked and a unit of blood should be immediately available since hemorrhage may necessitate returning the patient to the operating room. A patient can bleed to death in his chest if the drainage tubes are not functioning. If the tubes cannot be made to function, a chest x-ray may be needed.

A sudden release in drainage may also be seen if the patient has been allowed to lie on the tube and shut off the flow of drainage, or if a suddenly released clot has obstructed the chest tube. Nurses must continually guard against positioning the patient in such a way that the chest tubes become kinked. Milking or stripping the chest tubes is an essential postoperative procedure. It helps to prevent plugging of the tubes with fibrin and clots and, therefore, prevents pressure build-up and tension pneumothorax.

Caring for the patient who has had surgical treatment for lung cancer is truly a professional challenge for nurses. Thorough knowledge of the principles of postoperative treatment, expertise in carrying out procedures, and professional judgment are imperative. Patient-centered nursing dictates an individual plan of care for each patient designed to achieve his complete rehabilitation.

QUESTIONS AND ANSWERS

Q. Are people with healed tuberculosis likely candidates for lung cancer?

A. Yes, there is a slightly higher risk of lung cancer occurring in a patient who has had tuberculosis; and adenocarcinoma may develop in the area adjacent to the healed tuberculosis scar.

Q. Can cancer and tuberculosis coexist in the same patient?

A. Yes.

Usually the cancer is diagnosed too late to treat it satisfactorily because a person who has had tuberculosis is very likely to think that any symptoms he may have are due to a recurrence of that disease.

Anyone with healed tuberculosis should be suspected of having cancer whenever a change occurs in the person's chest x-ray films.

Q. Do chronic infections of the lungs predispose to lung cancer?

A. Not to the ordinary type of lung cancer. A rare form of cancer called "scar" cancer occasionally develops in people who have long-standing empyema with bronchopleural fistulas, and occasionally in people with healed tuberculosis. Most lung cancer is attributable to irritants such as cigarette smoke.

Q. Are patients whose tumors are found to be non-resectable advised to stop smoking altogether?

A. Usually they are advised to stop during the preoperative period. But often they go back to it after surgery and the physician leaves it up to the patient, although he may remind him that smoking never helps anyone.

Q. When a person who has been a heavy smoker for 10 or 15 years stops smoking, what are the chances of his developing cancer?

A. The small amount of data on this topic indicates that there is not much difference during the first five years after the person stops smoking. But after five years, the risk gradually diminishes and, theoretically, should eventually approximate that of the non-smoker after 13 years.

Q. Is it true that cancer has been produced experimentally in dogs?

A. Yes, cancers have been produced in the airways of dogs that have been subjected to carcinogenic agents. Dogs have also been taught to smoke cigarettes, and some of these animals produced rather typical cancers. However, most of the cancers that have been produced in experimental dogs have been the result of painting coal tars on the skin of the animals' backs.

Q. Are all patients taught coughing and deep breathing exercises before surgery?

A. Yes, and the instruction should begin as soon as it is known that the patient will be having surgery. The more practice he has before the operation, the easier it will be for him to deep breathe and cough afterwards.

Q. Are vibration and cupping done when deep breathing and coughing exercises are carried out and, if so, could not these maneuvers spread cancer to the other parts of the lung?

A. Some physicians think that this might happen, but cupping and vibration are done when the patient has pneumonia simply to help him recover. Sometimes the secretions are so thick and tenacious that the patient cannot deep breathe or cough, and he needs this assistance to loosen the secretions.

   It is probably not very likely that these maneuvers spread cancer.

Q. Is nitrogen mustard still used in the treatment of lung cancer?

A. Some patients with lung cancer develop a pleural effusion and, if the patient is not suitable for pneumonectomy, the fluid may be aspirated and nitrogen mustard instilled in the cavity. A tube is inserted for a few days and then withdrawn. This treatment causes adhesions to form between the parietal and visceral layers of pleura, and stops the fluid from forming.

   Nitrogen mustard is not used much in the systemic treatment of lung cancer.

Q. What is the advantage of arterial blood gases over capillary blood gases?

A. Capillary blood gases are not as accurate as arterial blood gases. They are done mainly on children. When the ear lobe is heated before taking the blood, a fairly well arterialized sample can be obtained, but it still is only an approximation of the actual arterial blood gases.

   The arterial blood gas report is the more accurate and, even when the femoral or radial artery is repeatedly punctured to obtain blood for this test, difficulties seldom arise. Sometimes the physician expects to take blood from one of these two arteries repeatedly and he puts an arterial line into one of the radial arteries so that a sample can be taken whenever it is desired.

Q. When a bronchoscopy is done, are routine washings taken for the acid-fast test for tubercle bacilli?

A. Yes. It is important to care for the patient as a whole—that is, the condition that is causing his symptoms may be cancerous or inflammatory, or both.

Q. How often should the tracheostomy cuff be released?

A. It is generally thought that it should be released every hour, or every two hours at the most.
There are several new types of cuffs on the market that cause less pressure and which can be left inflated indefinitely.

Q. Can the nurse maintain sterile technique while cleaning the inner cannula of a tracheostomy tube?

A. The nurse wears sterile gloves and a sterile disposable tracheostomy care set is used when carrying out this procedure. If the patient is on a respirator, an extra inner cannula is provided so that the patient does not have to be kept off the respirator for any length of time.

Q. Are patients taught how to use sterile technique for suctioning their tracheostomy tubes after they return home?

A. No. Sterile technique is used while the patient is in the hospital to prevent cross infection between patients. The lung patient is seldom sent home while he has a tracheostomy tube in.
An effort is made to get tracheostomy tubes removed from the lung patient as soon as possible because the tube can be a fertile area for the development of pneumonia.

Q. Is cold steam used in preference to warm steam for humidification and, if so, why?

A. Cold steam may be used (open or with a face mask) for a short time to humidify a room and to loosen up secretions.
Warm steam is used for patients on continuous ventilation to prevent fallout or condensation in the tubes.

Q. When are chest tubes clamped off?

A. A chest tube that is bubbling is never clamped off, nor is one in which there is an air leak.

A chest tube may be clamped while getting a patient out of bed or moving him from bed to a stretcher, but then it must be released immediately.

Q. How often are the chest bottles changed to minimize infection ascending through the tubes?

A. As long as the contents of the bottle stay clear and clean, it probably is not necessary to change the bottle. When the system is first hooked up, the equipment is sterile and closed, so that anything that enters the bottle comes from the patient's own lungs.
Every effort is made to remove chest tubes as soon as possible.

Q. How much does a disposable Pleur-evac cost?

A. The smaller one costs about $17; the larger one about $30.

Q. When using the Pleur-evac with 20 centimeters of negative pressure, how would the nurse reduce the pressure to 15 centimeters if the doctor orders this?

A. The atmospheric air vent is used for adding water to the suction chamber, so it would also be used for removing water. A sterile syringe attached to a sterile catheter could be used to aspirate the 5 centimeters from the chamber.

Q. Is it acceptable to add sterile water to the closed chest drainage system?

A. Nothing should be added to the bottle that would harm the patient if it accidentally got into the patient's chest. If something has to be added, saline would be better than water which could cause hemolysis.

Q. What is the usual setting on the Bennett MA 1 respirator, and who decides what the setting shall be?

A. Any setting above 60 that will give an acceptable PO_2 is used. The exact setting depends upon the patient's blood gases and is determined by the physician.

Q. How can one tell if a patient on a respirator is being assisted?

A. The respirator is set for a certain degree of sensitivity. As the patient's inspiratory effort increases, this is registered on the respirator's pressure gauge. The Bennett MA 1 respirator has a gas light that goes on when the patient is being assisted.

Q. What is the purpose of sighing a patient?

A. Sighing is simply taking a deep breath, but this is an important procedure for the patient on a respirator who is getting a constant volume of air. A sigh volume that is twice the normal volume for the patient will expand his lungs more completely and, hopefully, regular sighing will prevent atelectasis.

Q. What are some of the most common infections encountered in patients who are on respirators?

A. The most common infections that occur in patients on respirators are the various Pseudomonas. The various enteric bacteria are also troublemakers. Recent reports in the literature indicate that often these infections arise from using medications that have been contaminated in multidose bottles of such drugs as Mucomyst, Bronkosol, Vaponephrine, and Isuprel. (Pseudomonas and Serratiae organisms grow very well in these solutions.) Solutions should always be drawn from these bottles in a sterile manner as if they were going to be used for intravenous injections.

Q. What is an iatrogenic infection?

A. An iatrogenic infection is one that is introduced inadvertently by someone caring for the patient, or by erroneous treatment. This is an ever-present danger when a patient is on a respirator and is the reason for insistence upon sterile suctioning technique.

Q. How is the IPPB nebulizer cleaned after the use of such medications as Mucomyst?

A. The tubing is changed by the inhalation therapist, and the container is just rinsed with water.

Q. How often is the equipment on the ventilator changed?

A. When a patient is on continuous ventilation, the lines are changed every day down to the bacterial filter.
Because the patient has his own equipment for IPPB treatments, the equipment is changed every 48 hours, sometimes every 72 hours. If he has an active infection, however, it is changed every day.

Q. How is gas sterilization accomplished?

A. Gas sterilization is accomplished by putting a pellet of ethylene oxide in a closed container along with the articles to be sterilized, and letting them stay there for 24 hours.
The disadvantage of gas sterilization is that plastic or rubber items

must be aerated for at least 72 hours after sterilization before they can be used, unless the hospital has an aerator; then the time is reduced to 24 hours. At least half of the equipment is tied up at all times awaiting aeration, so a large inventory of these supplies is necessary.

Q. For how long are gas-sterilized articles considered to be sterile?

A. Gas-sterilized articles are wrapped in plastic bags and left in them for 72 hours before using. As long as they are kept in the bags they are sterile. If they are not used, they are resterilized after 30 days.

Q. In addition to explaining what follow-up care will be needed, what instructions are given to patients when they leave the hospital after thoracic surgery?

A. The patient must stop smoking or he is likely to develop cancer in the remaining lung.

X-rays of the chest should be taken every three months for the first two years, then every six months.

Frequent sputum tests are important—every six months, at least. The patient should report immediately any symptom such as pain in a bone, headache, a node or lump anywhere in the body.

SUGGESTED READINGS

Books

Arndt, von Hippel. *Chest Tubes and Chest Bottles.* Springfield, Ill.: Charles C Thomas, 1970.

Baum, G., Ed. *Textbook of Pulmonary Disease.* Boston: Little, Brown, 1965.

Bendixen, H. H., et al. *Respiratory Care.* Saint Louis: Mosby, 1965.

Best, C. H. and N. B. Taylor. *The Physiological Basis of Medical Practice.* Baltimore: Williams & Wilkins, 1961.

Blades, B., Ed. *Surgical Diseases of the Chest.* Saint Louis: Mosby, 1966.

Bouchard, Rosemary. *Nursing Care of the Cancer Patient.* Saint Louis: Mosby, 1967.

Clark, R. L., Jr. *Cancer Chemotherapy.* Springfield, Ill.: Charles C Thomas, 1961.

Craytor, Josephine and Margaret L. Foss. *The Nurse and the Cancer Patient.* Philadelphia: Lippincott, 1970.

Dubois, Rene J., Ed. *Bacterial and Mycotic Infections of Man.* Philadelphia: Lippincott, 1958.

Gibbon, J. H. *Surgery of the Chest.* Philadelphia: Saunders, 1962.

Hinshaw, H. C. and L. H. Garland. *Diseases of the Chest.* Philadelphia: Saunders, 1963.

Kinsella, T. J. *Tumors of the Chest.* Springfield, Ill.: Charles C Thomas, 1963.

Medical Clinics of North America. Modern Management of Respiratory Diseases. Vol. *51*, No. 2, Philadelphia: Saunders, 1967.

Nealon, Thomas F., Jr., Ed., *Management of the Patient with Cancer.* Philadelphia: Saunders, 1965.

Physiotherapy for Medical and Surgical Thoracic Conditions. London, England: Brompton Hospital, Physiotherapy Department, 1967.

Pulaski, E. J. *Common Bacterial Infections.* Philadelphia: Saunders, 1964.

Watson, William L., Ed. *Lung Cancer.* Saint Louis: Mosby, 1968.

Periodicals

Ahlstrom, Pearl. "Raising Sputum Specimens," *American Journal of Nursing,* *65*:109-119, March, 1965.

Bailey, A. J. "Lung Cancer and Smoking," *Canadian Nurse, 61*:285-286, April, 1965.

Baskfield, M. M. "Preoperative and Postoperative Care of the Patient with Cancer of the Lung," *Nursing Clinics of North America, 2*:609-622, December, 1967.

Betson, Carol. "Blood Gases," *American Journal of Nursing, 68*:1010-1012, May, 1968.

Boucot, K. R., D. A. Cooper, and W. Weiss. "Detection of Lung Cancer," *Hospital Medicine, 1*:28-32, September, 1965.

Creighton, Helen, and William Wallace Coulter, Jr. "The Whys of Pulmonary Function Tests," *American Journal of Nursing, 60*:1771-1774, December, 1960.

Dittbrenner, Sr. M. and W. M. Herbert. "Regimen for a Thoracotomy Patient," *American Journal of Nursing, 67*:2072-2075, October, 1967.

Dlouhey, A., et al. "What Patients Want to Know about Their Diagnostic Tests," *Nursing Outlook, 2*:265-267, 1963.

Drummond, Eleanor E. "The Respiratory Disease Campaign—Nursing Actions," *American Journal of Nursing, 63*:98-101, March, 1963.

Golbey, R. B. "Chemotherapy of Cancer," *American Journal of Nursing, 60*: 521-525, 1960.

Hadley, Florence and Katherine J. Bordicks. "Respiratory Difficulty-Causes and Care," *American Journal of Nursing, 62*:64-67, October, 1962.

Hanamey, R. "Teaching Patients Coughing and Breathing Techniques," *Nursing Outlook, 13*:58-59, August, 1965.

Harkins, H. P. "Aspiration Pneumonia," *Hospital Medicine,* 4:52-60, November, 1968.

Hedges, J. E. and C. J. Bridges. "Stimulation of the Cough Reflex," *American Journal of Nursing,* 68:347-348, February, 1968.

Horowicz, Clara. "Bronchoscopy as an Outpatient Procedure," *American Journal of Nursing,* 63:106-107, May, 1963.

Hueper, Wilhelm C. "Lung Cancer, Air Pollutants as a Cause," *American Journal of Nursing,* 61:66-68, April, 1961.

James, George. "A 'Stop Smoking' Program," *American Journal of Nursing* 64:122-125, June, 1964.

Kurihara, Marie. "Postural Drainage: Clapping and Vibration," *American Journal of Nursing,* 65:76-79, November, 1965.

Levine, E. R. "Inhalation Therapy-Aerosols and Intermittent Positive Pressure Breathing," *Medical Clinics of North America,* 51:307-321, March, 1967.

Mac Vicar, Jean. "Exercises Before and After Thoracic Surgery," *American Journal of Nursing,* 62:61-63, January, 1962.

Malinoski, Victoria F. "Air Pollution Research," *American Journal of Nursing,* 62:64-67, January, 1962.

Nett, Louise M. and Thomas L. Petty. "Acute Respiratory Failure," *American Journal of Nursing,* 67:1847-1853, September, 1969.

Pruitt, C. V., E. L. Westbury, and P. Hairston, "Nursing Care of Patients with Surgery of the Chest," *Nursing Clinics of North America,* 2:513-520, September, 1967.

Rodman, Theodore. "The Management of Tracheobronchial Secretions," *American Journal of Nursing,* 67:2072-2075, October, 1967.

Schwartz, William S. "Management of Common Pulmonary Diseases," *Journal of American Medical Association,* 181:134-141, July 14, 1962.

Sherman, R. S. "Pulmonary Cancer and the Hospital Radiologist," *Hospital Medicine,* 1:34-36, 1965.

Skinner, D. B. "Scalene Node Biopsy," *Hospital Medicine,* 1:34-38, 1965.

Turner, H. G. "The Anatomy and Physiology of Normal Respiration," *Nursing Clinics of North America,* 3:383-401, September, 1968.

Watson, W. L. and Elisabeth Loucks. "Oat-Cell Lung Cancer," *American Journal of Nursing,* 65:113-115, February, 1965.

Wolf, J. "Management of the Patient with Inoperable Bronchogenic Carcinoma," *Medical Clinics of North America,* 51:563-572, March, 1967.

Patients with Breast Tumors

Regional Medical Program — Oncology Nursing Seminar

on

NURSING MANAGEMENT OF PATIENTS WITH BREAST TUMORS

Seminar Leader

Guy F. Robbins, M.D.

Seminar Participants

J. Herbert Dietz, Jr., M.D., Consultant, Rehabilitation Program

Alfred A. Fracchia, M.D., Attending Surgeon, Breast Service

Frances Gutowski, R.N., B.S., Clinical Nursing Instructor

Sandra Holz, B.S., R.P.T., Physical Therapist

Guy F. Robbins, M.D., Director, Memorial Hospital Regional Medical Program and Acting Chief, Breast Service

Mary Sherry, R.N., Nursing Supervisor

Judith Trachtenberg, M.S.W., Social Worker

Breast cancer occurs in epidemic proportions in the United States. It is now the most common form of cancer in women and the leading cause of death from cancer in women in this country. Approximately seventy-one thousand new breast cancers occur every year and, unfortunately, about thirty-two thousand of them become metastatic before the patient is seen by a physician. Deaths from this disease were recently estimated at thirty-one thousand a year.

This dread picture could be changed if more women practiced breast self-examination, and if they sought medical advice at the first sign of a lump or other change in one or both breasts. In fact, half of them could be cured instead of one-third, as is the case at present. Lack of effective public education is undoubtedly the root of the problem. Strong health education programs need to be initiated as early as junior high school if our crisis-oriented approach to health is to be eradicated. In spite of all the publicity the American Cancer Society has given to the importance of breast self-examination, a large majority of women are still uninformed or careless about examining their breasts at least once a month. Since over 90 percent of the patients with breast cancer are themselves responsible for discovering the lump that proves to be cancer, it is vital that all women be trained in the technique of self-examination and that they develop a positive, healthy attitude toward the practice. (See Appendix A, p. 153.)

Breast cancer can occur in women of any age, although it does not usually occur in females younger than 19. There is one case on record in which the patient was 100 years old. However, the most common age is between 50 and 52, just after the menopause. There are eighty million women in this age group in the United States.

Although cancer can occur in just about anyone, some people appear to be more susceptible than others. For example, the incidence among Japanese and Eskimo women is very low, while it is quite high among Jewish women. Those most likely to develop this disease are usually women from the upper socioeconomic groups, those who have not had children, and those with relatives who have had cancer. Men also get breast cancer but more rarely than women; about 1 percent of all breast cancers occurs in males. The reason for the greater incidence in women may be that the increased amount of estrogen secreted during every menstrual cycle stimulates the breasts, and this repeated stimulation leads to breast cancer.

In addition to the estrogen theory, the viral theory is receiving considerable emphasis in connection with the cause of cancer in general. A number of recent studies have centered on the length of time this agent may be held in the body until a co-carcinogen enters the body and makes it effective. That co-carcinogen may be another agent; it may be nothing more than a reduction in the individual's resistance; it may be simply a source of irritation.

The first sign of breast cancer is usually a lump in the breast tissue. Sometimes a lump will appear just before the menstrual period and disappear postmenstrually, but any lump that remains after the period is over should be reported to the physician and investigated. Any other change in a breast, or unusual condition such as scaliness around the nipple or bleeding from the nipple should also be investigated promptly. After the doctor has made a physical examination, a mammogram may be a good aid to diagnosis, although only a biopsy will rule out cancer. However, even though the mammogram does not show cancer present, no localized lump should be allowed to remain in a breast in the hope that it will go away of its own accord. Watching and wating no longer applies.

Women who fall into the following high-risk groups should be especially careful to perform self-examination regularly, and to report immediately any lump or change in a breast: 1) women who have had one breast removed (there is a 20 percent chance that if the lesion occurred early in life, the woman will live long enough to have cancer in the other breast); 2) women who have had a benign lump removed from a breast; 3) women from families in which several members develop cancer; 4) women who have been on hormone treatment for a long period of time; and, 5) women who have been taking contraceptive pills for some time.

The most common site for breast cancer is in the upper outer quadrant of the breast. When it occurs in the medial or inner part of the breast, metastasis to the internal mammary lymph nodes, the sternum, and the ribs is a frequent development.

Several types of breast cancer are recognized. Most cancers occur in the ducts leading from the milk-producing glands, but they sometimes also appear in the tissue between the ducts and in the tiny alveoli near the edge of the breast. Sometimes a cancer that develops in one of the larger ducts near the surface bulges out and becomes an ulcerating lesion. Inflammatory cancer is characterized by redness of the area and a distinctly palpable raised edge. This is an acute cancer that responds to palliation but is rarely, if ever, cured; thus, primary surgery is not indicated even though only one breast is involved. Paget's disease is a form of cancer that occurs on the surface of the nipple; it may be manifested by just a tiny scratch, or the lesion may be quite large and extend underneath the breast tissue per se and into the axilla. An anatomical fact of importance in the latter case is the presence of lymph nodes in the axillary region that may become responsible for the dissemination of the disease.

DIAGNOSIS

The final diagnosis of breast cancer rests with the pathologist. Not all lumps or changes in breast tissue are indicative of cancer. Some of them are benign, removable fibrous tumors, and some are symptoms of cystic disease of the breast. The pathologist must examine tissue from the affected area microscopically to detect the presence of cancer cells. There are three ways of obtaining tissue for examination: 1) by removing a small wedge-shaped piece of the affected area by incision; 2) by aspiration of tissue cells with a needle; and, 3) by excising a portion of the lesion with the patient under anesthesia. At times, aspiration is done under local anesthesia the night before surgery; otherwise, the tissue is obtained in the operating room with the patient under general anesthesia. The first two methods save time in the operating room, but the greater accuracy of the third method accounts for its more frequent use. In about 95 percent of cases, the pathologist is able to identify cancer cells when they are present. The patient is kept anesthetized until a frozen section of the specimen can be made and examined by the pathologist and, if the biopsy is positive for cancer, the surgeon proceeds to perform a mastectomy.

Recently, reports have indicated that serologists have developed blood tests using a fluorescent technique that will show whether cancer of the breast is present, but the procedure has not yet been perfected to the point where it can be generally used.

COMPREHENSIVE MULTIDISCIPLINARY CARE OF THE MASTECTOMY PATIENT

The management of the mastectomy patient is based on the team concept. The doctor and the nurse, of course, are team members, but also important are the social worker, the physical therapist, the American Cancer Society volunteer, the anesthetist, and members of the patient's family. In fact, patients may ask questions of the housekeeping or dietary personnel that they hesitate to ask of the doctor, partly because these people often spend more time in the patient's room every day than the doctor does. Everyone who comes into contact with the patient is a member of the care team and must be made aware of how important it is to understand the suffering mastectomy patients experience, why they ask the questions they do, and why these questions must be answered in a way that will not increase the patients' anxiety.

Quality care, so badly needed by the mastectomy patient, should begin the first time she is seen by the nurse in the doctor's office. Actually, that is where rehabilitation also begins. From the very beginning, the patient needs to be reassured that everything possible will be done for her and that she will not be abandoned at any point in her illness. During the period of convalescence and adjustment, she will be particularly dependent on the rehabilitation team whose objective is the improvement of the patient's total survival. To rehabilitate means to restore to a former capacity. For the cancer patient, rehabilitation implies enabling her to return to her former life and activities. The team works toward three goals: 1) to restore the patient's external appearance; 2) to prevent loss of shoulder function by preventing lymphedema and giving proper care to the affected arm; and 3) to provide the emotional and psychological support needed to prepare the patient for a return to her normal setting and vocational activities. To help achieve these goals, the team at Memorial Hospital works with groups of mastectomy patients in postmastectomy classes.

So far, nothing has been found to take the place of surgery in the treatment of breast cancer. Success of the operation depends on complete ablation of the lesion but, even when this is done, about one-third of the patients have a recurrence within the next 20 years. Several recent articles in lay and professional journals have espoused the "lumpectomy plus radiation" treatment. However, it is impossible to tell which patients will have a recurrence, even when the original lesion is of the noninvasive type, because the disease may have already disseminated to the axillary lymph nodes and there is no way of knowing this until the nodes are removed and examined under the microscope. The results of a study carried out at Memorial Hospital during the years 1939-1952 furnish a case in point. Forty-six patients who had noninvasive (in situ) cancer of the breast were followed postoperatively. Six of them had had radical mastectomies; the other 40 had had only local incisions for the removal of a tumor. Fourteen of these 40 women later developed cancer in the remaining breast tissue; four were of the noninvasive type, but ten were invasive and in some cases fatal, although the original tumor had been of the noninvasive type. Thus it seems evident that patients with in situ cancer often do have a recurrence and that, in many cases, it is likely to be of the invasive type.

Preparation for Surgery

Entering the hospital for breast surgery can be a frightening experience for both the patient and her family. In addition to a booklet of instructions that is given to the patient who will have breast surgery at Memorial Hospital, a five-minute record entitled, "Advice to a Breast Patient," has been made to help her understand the various hospital procedures. The record tells her about the forms she will be asked to fill out, financial procedures, what to bring to the hospital, the kind of preoperative tests and examinations she will have, how long she can expect to be in the hospital if the operation turns out to be minor or extensive, and how soon, generally, she can expect to go back to work or take up her normal household activities. The patient may take this record home where she can replay it to refresh her memory and where her husband and family can hear it too. This has proven to be a very helpful procedure. The patient may not have been ready to receive the information at the time the doctor or nurse gave it to her, or she may have been worrying or thinking of something else. If she hears it several times, she is less apt to forget it and less apt to listen to misinformation offered by well-meaning but uninformed friends and relatives.

During the preadmission period, the sympathetic and understanding physician, nurse, and secretary can help to allay the patient's apprehensions about having a mutilating operation, of losing her femininity, or of possibly having a recurrence of the cancer. The patient will often ask: Do I really have cancer? How long will I live? How will my family take this? The nurse can probably be of greatest help when she listens intently and makes few positive comments herself, except to answer questions. This allows the patient to verbalize her feelings at a time when she has great need to talk. The nurse should be familiar with the various types of prostheses so that she can reassure the patient about her future appearance. Also, the nurse can honestly assure her that the operative risk is practically nil and that she will undoubtedly soon be able to resume her usual activities.

Although it would be helpful for the patient to meet and talk to all members of the care team before the operation, this is not generally advisable. She is probably nervous and apprehensive and cannot be expected to listen carefully and remember all the details these people might tell her. However, the staff nurse and the doctor should spend some time with her and her family before the operation so that their questions can be answered and the patient's emotional state observed. This might be the occasion for the physician and the nurse to tell the husband something about the operative procedure so that he will understand what has to be done. This will not only help to reduce his shock and distress but it will also help promote his wife's emotional and physical recovery. If there is time, and the patient seems emotionally composed, it might be well to tell her about some of the things she can expect to happen in the postoperative period. Such information might include facts about the immediate postoperative care in the recovery room, the reason for positioning the affected arm, for coughing and deep breathing, and for leg movements. The patient must even practice these exercises preoperatively.

To reduce postoperative psychological trauma, the patient should be told what the operation will conisst of—if that is known ahead of time—or what the possible alternatives are. She must be made aware that it will be necessary to remove the breast if the biopsy is positive. The surgeon is the proper person to give her this informaton, and it is he who obtains her signature on the consent form. The nurse may reenforce the doctor's explanation but it is best for her not to discuss biopsy reports with the patient because a negative report (frozen section) may subsequently be followed by a positive one (paraffin section).

The patient's own minister or the hospital chaplain can give the patient much comfort and can help her to sustain her courage and come to terms with her illness. This aspect of preoperative preparation should not be overlooked.

A complete medical history is taken, a physical examination is made, and routine and special diagnostic tests are carried out. A Papanicoloau test is done on all female patients. The evening before surgery an extensive skin "prep" of the entire hemithorax and axilla is done and the patient is instructed to bathe and shampoo with an antibacterial soap to reduce the bacterial flora on the skin to a minimum. In some instances Ace bandages are applied to the legs on the morning of surgery.

The Operation

If a biopsy has not been done in advance of surgery, one will be done in the operating room with the patient under anesthesia, and a frozen section is examined immediately. If the biopsy report is positive for cancer, the surgeon proceeds with the mastectomy.

For cancer of the noninvasive type, the mastectomy consists of removal of the breast, pectoral fascia, and the axillary lymph nodes. When the cancer is invasive and the lesion is in the outer half of the breast, the procedure carried out is a radical mastectomy which includes removal of the breast, pectoral muscles, and axillary nodes. For a cancer of the invasive type which is located on the inner or medial half of the breast, an extended radical mastectomy is done. This consists of the standard radical mastectomy plus the removal of part of the sternum, the rib ends, and the entire chain of internal mammary lymph nodes which, in these cases, are very likely to become sites for metastasis. The defect in the chest wall is repaired by an ox fascia lata graft.

When the amount of skin sacrificed is so great that the wound obviously cannot be closed, a skin graft from the abdomen or thigh will be done. A single sheet of split thickness skin is used. Skin grafting may also be necessary postoperatively if necrosis of the skin flaps occurs.

Many surgeons make it a practice to do a mirror biopsy on the second breast during the time the patient is in the operating room. The reason for this is that a considerable percentage of patients with cancer in situ in one breast are found to have a cancer in the second breast, even though there may be no objective clinical evidence of this at the time. In one group of patients who had in situ cancer in one breast and who presented no objective evidence of cancer in the other breast, biopsy of the second breast revealed 12 in situ cancers, one infiltrating cancer, and three atypical forms. In another group of patients who had infiltrating cancer of one breast, biopsy of the second one revealed 18 infiltrating cancers, 23 in situ cancers, and 30 precancerous lesions. Some of the atypical tumors do go on to develop into cancer. Since surgeons do not feel that this is inevitable, they do not do a bilateral mastectomy when cancer is found in one breast.

All breast specimens are subjected to paraffin section (permanent record) and, at Memorial Hospital, specimen radiography in addition to the frozen section examination. X-ray films are taken of the surgical specimen. After the operation the patient remains in the recovery room until she has fully reacted from the anesthetic and her vital signs are stabilized.

General Postoperative Care

The postoperative care of the mastectomy patient is based on three objectives: 1) the patient's emotional adjustment to the loss of the breast; 2) the healing of the wound; and, 3) the maintenance of function in the affected arm and shoulder. Today, postoperative complications are relatively rare and usually of a minor nature.

The affected arm should be kept elevated, with the elbow slightly higher than the shoulder, and supported on two pillows to reduce fatigue and pain, support venous return, and help prevent stasis edema. This position is based on the idea that water runs downhill and should be explained to the patient that way. When the patient lies on her side, the affected arm should be supported on two pillows placed in front of her body. Isometric exercises such as clenching and unclenching the fist a few times every hour are done (when the patient is awake) with the arm in the elevated position. The patient may hold a rubber ball or a roll of Kerlix in her hand while doing these exercises. The affected arm must never be used for intravenous or subcutaneous injections, skin tests, or blood pressure readings, and the patient must know the reasons for this restriction. However, she should be encouraged to use her affected arm as much as she can—for example, in bathing, feeding herself, combing her hair, and so on.

Approximately 50 percent of postmastectomy patients develop some degree of lymphedema on the operated side at some point in their postoperative experience, but in more than 90 percent of these patients it is not severe. There is marked variation in the area of the arm affected and in the persistence of the condition. The slight swelling that may occur early in the postoperative period usually subsides, but that which occurs weeks or months after the operation is likely to be persistent or progressive. The disability it causes is in proportion to the extent of the edema and the disfigurement resulting from it. Sometimes lymphedema develops a year or more after radiation therapy was instituted. Obese women are particularly prone to this complication, and they are advised to try to reduce their weight. Other aspects of treatment include keeping the arm elevated whenever possible and the use of a salt-free diet, diuretics, and massage. Mechanical devices for providing intermittent compression are available, but for this treatment to be effective it must be given frequently and regularly. The patient should also wear an elastic sleeve between treatments to keep the edema in check. If a subclinical infection is suspected, antibiotics or sulfa are prescribed. In a limited number of patients with long-term lymphedema, the transposition of the partially detached greater omentum into the axilla and upper arm has been helpful.

Prevention of infection is an important factor in preventing lymphedema. Antibiotics are started immediately at the slightest sign of infection in the affected arm or fluid beneath the skin flaps, or necrosis at the wound margins. Patients should be warned about the importance of avoiding burns and infections in the fingers or hand of the affected arm, and instructed to keep the arm covered when exposed to the direct rays of the sun. (See Appendix D, Do's and Dont's, p. 156.)

The knee gatch should not be used because it interferes with respiration and may lead to circulatory complications. Calf pain must be reported to the surgeon at once.

The mastectomy incision is large, and a tight dressing is applied to help prevent fluid from collecting beneath the wound flaps and to serve as a splint that helps reduce the pain associated with coughing and turning. This may cause some discomfort and, again, the reasons for its use must be explained to the patient. Although some drainage is expected, a large collection at the wound site can delay healing. Some surgeons insert Penrose drains during wound closure; others prefer to use Hemovac drains. The Hemovac is checked frequently to make sure it is functioning properly, is emptied every eight hours or as ordered by the surgeon, and an accurate record of the amount of drainage is kept. The resident checks the catheters and aspirates them in order to keep them patent. It is important that the Hemovac chamber be placed on a flat, firm surface to avoid breakage when compressing the chamber and to maintain negative pressure (suction). The patient should be instructed about the reasons for this and cautioned to call the nurse if the collecting chamber should suddenly become inflated. (See Appendix B, p. 154.) The Hemovac is pinned to the lower part of the dressing to prevent drag or pull on the catheter.

The first dressing change can be both a relief and a problem for the patient. It is a relief because the tight odorous dressing is removed and the patient can breathe freely again. It is a problem because she sees her deformity for the first time. She may be shocked by the extent of the surgery and by the concavity beneath the clavicle if the pectoral muscles were removed. Many patients prefer not to look for several days. The patient herself makes the decision about when to look, in her own way and in her own time.

The general nursing management for patients who have had extended radical surgery is the same as that for patients with a radical mastectomy except that after surgery underwater chest tube drainage is used for from one to two days to help reexpand the lung and to remove fluid from the pleural cavity. A routine postoperative chest film is taken of the patient before the chest tube is removed.

Frequently, throughout her hospital stay and for a long time afterward, the patient will continue to need emotional support. This is given by nurses. The patient may have postponed the surgery for several weeks or even years because she was fearful that losing a breast would mean losing her femininity, perhaps even her life. She may also have persuaded the surgeon to delay the operation for some reason or other—a wedding in the family, or a graduation, perhaps—and at the time this reprieve comforted her because she interpreted his acquiescence as an indication that her condition probably was not too serious. Now she feels guilty for having used such a ruse, or for having had an abortion and so interfered with nature's laws. She may feel that she is no longer an attractive sex partner—a most painful emotion—and need assurance that, in time, she can resume normal sexual activity. The depression that accompanies the loss of a breast is an expression of grief. This is a normal and natural reaction to mastectomy and it is up to the nurse to create an accepting and understanding environment wherein this grief can be expressed. The patient may withdraw, or she may become hostile, weep, talk incessantly, and express anger—especially toward the nurse. As her physical condition improves, so does her emotional adjustment and, throughout the postoperative period, the nurse must continue to listen and to give good psychological and emotional support as well as physical care. When she does so, it may be said that she is giving *total* care in the true sense of the word.

Routinely patients go to postmastectomy classes on the second postoperative day, barring complications. Patients who have had skin grafts or extended radical surgery do not go to class until the chest tube has been removed. Also, they do not exercise until the surgeon gives his approval.

Postmastectomy Group Therapy: The rationale for conducting classes for postmastectomy patients is based on the fact that these women have many common thoughts and problems, and adaptations to make. When these topics of concern are brought out into the open and discussed in a group, the patient's feelings of fear, anger, depression, and even mourning are lessened, and she is better able to quickly and productively begin to cope with the loss of a breast. Thus, patients frequently ask and discuss such questions as: What shall I tell my children? My husband? My friends? The people I work with? How will I react the first time I see my mastectomy? How will my husband react? Will this affect my sex life? What are my chances of having a recurrence? Of my dying of cancer?

The nurse is usually the first member of the rehabilitation team to see the patient. First she reviews the chart and places all pertinent data on a work sheet, including any abnormalities found by the doctor on his examination. For example, the patient may have a hearing or speech defect, a respiratory problem, heart disease, or arthritis, and any one of these conditions may affect her reactions and participation in the class. This work sheet is shared with all members of the team. (See Appendix C, p. 155.)

The nurse then interviews the patient at the bedside, tells her how she will benefit from attending the group sessions and what to expect. She ascertains how the patient feels about her surgery. Some patients are at first confused about what the team is trying to accomplish. The word "therapy" needs to be explained in lay language since some patients think of it in terms of psychotherapy only. Others, especially older women who have had a recurrence of cancer, think they will only be a burden to the rest of the class. Occasionally, much sophisticated persuasion is necessary to get some of these patients to come to class, but once they come they usually insist upon returning every day.

Classes are held five days a week from 10:30 A.M. until 12:00 noon.

Patients have a great deal of curiosity about their operations and want to talk about them, even though they are not yet ready to look at their incisions. During the class, the nurse discusses the operation and explains various aspects of the patient's physical care in general. She explains the reason for the tight dressing and the drainage system, for the feelings of numbness and tingling, and for the ecchymosis often seen in the affected arm. Bathing, the use of deodorants on the affected side, and breast self-examination are also discussed. Some patients express bitter feelings when self-examination is mentioned and sometimes make such comments as, "What's the use? Once you find a lump, you lose the breast anyway." Some patients, especially those with young daughters, ask if breast cancer is hereditary and wonder if they are carriers of the disease. Some ask about the possibility of breast reconstruction. Queries of this type are referred to the surgeon.

Brassieres and breast forms are discussed at length, and samples of them are passed around so patients can actually handle them; some patients are loathe to touch them until they see the others doing it. Handling the forms is an important step in the rehabilitation process. Ways of modifying one's own brassieres are described and patients are given a list of specialty shops where they may be properly fitted with a permanent breast form. The American Cancer Society volunteer will furnish a washable stretch brassiere for them to wear over the dressing in the meantime. Patients are advised not to be fitted with a permanent prosthesis until the incision is dry and the doctor or his office nurse say they are ready to be fitted.

The social worker acts as a coordinator of the group and keeps the discussions focused on reaching for and eliciting patients' feelings. When the patient realizes that the leader as well as the other team members and other patients are interested in listening and in helping her, she finds it easier to articulate many feelings that may be close to the surface but are initially so frightening that she is not able to verbalize them. With support and encouragement within the protected group setting, she can express her fear, anger, and embarrassment safely and therapeutically. In the group she begins to think constructively about her future. She gets some preparation for what the steps in her adaptation will be. At the same time, each woman's need or desire for denial about any aspect of her experience is respected by everyone in the group, provided the denial is not detrimental to her physical and emotional recovery. One sample of this type of interaction is provided by the experience of Mrs. M., a warm, young-looking 65-year-old woman who had recently had one breast removed and who was actively participating in the class when she learned (as a result of a paraffin section on the contralateral breast) that she would have to undergo a second mastectomy. That day she came to the group in tears and asked the others what she should do. They encouraged her to express her feelings, her fear of her life at needing surgery again in so short a time, and her fear that this might indicate that the cancer had already spread throughout her body. They understood what was at stake for her and what she was experiencing. They sensed that she wanted their approval and support to agree to the second operation, and they gave it—with warmth and understanding. Their reward, and the staff's too, came when Mrs. M. returned to the class after having successfully undergone the second mastectomy, to say thank you and to listen in turn to someone else.

If the social worker senses that any particular patient needs special help on either a practical or emotional plane, or if the patient asks for it, the worker will see her individually and work with her until the problem has been resolved.

The volunteer who assists with conducting the class is usually a member of a group called "Reach to Recovery." This organization, which started about 18 years ago as an independent group, became a division of the American Cancer Society in 1970. It is made up entirely of women who have had mastectomies. Its purposes are to provide advice, physical rehabilitation, information on prostheses and, perhaps most important of all, to give psychological support to women who have recently had extensive breast surgery. One may ask why such an organization is needed, considering the availability of doctors, nurses, and physical therapists today. The answer is that occasionally postmastectomy patients do not feel free to discuss their innermost thoughts and intimate problems with doctors or nurses. By her very presence, the Reach to Recovery volunteer encourages the patient to believe that she too will be able to live a normal and happy life again. Being able to talk to someone who has been through the same experience and who is obviously living a full, normal life helps dispel the fears and apprehensions of the woman who has just had a mastectomy. The volunteer does not demonstrate the exercises in class because this is the function of the physical therapist on the team. But she does participate in the discussions, answers questions, and goes to see each patient individually, thus giving patients a chance to ask questions that they might hesitate to pose to the entire group.

The volunteer realizes that it is the fear of the unknown that often causes anxiety in the postmastectomy patient, and the fact of her own full adjustment and return to life in the community is proof to the patient that life can still be full and interesting. One volunteer has also suggested that, particularly after this kind of surgery, the patient must be encouraged to hang on to her sense of humor even while she is being very realistic about learning to cope with her depression and other negative feelings.

At each postmatectomy class session, the physical therapist teaches five simple, nonfatiguing arm exercises. A physical therapist at Memorial Hospital perfected these exercises which have been refined over a period of several years until they are now easy for patients to learn and remember, do not allow for undesirable substitutions and, when done as directed, cause a minimum of pain and discomfort. The fact that these exercises can be done with little or no pain makes patients willing to do them five or more times a day.

"Wall climbing" is used as the first exercise. The second is of a "pendulum" type; it emphasizes relaxation of the shoulder and the entire arm within a comfortable range of motion. The third exercise consists of deep breathing; it stresses expansion of the anterior chest which is the key to success in making the exercises nearly pain-free since it relieves the feeling of tautness of the skin on the side of the surgery—a frequent complaint. Other benefits include lung expansion, improvement in posture, and assistance in bringing up secretions. The fourth exercise consists of lifting the clasped hands upward until beginning pain or a feeling of pulling at the site of the incision is felt, holding that position and breathing deeply until the pain or pulling sensation is gone, and only then proceeding to lift the hands higher. The fifth exercise, which is somewhat similar to the fourth, is of a "pulley" type and, again, as soon as the patient feels any pain or pulling at the site of the incision, she stops, holds the position while she does the deep breathing exercises, and proceeds to lift the arms higher only when all pulling or pain is gone. The exercises are all done in a sitting position, except the pendulum exercise, and in the proper order, starting with the simplest.

Although the exercises are demonstrated and practiced in the group, each patient is recognized as an individual whose medical background, type of incision, extent of surgery, emotional background and pain threshold is different from that of everyone else in the group. The nurse reviews each patient's chart every day before class for information on the status of wound healing, drainage, or any other facts that would affect the needs of the individuals in the group. Patients are encouraged to progress at their own rate, not to equal or surpass the performance of any other patient. So, while the exercises are done in the group setting, they are individualized on the basis of particular factors pertaining to each patient's status and her stage of recovery.

Many patients do not achieve full, unassisted, and comfortable range of motion by the time they leave the hospital. They are instructed to continue the four exercises at home—upon arising, before retiring, before or after their three meals, and at least two times a day to alleviate stiffness until they are able to carry on their normal activities and can reach equally high with both arms held close to the side of the head. They can then discontinue the exercises if they wish, or they may decide to continue them as needed to relieve any feeling of stiffness that may linger despite the return of full range of motion.

The rehabilitation team at Memorial Hospital sends a follow-up questionnaire to all patients one week after discharge from the hospital. The class leaders are informed of the patients' own evaluations of their progress as reported on the questionnaires. Three months later, a second questionnaire is sent out. This one is designed to gather information about the quality of the patients' survival, that is, information about their current level of functioning both at home and in the community. Returned questionnaires that contain queries pertaining to medical care are referred to the patient's surgeon. Approximately 85 percent of the questionnaires sent out to former Memorial patients have been returned and, by and large, the statements respondents have made about the postmastectomy classes have been gratifyingly positive.

Preparation for Discharge: Planning for the patient's discharge from the hospital should begin early in her stay and every member of the team should be involved in it. Perhaps the most important part of this preparation involves teaching the patient how to care for herself and, when this is not possible, teaching some member of the family how to give her the proper care. Particularly, the importance of following instructions regarding substitution therapy after ablative surgery cannot be overemphasized. It may be necessary to refer the patient to the visiting nurse in order to make sure that the medications are given properly and at the right times.

Before the patient leaves the hospital she is given a booklet that contains information on prostheses, clothing modifications, exercises, and the psychological adjustments she will need to make. In addition, Memorial Hospital patients receive a 16 rpm record ("Panel Discussion of Postoperative Breast Problems") that consists of a discussion by a nurse, a doctor, and three women who have had mastectomies. The experiences people usually have in the postmastectomy period are described, and the various problems the patient can expect to arise during her readaptation to society are discussed. This record has proven very helpful because most mastectomy patients are in more or less of a "fog" for two or three weeks after surgery, and the facts have to be repeated over and over. Having the record at home, they can play it as many times as necessary so that both they and their families can remember the things that are said.

The patient should be told that she and her husband should talk to the physician about their resumption of sexual relations and that it is he who decides when this is advisable. Couples often become emotionally upset because a considerate husband hesitates to suggest sexual intercourse, and the wife withdraws because she feels the loss of her femininity. Her husband's assurance that he loves her and that nothing has changed because of the operation are important in reestablishing normal relations.

If the patient has not already learned about prostheses in the postmastectomy class, she should be told that satisfactory external prostheses can be purchased in most department stores and corset shops. Immediately after the operation the patient can use a "leisure" or "sleep bra"—a stretch-type garment. Next in the postoperative period she can use a light dacron-filled breast form that is both comfortable and cosmetically acceptable. Finally, she can obtain a permanent prosthesis to match the remaining breast; there is a prosthesis for every type of figure. The small-breasted woman may wish to use a simple rubber form. A weighted type that simulates the heavier breast is also available. All patients can have an appropriate prosthesis for swim wear. (Swimming is one of the best exercises for the postmastectomy patient.)

The cost of a prosthesis ranges from a few dollars for a simple foam rubber pad to $75 and up for a silicone-filled form. It is not the cost that makes the prosthesis right for the person; it is whether it meets her individual needs. Funds can always be found, through some agency, to purchase a form, so this need not be a problem for the indigent patient.

Patients are advised not to wear a permanent prosthesis while the wound is still draining. However, if the woman is very upset about her appearance, and if her bodily image is such that she cannot accept the asymmetry, she may use a temporary prosthesis in the form of a simple pad (a Kotex, for example, or the dacron-filled breast form supplied by Reach to Recovery) placed in the empty cup of the bra that she is wearing to support the unaffected breast. This will give her contour and the feeling of having a prosthesis even though she is still wearing a dressing.

The patient is encouraged to wear the dacron-filled washable prosthesis and stretch bra given her by the Reach to Recovery volunteer while she is still in the hospital. Patients with a heavy remaining breast are more comfortable in their own brassieres which may be enlarged to fit over their dressing by using a brassiere enlarger. These extenders hook onto the brassiere without sewing and are available in many department and "Five-and Ten-Cent" stores.

After her discharge from the hospital, the postmastectomy patient is closely followed by the doctor and nurse, either in the doctor's office or the clinic. The clinic nurses have attended the classes so they are able to check on whether the patient is doing the exercises properly at home and whether the affected arm has a good range of motion. They also often need to teach the technique of breast self-examination, since the patient had no opportunity to learn this while in the hospital when both breasts were bound up by a tight dressing. For the weak or debilitated patient who needs assistance with the exercises, arrangements may need to be made for her to be seen by the visiting nurse. Throughout her follow-up care, the patient will continue to need emotional support.

ADVANCED BREAST CANCER

Breast cancer grows slowly and manifests itself in many different ways. Probably no disease stirs the imagination and taxes the ingenuity of the physician more than advanced breast cancer. Often metastases do not show up for several years after the primary cancer has been treated; therefore, periodic follow-up of all patients is necessary. Some patients do not see a physician at all until after metastasis from a primary lesion has occurred and the condition has become inoperable. The entire internal mammary chain of lymph nodes may be involved, any or many bones of the skeleton, the lungs, the liver, the brain, and so on. One of the most common sites of recurrence is the chest wall—a local recurrence. The patient may present with a small nodule or massive involvement and ulceration, depending on how soon she seeks medical advice. Often the inoperable cases occur in reclusive women who do not present themselves to a physician until the disease is widespread, sometimes fungating, and involves all of one and sometimes part or most of the other breast, as well as the axilla.

Skin care is most important. Power spraying with half-strength hydrogen peroxide followed by saline solution can be quite effective. Half-strength Dakin's solution or half-strength acetic acid soaks may be applied after the wound spray to clean out the affected area and cut down on odor. Telfa dressings, which prevent adherence and consequent bleeding, may be utilized to advantage in these cases. If the area is being radiated, the skin must have even more meticulous care; the patient should be observed for nausea and vomiting; and intake and output is to be carefully recorded.

As to medical treatment for advanced breast cancer, various palliative measures are employed including radiation, hormonal therapy, adrenalectomy, oophorectomy, hypophysectomy, and chemotherapy.

Radiation Therapy

Radiation is the most frequently employed and most effective agent used to relieve the pain experienced by patients with inoperable advanced breast cancer. It furnishes palliation for approximately 70 percent of the patients in whom it is used. Many types of radiation-producing machines are employed—low voltage, high voltage, supervoltage, cobalt units, and the betatron for instance. Radiation can also be used intracavitarily as radioactive gold (Au^{198}) or radiophosphorus (P^{32}), or interstitially as radon seeds, iodine seeds (I^{125}), or radioactive yttrium (Y^{90}). The contraindications for its use are obvious—previous x-ray therapy or widely disseminated cancer which can be controlled only locally.

Radiation is also used in patients with advanced breast cancer to produce therapeutic castration and thus eliminate estrogen production but, unless the patient is considered a poor surgical risk, surgical castration is the better procedure. It not only removes the hormones more quickly; it is also more dependable. Forty percent of patients so treated show improvement, and duration of life thereafter averages about nine months.

Hormonal Therapy

Recently, alteration of the patient's hormonal environment has become a widely used modality in the treatment of advanced inoperable breast cancer. This treatment is based on the theory that the development of the female breast is the result of activity of the female sex hormones (estrogens) and that, naturally, the growth and development of cancer cells in the breast tissue will be affected by the administration of sex hormones. Alteration of the hormonal environment may be accomplished in either of two ways: addition or deprivation.

When addition is the method chosen, either male or female hormones may be used. The male hormones, the androgens, are particularly effective. Testosterone propionate can be given intramuscularly, usually 100 mg three times a week; or fluoxymesterone (Halotestin) or Metandren may be given orally. The androgens are particularly useful in premenopausal women who have had a therapeutic castration and then relapsed, or in postmenopausal women who have had an oophorectomy or adrenalectomy and then relapsed. Contraindications for their use are edema, cardiorenal disease, or hypercalcemia. Response to treatment with androgens varies with the part of the body to which the disease has metastasized; 19 percent of patients with cancer of the skeleton, 22 percent of those with cancer of the soft tissues and, unfortunately, only 4 percent of those with cancer of the lung, show improvement. The duration of life with this treatment is usually about eight months.

The female hormones (estrogens) are most effective in women who are five or more years postmenopausal, preferably ten years. Stilbestrol, 5 mg three times a day is the usual order, but ethinyl estradiol and estradiol benzoate are also used. Contraindications for use of the estrogens are the same as those for the androgens (mentioned in the foregoing paragraph), but the response rate is somewhat higher—28 percent of patients with carcinoma of the skeleton, 41 percent of those with carcinoma of the soft tissues, and about 33 percent of those with carcinoma of the lung, show improvement. The average life duration for patients receiving this therapy is about nine months.

When androgens, estrogens, or corticosteroids are administered as additive therapy, the patient must receive the ordered dose daily, if not by the oral route, then by intramuscular or intravenous injection, until the physician decides to taper the dosage. (Cortisone is tapered, never abruptly discontinued.) The nurse must be aware of such possible side-effects as nausea, edema, deepening of the voice, hirsutism, acne, hypercalcemia and, in the case of cortisone, steroid-induced diabetes mellitus, steroid ulcer, and such other side-effects as "moon-face" and changes in bodily contour.

The second method of altering the hormonal environment, deprivation, is accomplished through ablative surgery. It may be an oophorectomy (in male patients, an orchiectomy), adrenalectomy, or hypophysectomy, all of which are drastic procedures indeed. The patient's life thereafter depends on hormonal replacement. For the premenopausal woman, oophorectomy is often the choice. Improvement is marked and may last for several years. This period is referred to as the free interval period.

Approximately 20 years ago, adrenalectomy came into use as a method of treatment for patients with inflammatory or disseminated carcinoma who, after a long period of remission, have responded well to castration but less well to androgens and corticosteroids, or for those whose cancer may have been aggravated by estrogens. This operation removes the other source of estrogen production in the body. About one-third, or 35 percent, of patients treated by adrenalectomy show improvement, and the life duration thereafter ranges from a low of eight months to an average of 22 months. There is one recorded instance of a patient having lived for 14 years after the operation. Following adrenalectomy, the patient must receive daily supplements of cortisone and salt.

Hypophysectomy, which eliminates all estrogen production in the body, is indicated for patients who might be considered for adrenalectomy except that removal of the pituitary gland seems to give better results in patients who have pulmonary or cardiopulmonary disease in addition to advanced breast cancer. The surgical approach to the gland may be transcranial, transsphenoidal, transfrontal, or stereotaxy. In the last named approach, the gland is destroyed by the application of intense heat or cold via a wire that is inserted into it. The primary reason for doing a hypophysectomy is that it abolishes the gonadotrophic hormone (sexual gland) stimulation, and also abolishes the adrenocorticotrophic hormone, somatotrophin (the growth hormone), and prolactin. Disadvantages of this operation are primarily the complications that may follow it—visual disturbances, spinal fluid leak, meningitis and, occasionally (when the transfrontal approach is used), convulsive seizures. These patients must take cortisone daily as well as thyroid extract for the rest of their lives, and they also need to take pituitary extract temporarily. The results as far as improvement and duration of life are concerned are similar to those after adrenalectomy.

The nursing care of the patient who has ablative surgery includes the preoperative care necessary for any operation; i.e., seeing that the ordered diagnostic tests are carried out, and preparing the patient for the operating room. Postoperatively, the care includes monitoring the vital signs, encouraging coughing and deep breathing, exercising and ambulating as ordered, measuring intake and output, and maintaining proper nutrition as well as bowel and bladder function. If the patient has had an adrenalectomy, the nurse carries out all the procedures listed above but, in addition, she must observe the patient closely for signs and symptoms of adrenal crisis—lethargy, hypotension, progressive weakness, nausea, vomiting, and a rise in temperature with no apparent infectious cause. The fact that cortisone replacement is necessary for the rest of the patient's life cannot be overemphasized; comparing it to a diabetic's need for insulin may help the patient to understand this better. She should also be alerted to the fact that under any sort of stress, physical or emotional, she may need more cortisone than her maintenance dose. And in the event that she does not take it orally, she must inform the doctor at once so that he can give it to her by injection. She should be advised that if she moves to a different area she should immediately place herself under the care of a nearby physician. She is given an instruction sheet containing these and other facts she needs to know regarding her care on discharge from the hospital. She also carries a plasticized instruction card with her at all times. On one side there is information for the patient and on the opposite side information for the physician. (See Appendix E, p. 158.)

If the physician has chosen to do a hypophysectomy, the nurse gives the usual postoperative care but she must also observe the patient closely for signs of diabetes insipidus, rhinorrhea caused by spinal fluid leak, hemorrhage, changes in vision, and other signs of alteration in the patient's neurological status. Diabetes insipidus is manifested by excessive thirst and urinary output; extreme care must be taken in recording intake and output and the urine should be monitored for specific gravity. Intramuscular Pitressin will be prescribed by the physician to reverse this situation. This medication is suspended in oil; therefore, the ampule must be warmed and well shaken before the suspension is drawn up. As the patient convalesces, posterior pituitary extract in powder form (Pitressin snuff) may be administered into the nares by insufflation as the patient exhales; this is to be absorbed through the nasal membrane and is not to be inhaled.

Following hypophysectomy, the patient will receive cortisone as after adrenalectomy but, in addition, she will receive the thyroid hormone for life, usually by mouth in the form of Cytomel. Again, the nurse has the responsibility for teaching the patient the absolute necessity of taking her medications. The manner of administration is as important as the drug; if the order is for intramuscular injection, it must be given that way; if for intravenous, that must be the mode and no substitutions are allowed. Patients who have had an adrenalectomy or hypophysectomy are encouraged to wear medical alert bracelets in case of accident away from home.

Chemotherapy

Chemotherapy involves the use of non-hormonal chemicals that attack the dividing and growing cancer cells directly. Nitrogen mustard was the first of these chemicals and, for a time, was widely used. Today, chlorambucil, (Leukeran), cyclophosphamide (Cytoxan), Thio-Tepa, methotrexate, and 5-fluorouracil are the ones most often employed. The best choice for metastasis to the liver is 5-fluorouracil, but methotrexate and Leukeran are also helpful. Velban (vinblastine) is useful in cases of metastasis to the lung.

The results of chemotherapy for breast cancer are still somewhat disappointing and research for a better drug continues. Nevertheless, objective improvement for two months has been noted in 15 percent of patients treated with chemotherapy, for six months in 10 percent, and for one year in 2 percent. Consequently, medical opinion seems to be that chemotherapy should be used as a supplement for—and subsequent to—other methods of hormonal manipulation or palliative therapy rather than as a primary method of treatment.

Symptoms of toxicity from use of these chemicals include stomatitis, mouth ulcers, vomiting, diarrhea, skin rash, hemorrhage, leukopenia, and alopecia.

Nursing care of the patient on chemotherapy includes careful observation and recording of intake and output, since the patient is frequently subject to nausea and vomiting. Other signs of drug toxicity must also be carefully watched for. Bleeding may occur from any site as a result of bone marrow depression including a lowered leukocyte count. Hence, the patient's personal hygiene must be closely supervised and extra precautions taken to prevent her from being exposed to individuals suffering from some infection.

Treatments of Choice for Metastatic Cancer of the Breast

Metastasis to the bones occurs frequently in advanced breast cancer. In 70 percent of patients, radiation will result in improvement. When skeletal dissemination is diffuse, estrogens are used for the older patients, and for others androgens, castration, oophor-adrenalectomy, and hypophysectomy are employed. Chemotherapy has not been effective in these cases.

Whether she is confined to bed or ambulatory, precautions must be taken to immobilize the patient (using such devices as the surgical collar if indicated), and to protect her from pathological fractures of the extremities or trauma to the lungs from fractured ribs. A pull sheet may be used to help turn and move the patient safely in bed.

The nurse must be alert for such symptoms as lethargy, confusion, nausea and vomiting—all signs indicative of hypercalcemia. The most important means of combatting this condition is good hydration. Fluids should be forced, orally if possible, but if the patient is nauseated, vomiting, or has an uncooperative attitude, the parenteral route must be used.

Since radiation is a frequent method of treatment for these patients, skin care must be meticulous.

When metastasis to the lungs has occurred, castration, oophor-adrenal-ectomy, or hypophysectomy are the usual methods of treatment unless the patient is in the older age group for whom estrogens are used and, finally, chemotherapy. Chemotherapy seems to be more effective in metastasis to the lungs than in metastasis to other sites.

Nursing care of these patients involves close observation for respiratory embarrassment. The patient may become apprehensive when she experiences shortness of breath or dyspnea on exertion. Nursing measures that will help relieve dyspnea and its consequent apprehension include changing the patient's position frequently, keeping the head of the bed elevated, re-arranging the pillows, opening windows (an air-conditioned room is highly desirable), having the patient sit up in a chair for meals if she is able, anticipating her needs, and keeping necessary items, especially the call bell, within easy reach.

The patient may be treated by radiation and a chest tap, or a closed thoracotomy may be done to relieve symptoms caused by pleural effusion. During withdrawal of fluids from the pleural cavity, the patient's blood pressure and pulse should be monitored carefully because of the possibility that hypovolemia will occur. Radioactive phosphorus (P^{32}) may be injected intrapleurally through the tube after the removal of the effusion. The nurse should be aware of the precautions to be taken when this treatment is used, and know what side-effects may be manifested after the procedure. Phosphorus-32 is a beta emitter and the patient's own body acts as an effective shield; therefore isolation is not necessary.

Seepage can be detected by the presence of a blue stain on the dressing. One of the nurse's important responsibilities is the careful handling of contaminated dressings, as well as linens; these are carefully collected in a plastic bag and saved for monitoring and disposal by health physics personnel.

When disseminated mammary carcinoma involves the liver, nausea and vomiting may be quite severe, and jaundice is often present as well as ascites. The patient must be closely observed for signs of hepatic coma, metabolic changes, asterixis, lethargy, euphoria, apathy, or any other change in the neurological status. The physician usually orders a low protein, high carbohydrate diet. Neomycin may be given orally or as a retention enema to prevent the absorption of nitrogen products from the colon. When irradiation therapy is used, nausea and vomiting will become most intense, and diarrhea may also be a problem. Very careful observation and recording of intake and output is stressed. Rest is even more important for these patients than for those who are under treatment by irradiation for metastasis to other areas. Sometimes a paracentesis is done to relieve the symptoms caused by ascites, and then the patient's vital signs must be carefully monitored during the procedure and the patient observed for signs of shock due to hypovolemia. Phosphorus-32 is sometimes used for treating patients with metastasis to the liver when it is accompanied by ascites.

For metastasis to the brain, irradiation plus the administration of corticosteroids is the current treatment of choice. Nursing care includes very careful observation of the patient, because changes in her mental status make her likely to be disoriented and subject to such accidents as falling.

Irradiation is the usual treatment for a local recurrence of breast cancer and for localizing inflammatory carcinoma, but if the lesion is too diffuse, ablation by adrenalectomy or hypophysectomy is the treatment of choice.

For disseminated cancer that is accompanied by the accumulation of fluid in a body cavity, centesis followed by chemotherapy is the usual mode of treatment. Ascites may be treated by paracentesis followed by instillation of phosphorus-32; pleural effusion by thoracentesis followed by nitrogen mustard (HN_2); and pericardial effusion by pericardial tap followed by external radiation and phosphorus-32.

Neurological deficits such as paralysis and pain due to brachial plexus involvement should receive sling support and assistive exercise prescription. Patients with paraplegia or paralysis from spinal cord compression by metastatic lesions may respond to training in transfer activities and wheelchair independence, and whatever ambulation remains possible with the assistance of parallel bars, walkers, crutches, or canes. Extensive bracing is not generally recommended for patients with metastatic cancer of the spine.

COMPREHENSIVE CARE OF THE PATIENT
WITH ADVANCED BREAST CANCER

Because advanced breast cancer manifests itself in many different ways, and because of the connotation of the words "inoperable cancer," patients with this condition have particularly trying social, emotional, physical, and economic problems. How these problems are handled varies according to the emotional and psychological stability of the patient. Factors that contribute to her acceptance or rejection of her status include how much she knows about her condition, and previous experience she may have had with cancer in members of her family or friends, and her family responsibilities. Her emotional reactions depend, to a large degree, on the attitudes and actions of the physician, nurses, and other professional members of the health team.

The need of individual social work for patients with advanced breast cancer is always evaluated since this is a long-term disease that often covers several years. Throughout these years, varying crises may arise which can best be handled by the intervention of a social worker. For example, if the patient is the mother of a family her increasing disability may make it necessary to obtain the services of a homemaker in order to keep the family intact and functioning. At the same time, the whole family can benefit from the availability of the social worker as a person with whom they can share their grief, sorrow, and anxiety about the patient. Even after the patient dies the family may continue to need psychological support and practical help.

The Nurse's Role

The nurse's role in the care of patients with advanced breast cancer is particularly important because she must not only be sensitive to the patient's physical needs but also to her emotional needs which, in these cases, are often multiple and serious. She acts as intermediary between the doctor and the patient and, as such, she can be a source of comfort during the patient's long illness. The importance of supportive nursing for the patient who must be re-admitted to the hospital several times, or remain there for a long period of time, cannot be overemphasized.

Keen nursing judgment is essential. For example, some nurses may be inclined, because of empathy, not to disturb the patient while, on the other hand, some may push the patient too hard and too far. The nurse must be able to judge how much activity the patient is capable of and then encourage her to move about and do what she can. If she is unable to stay up for long periods of time, she should be gotten out of bed often and helped to walk, if possible, not just put in a chair. If she cannot be out of bed at all, she should be turned frequently; sometimes she can turn herself with less pain, especially if there is a trapeze bar over the bed that she can grasp. If she is able, she should be helped to sit up in bed, or on the edge of the bed occasionally. Passive range of motion exercises may be done if there are no contraindications such as metastasis to the bones.

Because prolonged bed rest may lead to pneumonia, thrombophlebitis, and poor elimination, the patient should be encouraged to cough and practice deep breathing, and the nurse should see that good nutrition and hydration are maintained.

Vomiting and nausea lead to anorexia, and the poor state of nutrition that results often leads to serious skin problems; consequently good skin care is of the utmost importance. General measures include careful attention to intake and output, frequent turning of the patient, avoidance of soap and water on skin areas that have been exposed to radiation, the application of A & D ointment or cornstarch if ordered, and frequent inspection of the skin to detect any reddened or inflamed areas. Early detection of trouble spots is important because it may be possible to avoid the development of decubiti by the application of benzoin and thymol iodide, or the use of a flotation pad or alternating pressure mattress.

Many of these patients are treated by radiation and this usually leads to nausea and vomiting. Thus, intake and output should be carefully observed and recorded. Patients should rest as much as possible, especially after their return from daily treatment.

Lymphedema may present a problem in either the postmastectomy patient with recurrent disease or the inoperable patient. Again, good skin care is necessary and precautions must be taken to prevent infection. For example, when the patient's nails are clipped or manicured, caution must be exercised to avoid causing a break in the skin. Use of the elastic sleeve and elevation of the arm may be effective in reducing swelling due to lymphedema. As is the case when there is no lymphedema present, the arm on the affected side should never be used for skin tests, subcutaneous injections, finger-sticks, venipuncture, or for monitoring blood pressure.

The control of odors arising from open lesions often presents a nursing problem, especially in the case of fungating chest-wall lesions. Some control measures that may be taken include frequent, meticulous cleansing and re-dressing of the wound, removing soiled dressings from the room immediately instead of dropping them into a wastebasket at the bedside, and spraying the room with a deodorant spray. A few drops of essence of peppermint or Nilodor applied to the outer dressing and along the top and bottom of the bed frame can be quite effective in overcoming offensive odors.

Pain is almost always a symptom in the patient with advanced breast cancer. Every effort is made to keep the patient as comfortable as possible, but it is important that the nurse keep the physician informed as to the location, quality, and intensity of the pain so that he may, if he wishes, institute therapy to alleviate the disease manifestation that is causing the pain. For example, pain may occur when the venous return is obstructed due to a nerve being compressed as a result of the extension of the tumor, by metastatic disease of the bone, or by inflammation, infection, or ulceration at the tumor site.

Potent narcotics are reserved for use in the later stages of the disease. Whenever possible, pain medications should be given by mouth, especially if the patient is to be transferred to her home. (Tranquilizers often enhance the effect of the narcotic.)

Many of these patients will have been in the hospital previously for ablative surgery and have been re-admitted for another reason. In these cases, the nurse must be particularly alert to the patient's need for hormonal replacement such as cortisone and thyroid. She should watch for signs of adrenal crisis, thyroid crisis, and diabetes insipidus, and should keep careful intake and output records.

In the relatively new field of clinical immunology, the nurse's responsibilities include close observation of the patient, giving the necessary care to the injection sites, reinforcing the doctor's explanation about immunotherapy, and carrying out the physician's orders in regard to blood sample collections.

Some patients with advanced breast cancer, particularly if they have been ill for a long time, become careless about their personal hygiene and appearance and need to be encouraged to "spruce themselves up." If the patient cannot afford to pay for a professional hairdresser, the nurse might wash and set her hair for her or, if she has lost her hair arrange for her to get a wig or wiglet. A depilatory or razor will take care of the problem of hirsutism. Wearing makeup and her own gowns and robes will help her to feel more attractive. Many of these patients are mothers, some with young children, and they enjoy hearing nurses chat about their own families, current events, or fashions. But, more importantly, the nurse needs to be a good listener. Some form of recreational or occupational therapy, a radio, television, or a good book may help the patient to pass the time. It is important to keep her alert and occupied for as long as possible.

Nursing the patient with advanced breast cancer is not only time-consuming, it is physically exhausting. Job satisfaction is difficult to achieve and the nurse may have to readjust her thinking in terms of goals. For example, she might have to settle for helping the patient find ways to be more comfortable and reasonably adjusted during her illness, rather than aiming for total rehabilitation for maximum health. True, many patients die of cancer, just as they do of other diseases, but at the same time many people lead useful and productive lives with their cancer under control. This fact should help the nurse to maintain a positive attitude toward cancer, to believe that every life is worth living and every cancer patient worth treating, and to encourage her patients to do everything they can for themselves in order to avert loss of hope. Cancer is not a hopeless condition; there are only those who have become hopeless about it.

QUESTIONS AND ANSWERS

Q. To what extent does early diagnosis affect the mortality rate in breast cancer?

A. Every decade there is a 5 to 10 percent reduction in the mortality rate for breast cancer. This is apparently the result of a definite trend toward earlier discovery of the disease by both physicians and patients.

Q. Should all breast lumps be biopsied?

A. Not necessarily. If a patient has chronic cystic mastitis, or a fibrous mastopathy, a biopsy is not usually done.
The physician relies on the secondary clinical signs when determining whether to do a biopsy. When a mass appears suddenly, is firm, hard, or irregular and if, in addition, fixation has occurred and the skin is indented, or if the mass is pointing and ulcerated, then a biopsy is done. When there are multiple masses, the physician sometimes has a difficult time deciding which one to biopsy. In such a case, a mammograph may be helpful in locating the most suspicious or occult one.

Q. If a person is having a physical examination postmenstrually, and is told that her breast feels lumpy, should she pursue it or forget it?

A. She should pursue it with a general surgeon or breast specialist and be very careful about self-examination. The American Cancer Society has an excellent film on self-examination as well as an illustrated leaflet that is printed in both English and Spanish.

Q. Is prophylactic castration recommended for patients who have had a radical mastectomy?

A. Only for those whose cancer is very extensive at the time of primary surgery.

Q. What is the cause of recurrence of cancer after mastectomy?

A. Incomplete or inadequate removal.

The term incomplete usually describes an operation in which not all of the diseased area was removed and this usually correlates directly with the amount of disease present; in other words, the more advanced the primary disease, the more likely it is to recur after surgery.

The term inadequate usually refers to a simple mastectomy that was performed on a patient who should have had a radical mastectomy.

Q. What is the ratio between nonnursing and nursing mothers in regard to the incidence of breast cancer?

A. The incidence is higher in women who have not nursed an infant, never had a lactating breast, or never been pregnant.

Q. Why are not more simple mastectomies done, rather than radical?

A. Simple mastectomy is advised only when the cancer is caught very early and is in situ. The axillary nodes are involved in 25 to 50 percent of patients with infiltrating cancer and, in these cases, mastectomy with removal of axillary contents is the treatment of choice.

Q. Is there any truth in the claims made in recent magazine articles that radical mastectomy is often done when it is not necessary and that simple mastectomy and radiation therapy is all that is needed?

A. Probably not.

Studies have shown that more often than not breast cancer develops in multiple areas of the breast; many patients will have a recurrence if only a single mass is removed.

Some cancers are resistant to radiation and there is no way of knowing this before trying it; also there are cases on record of cancers having occurred in areas that *had* been subjected to prophylactic radiation.

Q. Would most patients with breast cancer live longer without surgery?

A. There is no guarantee of longer life without surgery.

Studies done in the past, before radical mastectomy was introduced, indicated that 18 percent of patients who had simple mastectomies lived for five years. About the same percentage will survive that long without treatment.

At Memorial Hospital clinic, 70 percent of patients who have radical mastectomy are alive after five years, and over 55 percent of them are free of disease.

Q. If a patient between 20 and 40 years of age receives estrogen therapy for treatment of fibrocystic disease of the breast, and then develops cancer at menopause or postmenopausally, can the estrogen therapy be implicated?

A. Probably.
It is thought that fibrocystic disease is actually caused by estrogens. There are cases on record that report patients with this diagnosis as having had a remission of symptoms after having received estrogens. Then, at menopause, because of hot flashes or other symptoms, estrogens were given again and the symptoms of fibrocystic disease recurred. This would seem to implicate estrogens as a cause of the recurrence of fibrocystic disease. It would also seem to implicate it as a cause of cancer in these patients.

Q. Is thermography helpful in making the diagnosis of breast cancer?

A. Yes, but only when the environmental conditions are ideal—the room must be perfectly balanced as to heat, for example.
Thermography is most useful when superimposed on clinical impressions plus mammography.

Q. How do most husbands react to their wife's mastectomy?

A. A very small percentage of husbands reject their wives because of the mastectomy. If any kind of marital problem existed before the mastectomy, this may become exacerbated by the operation.
In many instances, the relationship the couple had before the operation will be made stronger by it.
In the beginning, a husband is naturally upset by the fact of his wife's illness, that she has cancer, and that sometimes she cannot cope with her feelings about it. Many of them become stronger for a while and are able to help the patient make the necessary adaptations. Basically, the reaction depends in a large measure on how the wife herself feels about it. If she can look at herself and still feel that she is a whole person, it will affect her husband's reaction as well as her own.
As to marital intimacy after the operation, this again depends on the type of person the husband is, the couple's former relationship, and the woman's own views of herself.

Q. How are radical mastectomy patients advised about future pregnancies?

A. This depends on the status of the pathology at the time of the operation. If the nodes were not involved, the patient is advised to wait a minimum of three to five years before becoming pregnant. If the nodes were involved at the time of surgery, most physicians would advise against any future pregnancies.

For the majority of these women, the contraceptive of choice is the IUD.

Q. What advice is given when breast cancer is detected in a young girl who is pregnant?

A. The medical advice is the same as though she were not pregnant. That is, a radical mastectomy should be done.

Q. Are women who have an oophorectomy when young less likely to get cancer of the breast when they are older?

A. A recent study showed that the incidence of breast cancer is lower in older women who had oophorectomies while still under the age of thirty-five.

Q. What should the social worker do if a patient tells her that she will commit suicide the first chance she gets?

A. First, appreciate the fact that the patient is asking for help. Encourage her to talk about her feelings—what she is thinking about, what she is reacting to, what the mastectomy meant to her. Do this in one or as many sittings as needed.

Inform the surgeon and the head nurse on the unit (or the team leader) of what the patient has said and what you have done. The surgeon will ask a psychiatrist to see the patient if he thinks this is necessary. At Memorial Hospital it has been found that cancer patients who threaten suicide, or who actually commit suicide, are almost always those who have been on large doses of cortisone which sometimes causes severe personality changes. It is well to keep this in mind when caring for patients who are receiving large doses of cortisone.

Q. Is it necessary for the patient to take Pitressin after hypophysectomy?

A. Yes, but temporarily. After a time vasopressin is again produced in the hypophyseal stalk.

Q. Is administration of thyroid started immediately after a hypophysectomy?

A. Usually it is not started for about one to two months because the thyroid gland stores the thyroid hormone for approximately a two-month period. It is generally conceded that the greater the symptoms of hyperthyroidism that appear when the thyroid extract is withheld, the more complete the hypophysectomy is presumed to be. In one series of about 7,000 hypophysectomies (transfrontal), about 10 percent were found at autopsy to have been incomplete.

Q. Are the personality changes that occur after hypophysectomy due to physiological or psychological factors?

A. No doubt a great psychological change takes place after hypophysectomy in that the patient becomes myxedematous unless the thyroid hormone is replaced, or adrenally insufficient unless cortisone is replaced. There are also psychological changes caused by the fact that the operation involved what amounted to a minute prefrontal lobotomy. One important point for the nurse to remember is that the patient who has had an adrenalectomy or hypophysectomy has a built-in method of suicide; that is, life depends on taking the ordered medications, and sometimes it is impossible to make the patient completely aware of this. A patient can purposely commit suicide by not taking the prescribed cortisone.

Q. Are hormones of the opposite sex useful in treating cancer of the breast?

A. At times they are.
Improvement is seen when estrogens are given to men with breast cancer. Improvement is seen when male hormones are given to women with breast cancer 1) immediately after an oophorectomy; 2) during a recurrence of cancer; and 3) when the patient is one to five years postmenopausal. In female patients five or more years postmenopausal, the rate of improvement with the use of estrogens is higher than when androgens are used.

Q. What is the physiological rationale for the use of estrogens in postmenopausal women?

A. The purpose is to get rid of the cyclomotor symptoms that occur—hot flashes, insomnia, etc. Also because estrogens cause a return of tissue turgor; the vagina becomes more moist—youthfulness returns. One of the most undesirable features of the use of estrogen in postmenopausal women is that if the patient had chronic cystic mastitis before menopause, she would probably develop it again with the use of estrogens. Also, the physician must be sure there is no dormant cancer in situ present. The patient should have a thorough examination, probably including a mammogram, before starting estrogen therapy and every year thereafter.

Physicians are usually reluctant to prescribe estrogen for postmenopausal women in whose families there is a high incidence of cancer.

Q. If hormones are not very effective and if they may cause chronic cystic mastitis, why use them?

A. Because it is the best treatment we have at the moment for advanced breast cancer.
Estrogens have been effective in about one-third of aged patients treated; testosterone in about 20 percent.

Q. When is radiation therapy indicated after mastectomy?

A. In general, radiation therapy is not thought to be necessary if the nodes are negative and the lesion is in the outer half of the breast. Often, patients whose lesions are on the inner (medial) half of the breast are given radiation therapy after surgery, even when the nodes are negative.

Q. What is the best way of handling the nausea and vomiting that often follow radiation therapy?

A. Have the patient eat a good breakfast 1-2 hours before the treatment so she will get a large share of her daily caloric requirement; then give her smaller meals the rest of the day.
Compazine and Tigan are often used to help control nausea and vomiting; they have been found to be quite effective.

Q. Is there any benefit to be derived from a partial dose of radiation when the patient cannot take the full amount she is scheduled for?

A. Probably not. Breast tumor is only partially radiosensitive—much less so than other tumors—and requires high dosage. For primary treatment it runs from 6,000 to 8,000 rads.

Q. Is chemotherapy useful in prolonging the life of patients with breast cancer?

A. There is no guarantee that chemotherapy will prolong life in cases of breast cancer. Chemotherapy is a palliative treatment.
No drug has yet been found that is totally effective in breast cancer.

Q. Why is it not possible to get a positive biopsy on every specimen the first time around?

A. Because it is not always possible to hit the area where cancer cells are present, especially in an aspiration biopsy.

Q. What emergency situations might arise in patients with large, fungating breast ulcers?

A. The most important emergency would be hemorrhage. Pressure should be applied immediately and continuously over the bleeding site and help summoned without leaving the patient. It may not be possible to get help for the patient in time to save her life. If the hemorrhage is from a major vessel a pneumothorax could develop from the lesion invading the pleural cavity.

Q. Is it dangerous for a nurse who has had a radical mastectomy to work in isolation?

A. Not if the incision is healed and there is no drainage. There is no danger either to herself or the patient.

Q. Is there a class for husbands of mastectomy patients at Memorial Hospital?

A. Such a class was started in August, 1971, and is quite successful.

Q. How do most patients feel about attending postmastectomy classes?

A. They start out with both positive and negative feelings. At first it is hard for them to talk to someone they scarcely know about their thoughts, feelings and actions. The group leader tries to elicit facts about patients' normal patterns of living and uses that information to facilitate discussion. It often takes a lot of time and patience on the part of the leader before patients open up and discuss their feelings freely.

Q. Are patients who have been in the class for several days generally supportive to the new patients?

A. Yes, very much so.
   In some ways, the class approach resembles the Alcoholics Anonymous approach, since it is based on the idea that people who have had the problem know the most about it and about how to be helpful. However, the group is not promoted as a club of any sort, and, although some patients come back to the class once or twice after recovery, this is not stressed because every patient should get back into living a normal life as soon as she feels up to it.

Q. Why was a particular set of exercises developed for use at Memorial Hospital instead of those which have been in vogue for years?

A. Because of what the team members learned from watching patients doing exercises and the belief that exercises could be devised that would help women return to their jobs and household activities earlier. These exercises actually "zero in" on the use of the shoulder when exercising, whereas the older exercises allowed for substitutions. For example, if a person doing the old exercises is asked to make a circular motion with her arm while holding a string tied to a doorknob, she could keep the arm close to the side and use only the forearm to make the motion. The objective of the Memorial exercises is to make sure the patient is exercising the arm in such a way that normal shoulder movement will be reestablished.

Q. What exercises are patients with simple mastectomies taught?

A. They are taught the same exercises as patients who have radical mastectomies, but their rehabilitation is simpler and faster.

Q. Are family members encouraged to help the patient with her exercises?

A. There is no reason why family members should not come to the class and learn how to do the exercises, but classes are usually held in the morning when most people are at work.

The patient can usually learn to do them properly by the time she goes home. Also, she is given a list of the exercises, written out in great detail, to take home and refer to if necessary.

Translators should be provided for patients who do not speak English, so that they can learn in class how to do the exercises properly. (Exercise information is available in Spanish.) Staff nurses routinely check the patients' exercises to make sure they are being done properly. The volunteer often visits the patients in their rooms while their families are there and teaches them also how the exercises should be done.

Q. Can exercises sometimes cause damage to skin flaps?

A. Obviously, yes. However, if given under careful supervision, the new exercises will usually not result in damage to skin flaps. Patients are instructed to stop the exercise as soon as they feel any pulling or pain in the incision area and to do deep breathing which, in a gentle fashion, eases the tension on the skin flaps. Also, the patient's charts are checked before each class for any notation about elevation of the flaps, or dusky areas on the flaps near the incision, and these patients are told to do the exercises more carefully.

Q. How soon should a patient who is discharged from the hospital with a still draining wound start the exercises?

A. The physician decides this in each individual case. If there is a great deal of fluid accumulation he would probably say to defer exercises until this situation has been corrected. The biggest healing problems occur in the axillary area. Some patients discharge a lot of serum from the wound here and this, plus exercise, keeps the skin flaps from becoming fixed to the chest wall. In these cases, exercises probably should be deferred until fixation takes place and the wound is at least partly healed.

Q. Do patients ever have problems such as pain and swelling in the affected area from over-exercising after they get home?

A. Patients are taught in the class, and it is repeated in the booklet they are given, that they must avoid over-exercising. Injury is more of a problem. Any injury such as a burn or bruise, or an infection in the arm, will increase the possibility of lymphedema. If a woman does gardening or heavy house work, she should cover the arm and hand so as not to get thorns, steel wool bits, etc., in the skin. Also she should use good judgment about not doing too much with that arm.

Q. Does the volunteer go to a patient's home if the patient was not seen in the hospital and has been referred by the visiting nurse?

A. Sometimes. The patient can go to the Reach to Recovery office if she needs help, but if she can't get there a volunteer may go to her. The volunteer makes one follow-up visit to the patient's home (even if she has seen her in the hospital) to check the prosthesis and answer any questions the patient may have. If the patient needs still further help and cannot get to the office, the vounteer may make a second home visit.

Q. Is it true that the Papanicolaou test is used in the diagnosis of breast cancer?

A. A Pap smear does not have to come from the cervix. It is possible to use the test on discharges from the nipple or on fluid aspirated from the breast. However, because cancer cells are so seldom picked up by this method, it is not frequently used.

APPENDIX A

A Breast Check—so Simple . . . so Important*

Bathing. Showering. Your moment to take care of yourself. Time to begin your breast self-examination.

Your fingers slide easily. As you wash you can do a simple check that will require practically no time.

Examine your breasts. Keep your fingers flat and touch every part of each breast. Feel gently for a lump or thickening. The fact that your skin is slippery makes it easy.

Why should you do this? It can save your life. After all, it's what you don't know that can hurt you.

Most women discover breast changes by themselves. But some of them are late in making the discovery.

It's important to see your physician as soon as you discover a lump or thickening. That discovery most often represents a perfectly harmless condition. In fact, most women are told by their physicians, "You have no need to worry. Everything is fine. But you were wise to see me as soon as you did."

You can avoid that mistake by checking your breasts once a month after your menstrual period. Be sure to continue these checkups after your change of life.

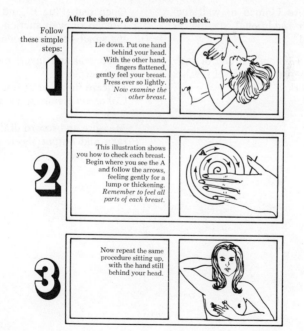

After the shower, do a more thorough check.

Follow these simple steps:

1 Lie down. Put one hand behind your head. With the other hand, fingers flattened, gently feel your breast. Press ever so lightly. *Now examine the other breast.*

2 This illustration shows you how to check each breast. Begin where you see the A and follow the arrows, feeling gently for a lump or thickening. *Remember to feel all parts of each breast.*

3 Now repeat the same procedure sitting up, with the hand still behind your head.

*From a pamphlet distributed by the American Cancer Society.

APPENDIX B

MEMORIAL SLOAN-KETTERING CANCER CENTER
DEPARTMENT OF NURSING

Hemovac

Purpose: To remove wound exudate by application of gentle suction through catheters which are inserted under the wound flaps.

Care of Hemovac

Steps: What to do	*Points: How to do it*
1. Compress Hemovac and close Plug B to establish suction.	Place Hemovac on firm, flat surface; compress with palm of hand and seal.
2. Secure Hemovac in place.	Fasten Hemovac with safety pin to draw sheet or patient's gown.
3. Maintain proper functioning.	*Keep Hemovac compressed or suction will be lost and Hemovac will be of no value.*
4. Attach to Gomco or wall suction for additional suction as ordered.	Open seal (Plug B) and connect to Gomco or wall suction tubing, using small-size glass connector.
5. Empty Hemovac at end of each tour or when fluid level reaches line marked "FULL."	Open seal and invert over measuring receptacle. Squeeze fluid out of opening. Compress Hemovac as described in Step 1. Measure and record drainage on intake and output sheet, and on patient's chart.

APPENDIX C

BRA   ROOM

MEMORIAL SLOAN-KETTERING CANCER CENTER
POSTMASTECTOMY REHABILITATION CLASS RECORD

ADMISSION DATE:
INTRODUCTION DATE:
DIAGNOSIS:
DATE OF SURGERY:
SURGERY:
COMPLICATIONS:
OCCUPATION:
MARITAL STATUS: S M W D SEP.
CHILDREN:
CLASS ATTENDANCE DATES: ADDRESS:
DATE OF DISCHARGE:

                                                 TEL.

NURSE: VITAL SIGNS
                                       E.B.L.
                                       REPLAC.
                                       HG. & HCT.
                                       CHEST X-RAY
                                       EKG
                                       HANDEDNESS L, R, AMBI.

APPENDIX D

Do's and Don'ts For Hand and Arm Care

Sometimes after a mastectomy one's arm may swell. This initial swelling will gradually disappear and the affected arm will return to near normal size, provided some simple precautionary measures are strictly adhered to. Black and blue areas occasionally occur following mastectomy. These develop as the result of surgical injury to the capillaries, which are minute blood vessels. Within a relatively short time they gradually disappear. As the result of the removal of the lymph nodes and channels in the armpit, the arm becomes less able to combat infections.

1. Every effort must be made to avoid breaks in the skin as these may lead to possible infection.
    a. Avoid injections and vaccinations in operated arm.
    b. Be careful when manicuring nails—use a cuticle cream or cuticle remover instead of scissors.
    c. Wear canvas gloves when gardening—avoid thorn pricks.
    d. Wear protective gloves when using steel wool.
    e. Wear a thimble when sewing—avoid needle and pin pricks.
    f. Take care of cuts and scrapes. Wash area and cover with a protective dressing.
    g. Avoid harsh detergents which may cause chapped hands—use a good hand cream several times a day.

2. Avoid any constriction which may cause swelling.
    a. Avoid having blood pressure taken on affected arm.
    b. Wear loose jewelry—loose dress sleeves—avoid pressure and swelling.
3. Avoid burns—they can lead to possible infection.
    a. If you must smoke, hold cigarette in the hand of your unaffected arm—and—close match cover when striking matches.
    b. Avoid reaching into hot oven with affected arm. Use a padded glove.
    c. Get your tan gradually—avoid sunburn.

4. Inform your doctor of any new development promptly.
    a. If the affected arm suddenly swells or becomes reddened—contact your doctor immediately. This usually signifies a low-grade infection and you should not treat this condition yourself.

5. To avoid drag or pull—carry heavy packages and pocketbooks in your unaffected arm.

6. Avoid hormone beauty creams and hormone drugs. Consult your surgeon for his approval first.

7. Examine your remaining breast or skin over your chest area once a month and report any changes to your surgeon. (See breast self-examination leaflet enclosed.)

8. Keep your follow-up appointments. This is most essential to your well-being.

Post-Mastectomy Classes

Held daily at 10:30 sharp Mondays through Fridays in Room 236 Memorial. Each group of exercises is to be done at least 5 times a day

a. Upon arising
b. Upon retiring
c. Before or after meals (3)
d. As often as necessary if you feel any stiffness

The exercises are all done in the sitting position with the exception of the pendulum exercise. Exercises are done in the following order:

a. Wall climbing for measurement and exercise (standing position)
b. Pendulum (across the body, circling, back and forth—standing position —bent over)
c. Deep breathing with unaffected arm on center of chest
d. Clasped hand raised (seated)
e. Pulley (seated)

Evening Session

There is a group for *couples* (the patient and her husband or male friend) which meets every Wednesday evening, Room 236 Memorial between 6:30 and 7:30 P.M. You are invited after you have been discharged as well as while you are still in the hospital. Coffee is served.

APPENDIX E

Patient's Wallet Card

(Front Side)

MEDICAL INFORMATION FOR PATIENTS WITH ADRENAL INSUFFICIENCY

During any illness:
1. Double the dose of cortisone or prednisone (Meticorten).
2. Consult your physician.
3. Take salty broth or soup.

If you cannot take your medicine because of nausea or vomiting:
1. Call your doctor at once!
2. Take four times your usual dose of cortisone or prednisone as soon after vomiting as possible. Some of the medication will stay down.
3. Take salty soups as soon as condition permits.

(Reverse Side)

MEDICAL INFORMATION FOR PHYSICIANS

This patient has undergone total hypophysectomy and is under care for adrenal insufficiency. In emergency:
1. Treat for adrenal crisis with I.V. and I.M. hydrocortisone or cortisone.
2. Administer I.V. isotonic saline.
3. Continue I.M. cortisone until oral medication is tolerated.
4. Conditions which must be treated promptly: blood loss, fluid and electrolyte loss, infection, severe diarrhea.

For further details:
1. Private patients: Call patient's private physician's office.
2. Clinic patients: Call Memorial Hospital, TR 9-3000, ask operator for "doctor on call for endocrine service." If necessary, phone Dr. E. Greenberg, RE 7-9521.

SUGGESTED READINGS

Books

Ackerman, Lauren W. and J. A. del Regato. *Cancer: Diagnosis, Treatment, and Prognosis.* St. Louis: Mosby, 1969.

American Cancer Society. *Cancer Management.* Philadelphia: Lippincott, 1968.

Bouchard, Rosemary. *Nursing Care of the Cancer Patient.* St. Louis: Mosby, 1967.

Brauer, Paul H. "Should the Patient be Told the Truth?" *Social Interaction and Patient Care.* Philadelphia: Lippincott, 1965.

Breast Cancer: Early and Late. Chicago: Year Book Medical Publishers, 1970.

Brunner, Lillian Sholtes, and others. *Textbook of Medical Surgical Nursing.* 2nd ed. Philadelphia: Lippincott, 1970.

Carlson, Carolyn E., Coordinator. *Behavioral Concepts and Nursing Intervention.* Philadelphia: Lippincott, 1970.

Ecology of the Cancer Patient. Washington, D.C.: Interdisciplinary Communication Associates, Inc., 1970.

Engel, George L. "Grief and Grieving," *A Sociological Framework for Patient Care.* New York: Wiley, 1966.

Herberger, Winfried. *Treatment of Inoperable Cancer.* Baltimore: Williams & Wilkins, 1966.

Hickey, Robert C., Ed. *Palliative Care of the Cancer Patient.* Boston: Little, Brown, 1967.

Leis, Henry P., Jr. *Diagnosis and Treatment of Breast Lesions.* Flushing, L. I., New York: Medical Examinating Publishing Company, 1971.

Moore, F. D., et al. *Carcinoma of the Breast.* Boston: Little Brown and Company, 1968.

Nealon, Thomas, Ed. *Management of the Patient with Cancer.* Philadelphia: Saunders, 1965.

Shafer, Kathleen Newton, et al. *Medical-Surgical Nursing,* 4th ed. St. Louis: Mosby, 1967.

Periodicals

Bruce, J. "The Enigma of Breast Cancer," *Cancer, 24*:1314-8, December, 1969.

Crile, G., Jr. "Possible Role of Uninvolved Regional Nodes in Preventing Metastases from Breast Cancer," *Cancer, 24*:1283-5, December, 1969.

Egan, R. L. "Mammography," *American Journal of Nursing, 66*:108-111, January, 1966.

Farrow, J. H. "Rehabilitation Following Breast Surgery," *Ca; A Cancer Journal For Physicians, 16*:22-23, November/December, 1966.

Farrow, J. H. "Current Concepts in the Detection and Treatment of the Earliest of the Breast Cancers," *Cancer, 25*:468-77, February, 1970.

Gershon-Cohen, J., et al. "Modalities in Breast Cancer Detection, Xeroradiography, Thermography and Mammography," *Cancer, 24*:1226-30, December, 1969.

Gould, Mitchell A. "Causes of Patients' Delay in Diseases of the Breast," *Cancer, 17*:564-577, May, 1964.

Gribbons, C. A., and Aliapoulios, M. A. "Early Carcinoma of the Breast," *American Journal of Nursing, 69*:1945-50, September, 1969.

Gribbons, C. A. and Aliapoulios, M. A. "Treatment for Advanced Breast Carcinoma," *American Journal of Nursing, 72*:678-682, April, 1972.

Harrell, Helen C. "To Lose a Breast," *American Journal of Nursing, 72*:676-677, April, 1972.

Martley, I. O., and Brandt, E. M. "Control and Prevention of Lymphedema Following Radical Mastectomy," *Nursing Research, 16*:333-336, Fall, 1967.

Holleb, A. I. "Breast Cancer and Pregnancy," *Ca; A Cancer Journal For Physicians, 15*:182-3, July/August, 1965.

Holleb, A. I., et al. "Cancer of the Male Breast," *New York Journal of Medicine, 68*:656-63, March, 1968.

Kennedy, B. J. "Hormone Therapy for Advanced Breast Cancer," *American Journal of Surgery, 18*:1551-57, December, 1965.

Kennedy, B. J., and French, Lyle. "Hypophysectomy in Advanced Breast Cancer," *American Journal of Surgery, 110*:411-415, September, 1965.

Kerr, I. F., et al. "Breast Cancer and Heredity," *Lancet, 1*:1322-3, January 17, 1967.

Leis, H. P. "Prophylactic Removal of the Second Breast," *Hospital Medicine, 4*:45-55, January, 1968.

Lemon, H. N. "Endocrine Influences on Human Mammary Cancer Formation— A Critique," *Cancer, 23*:781-90, April, 1969.

Lewison, E. F. "The Nurse's Role in the Early Detection of Cancer Of The Breast," *Nursing Forum, 4*:82-86, No. 3, 1965.

Lewison, Edward F. "The Treatment of Advanced Breast Cancer," *American Journal of Nursing, 62*:107-110, October, 1967.

Lewison, E. F. "The Total Care of Your Mastectomy Patient," Revised 1967, *Identical Form, Inc.,* 17 West 60th Street, New York, N. Y. 10023.

MacMahon, B., et al. "Endocrinology and Epidemiology of Breast Cancer," *Cancer, 24*:1146-54, December, 1969.

Mayo, P. and Wilkey, N. L. "Prevention of Cancer of the Breast and Cervix," *Nursing Clinics of North America, 3*:229-241, June, 1968.

Papadrianos, E., et al. "Cancer of the Breast as a Familial Disease," *Annals of Surgery, 165*:10-19, January, 1967.

Quint, J. C. "Mastectomy: Signpost in Time," *Journal of Nursing Education,* 2:3, September, 1963.

Quint, J. C. "The Impact Of Mastectomy," *American Journal of Nursing, 63*: 88-92, November, 1963.

Robbins, G. F. and Berg, J. W. "Bilateral Primary Breast Cancer," *Cancer, 17*: 1501-1527, December, 1964.

Rosemond, G. P., et al. "Postoperative Care and Rehabilitation in Breast Cancer after Surgery," Cancer, *24*:1307-9, December, 1969.

Ross, W. L. "The Magnitude of the Breast Cancer Problem in the U.S.A.," *Cancer, 24*:1106-8, December, 1969.

Snyderman, R. K., et al. "Breast Reconstruction," *Surgical Clinics of North America, 49*:303-11, April, 1969.

Sokol, E. S., et al. "Role of Mammography with Palpable Breast Lesions," *Surgery, 67*:748-53, May, 1970.

Strax, P., et al. "Mammography and Clinical Examination in Mass Screening for Cancer of the Breast," *Cancer, 20*:2184-8, December, 1967.

Thornblad, Inga. "Hormonal Ablative Therapy for the Premenopausal Patient with Advanced Cancer," *Nursing Clinics of North America, 2*:659-669, December, 1967.

Urban, J. A. "Extended Radical Mastectomy for Breast Cancer," *American Journal Surgery, 106*:399-404, September, 1963.

Urban, J. A. "Biopsy of the Normal Breast in Treating Breast Cancer," *Surgical Clinics of North America, 49*:291-301, April, 1969.

Urban, J. A. "Bilateral Breast Cancer," *Cancer, 24*:1310-13, December, 1969.

Urban, J. A. "Therapy of Primary Breast Cancer," *California Medicine, 112*: 10-3, April, 1970.

Wolf, E. S. "Nursing Care of the Patient with Breast Cancer," *Nursing Clinics of North America, 2*:587-598, December, 1967.

Wynder, E. L. "Identification of Women at High Risk for Breast Cancer," *Cancer, 24*:1235-40, December, 1969.

Zimmer, T. S. "Pitfalls and Limitations of Breast Examinations," *Hospital Medicine, 4*:13-18, August, 1968.

Patients with Tumors
of the Liver

Regional Medical Program — Oncology Nursing Seminar

on

NURSING MANAGEMENT OF PATIENTS WITH TUMORS OF THE LIVER

Seminar Leader

Joseph G. Fortner, M.D.

Seminar Participants

Noreen Byrne, R.N., B.S., Head Nurse

Joseph G. Fortner, M.D., Chief, Gastric and Mixed Tumor Service
and Chief, Transplantation Service

David W. Kinne, M.D., Clinical Assistant Surgeon, Gastric and
Mixed Tumor Service

Patricia Mazzola, R.N., B.S.N., Clinical Nursing Instructor

Sandra Nehlson, R.N., Ph.D., Assistant Immunologist,
Transplantation Service

Donna Vermes, R.N., Assistant Head Nurse

Primary hepatoma is relatively rare in the United States and Europe. Comparatively, it is more common in southeast Asia, in southern India, and in the part of Africa that is south of the Sahara. Probably the highest incidence rate in the world occurs in Mozambique where the rate among Negro men between the ages of 25 and 35 is 500 times that in the United States. The rate is also high among the African Bantus many of whom leave their native homes to seek work in the gold mines of South Africa where their disease is discovered and where cancer of the liver has been intensively studied.

The wide variation in incidence of primary cancer of the liver among the peoples of the world is not the result of differences in race or heredity, but of environmental factors. What these specific factors are is not definitely known although researchers have suggested several clues. One clue is that a mold found on nuts that are a staple in the diet of certain African tribes causes hepatoma when given to rats experimentally, and may also cause the disease in man.

Of greater importance perhaps is the possibility that a viral infection is the causative agent. In a study of 200 Sengali with primary liver cancer, 42 percent had SH antigen in their blood serum. In a series of 28 cases of primary hepatoma studied at Memorial Hospital, only 6 percent had this virus related antigen in their serum, but this is still about three times the percentage one would expect to find in the general population. Had the improved methods of detecting the virus that are now available been used, this latter study might have shown the percentage to have been higher. An important fact is that when the pathologist examines the liver of a patient who had primary cancer of the liver, he often sees evidence that the patient also had hepatitis. Of interest also is the fact that about 60 percent of patients with hepatoma have cirrhosis too—not the alcoholic or nutritional type, but the post-necrotic type that usually results from a previous infection. Thus, there is considerable indirect evidence at present to suggest that a virus may be the causative factor in primary cancer of the liver.

Another fact of importance in the diagnosis of this particular tumor is that in a fairly large percentage of cases a certain protein, alpha feto globulin, is found in the circulating blood. This protein, which is produced by the cells of a hepatoma, can be detected by the use of a very sensitive test.

About 80 percent of African patients and about 25 to 30 percent of English and American patients with hepatoma (including those in the Memorial Hospital series) have had a positive reaction to this test.

A significant breakthrough in the study of liver tumors is that radiologists, through the use of selective angiography, have become expert in defining the extent as well as the location of the tumor. In this procedure, a catheter is put into an arm or leg artery and threaded up to the celiac plexus where the hepatic artery branches off. Not only is it possible then to visualize the location and size of the tumor, but the surgeon can also see the anatomical arrangement of the blood vessels.

TREATMENT

The usual treatment for hepatoma is surgery. The newer concepts of surgical treatment are based on the location of the tumor. A bilateral subcostal incision is made and the tumor located. If only the right lobe is involved, a right hepatic lobectomy is done. Similarly, if only the left lobe is involved, a left hepatic lobectomy will be done. A right lobe tumor that extends over into the vena cava can now be safely resected by using our cold perfusion technique. A tumor that involves both right and left lobe but no other structures may be treated by removing the entire liver and replacing it with a liver transplant. Should the tumor involve both lobes and other structures, the preferred treatment is to tie off the hepatic artery and infuse a chemotherapeutic agent directly into the liver.

Preoperative Care

The nurse must be knowledgeable about the several functions of the liver in order to understand the various needs of the patient who undergoes liver surgery, and the treatments he will receive. Briefly, the three outstanding functions of the liver may be classified as blood-related, metabolic, or detoxifying. One of the blood-related functions is removing the bilirubin that results from red blood cell breakdown, and conjugating it into water-soluble bilirubin. When this function is impaired, the degree of alteration in the liver's ability to handle bilirubin can be ascertained by determining the serum bilirubin level. An important metabolic function is to convert glucose into glycogen, store it, and then convert it back into glucose and release it into the bloodstream when the body needs glucose. The liver also converts ammonia into urea and excess amino acids into carbohydrate. It manufactures fibrinogen, prothrombin, albumin, and globulin. It forms antibodies and heparin. Impairment of any of these functions will be reflected in signs and symptoms that the nurse should be able to recognize and which she should carefully observe and report.

The patient who faces a lobectomy or hepatic artery ligation has all the anxieties of any hospitalized person, plus many additional worries. The thought of the major surgery which he must undergo is quite overwhelming because, in most cases, the reason for it is primary or metastatic cancer of the liver. The prognosis in these cases is guarded and may well be sensed by the patient. During the preoperative period, both the patient and his family need strong emotional support to reduce some of the tensions with which they are trying to cope. They should be encouraged to verbalize their feelings so that the nurse can help allay their fears. She should spend as much time as needed to explain tests and procedures that are being done. Increased understanding of these procedures will help to minimize the patient's fears and strengthen his ability to tolerate his many discomforts. He is generally uncomfortable, and the extensive preoperative workup can increase his discomfort and anxiety.

The general nursing activities involved in the preoperative care of the patient with liver disease are directly related to his problems and symptoms. Jaundice, due to increased bilirubin in the blood, calls for good skin care, especially if the jaundice is accompanied by pruritus. The patient may find his icteric sclera both frightening and repulsive. Therefore, keeping the room softly lit and mirrors to a minimum may help to prevent the patient from becoming upset about his appearance.

Careful attention should be given to building up the patient's nutritional state. Some degree of anorexia may be present and, to help improve his appetite the patient should be given good mouth care, be comfortably positioned, and have his room well ventilated before meals are served.

Since the prothrombin time may be increased in patients with liver damage, there could be a tendency toward bleeding. The site of any injection should be watched closely and pressure applied if any bleeding should develop. Urine and stools are checked for blood; guaiac tests may be ordered on all stools. Accurate collection of all specimens in regard to time is very important.

The preoperative workup includes various liver function tests. Chest x-rays are done to disclose any possible metastasis to the lung. When metastasis is suspected, tomograms may be ordered, and the findings may constitute a contradindication for hepatic lobectomy. Other radiographic studies include a skeletal survey, gastrointestinal series, and IVP. Of course, a cardiogram is also done. A liver scan to determine the location of the tumor is required and, for best visualization, a celiac angiogram is usually employed. For this procedure, a catheter is threaded through the femoral artery up into the celiac or hepatic artery and a radiopaque dye introduced through the catheter to outline the vascularization of the liver. When all these tests and the procedures that precede them are carefully explained to the patient, some of the anxiety and irritability they cause may be considerably decreased.

In preparing the patient for lobectomy, it is important to improve liver function as much as possible. Although the liver can regenerate with as little as 20 percent of it remaining after surgery, that 20 percent must be functioning optimally. A thorough alcoholic and dietary history is taken and if any nutritional deficiency is found, the patient is placed on a diet rich in carbohydrate, protein, and vitamins. Serum proteins can be supplemented, if necessary, with human serum albumin. Blood volume is checked and it, too, can be supplemented with whole blood or blood constituents. Vitamin K may be given to assist the liver in the production of prothrombin.

A bowel preparation is done because the bowel may have to be opened during surgery and also because the breakdown of protein in the intestine may lead to postoperative ammonia intoxication. The patient is given an antibiotic, usually neomycin or sulfasuxidine. The bowel is cleansed mechanically by such cathartics as magnesium sulfate or castor oil, and a daily colonic irrigation. All this may make the patient very uncomfortable and dehydrated and may also deplete his blood potassium. The nurse must encourage him to take fluids, and potassium chloride tables may be ordered. The patient is given a low residue diet on the third preoperative day, a full liquid diet on the second preoperative day, and a clear liquid diet the day before surgery. The patient's chest and abdomen are "prepped" for surgery. Most importantly, the patient is taught deep breathing and coughing exercises.

Hepatic Artery Ligation

Hepatic artery ligation and infusion with a therapeutic agent is considered when the patient has a liver tumor, either primary or secondary, that extends outside of the liver and is not resectable by hepatic lobectomy or total hepatectomy followed by a liver transplant. Although the patient still has cancer outside of the liver, it is the extensive disease in the liver that is his major problem, and hepatic artery ligation is done as a palliative measure.

It is an extremely useful procedure in cases of non-resectable cancer and the rationale for trying it is based on several pieces of evidence. Angiographic studies as well as corrosive cast studies of tumors removed at autopsy show that the hepatic artery is the almost exclusive source of blood supply to both primary and metastatic liver tumors. The portal vein, which normally brings about 75 percent of the liver's oxygen supply, probably is the almost exclusive source of blood supply to the remaining normal parenchyma.

This procedure was first tried on experimental animals, mainly rats, with liver tumors and it was found that ligation of the hepatic artery resulted in selective necrosis of the tumor; the surrounding parenchyma survived and did not necrose. Then it was tried on humans and the same selective necrosis of the tumor and preservation of the normal parenchyma occurred. The reports of several series of patients on whom the procedure has been performed are now available. In Sweden, one surgeon reported significant objective palliation of up to two months in patients with metastatic cancer of the liver, and one in Thailand reported palliation for the same length of time in 12 out of 40 patients. An even more encouraging report has come from Great Britain where ten patients with either primary or metastatic cancer of the liver have undergone hepatic artery ligation with simultaneous placement of a catheter in the distal hepatic artery for infusion of cytotoxic agents to treat any surviving cancer tissue. All of these patients have had significant palliation for up to eight and ten months. Both primary and metastatic cancer was represented in 23 patients in a series of Memorial Hospital patients who were treated by hepatic artery ligation, and in whom palliation was achieved for varying lengths of time.

A study of the preoperative and postoperative arteriograms done on patients in the Memorial Hospital series disclosed one of the reasons why greater therapeutic benefit was not achieved through hepatic artery ligation; that is, collateralization between other blood vessels and the hepatic artery. In one series of arteriograms on the same patient, the right hepatic artery was shown to be receiving significant amounts of blood from the phrenic arteries, from the superior mesenteric artery, and from the retroduodenal artery. Thus, the tumor was getting a significant supply of blood, although the hepatic artery per se was occluded. One of these patients was studied by arteriography immediately after the operation and again six weeks later and the two arteriograms were identical, indicating that collateralization occurs rapidly and that it persists.

Postoperative values in Memorial Hospital patients who have had the hepatic artery ligation operation have been quite consistent. In most of them, the preoperative total bilirubin was within normal range; after the ligation there was some elevation (two had marked elevation); and by two weeks postoperatively it had returned to normal. The alkaline phosphatase value, which is a measure of obstructive phenomena in the liver, was mildly or significantly elevated preoperatively, rose markedly after operation, and then drifted down toward the preoperative range. Enzymes that are indicative of hepatocellular change rose markedly after hepatic artery ligation and then rather rapidly returned toward normal. Another index of hepatocellular dysfunction, LDH, also rose rapidly after operation and then returned toward normal. Postoperative liver scans were no different from preoperative scans with one exception and, in that case, the change was due to the fact that the tumor had occluded the left branch of the portal vein so that when the hepatic artery was ligated the left lobe was deprived of its entire blood supply and this resulted in necrosis of that lobe. Postoperative flow studies, done with the radioisotope technetium-99, have shown that the flow to both right and left hepatic lobes is diminished while that to the spleen, via the splenic artery, is increased.

Other parameters that were measured pre- and postoperatively were fever, appetite, pain, liver size, and duration of the response. Only one patient had fever preoperatively and that disappeared after the operation. All of the patients experienced an improvement in appetite postoperatively, especially for meat, and this occurred even in those who had had an intolerance for meat before the surgery. The most significant subjective change that occurred in all patients was the relief of pain. This probably was related to a reduction in the size of the liver and in the amount of stretching of the liver capsule after the hepatic artery ligation since, in all patients, the liver either diminished in size or at least did not increase. Fifty percent of patients showed an objective improvement which lasted an average of 20 weeks. It should be noted that these patients were unresponsive to systemic chemotherapy.

Currently, the technique being used at Memorial Hospital for patients with inoperable liver cancer consists of hepatic artery ligation and simultaneous infusion of a cytotoxic chemotherapeutic agent through a catheter inserted into the hepatic artery. This catheter, which is left in place after the operation, is attached to a small pump and thus the chemotherapeutic agent can be delivered to the hepatic artery (at intervals) for a period of several weeks postoperatively, even after the patient goes home. It is expected that this procedure will result in a longer period of palliation for the patient.

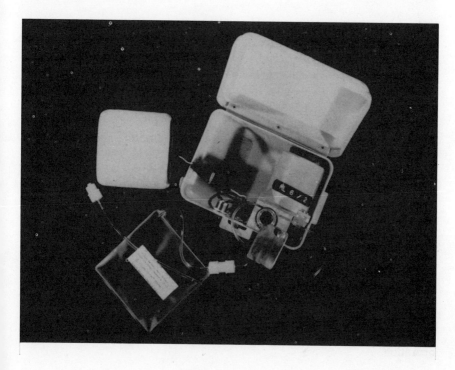

Figure 1. Perfusion pump used to infuse cytotoxic chemotherapeutic
agent through catheter inserted into hepatic artery

Hepatic Lobectomy by Isolation and Cold Perfusion

When the standard techniques of the past have been used, the operative
mortality for left hepatic lobectomy has been 11 percent, and that for right
hepatic lobectomy 32 percent. It is now thought that these high rates were
the result of attempting to remove tumors that were too large for such treatment. Now an operation has been designed that will make lobectomy safer.
Because the entire procedure is done under controlled conditions, extensive
resections that formerly would have been impossible can now be done. This
operation is referred to as hepatic lobectomy by isolation and cold perfusion
technique.

Instead of a paramedian incision which has been used in lobectomy procedures in the past, a bilateral, subcostal incision is used to give better exposure of the area involved. The abdomen is opened and the liver exposed.

Once it is determined that a tumor is present and that it is operable, the chest is opened through a convenient interspace, the peritoneal reflections between the liver and kidney are severed, and the liver is retracted upward and to the left. The adrenal vein is doubly ligated because the liver must be completely isolated. Other structures are severed or ligated as necessary to completely free the liver. The porta hepatis containing the portal vein, hepatic artery, and bile duct is dissected. When the right lobe is removed, the right hepatic artery is tied off and a catheter is inserted into the cut end. Perfusate will then flow into the left lobe and chill it. The portal vein is treated in a similar fashion. The hepatic artery and portal vein are occluded and the liver portion is then perfused with chilled lactated Ringer's solution. The vena cava above and below the liver is clamped and an opening made in it so that the perfusate that is being introduced through the hepatic artery and portal vein catheters can run through the lobe.

This technique can be very useful in the treatment of hepatoma because conditions in the operative area can be controlled making it possible for the surgeon to take the time he needs to perform a very precise operation. The technique can also be useful to the trauma surgeon in repairing a fractured or lacerated liver because it makes possible the isolation of the liver from the circulatory system for as long a time as is needed to complete the repair operation.

Postoperative Nursing Care Following Hepatic Ligation or Lobectomy

The vital signs of patients who have had a hepatic artery ligation or a hepatic lobectomy must be checked frequently. Chest tubes which are connected to underwater drainage must be kept free from any obstruction. They are usually removed by the fifth postoperative day. All dressings should be checked frequently and the color, amount of drainage, and any change in the amount reported to the physician.

The patient returns from the operating room with both a Levin tube and a Foley catheter in place. The Levin tube, which is attached to low suction, is irrigated with normal saline every three hours to maintain patency. The patient will be receiving intravenous fluids and serum albumin daily. Strict intake and output records must be kept.

The patient will be given a broad spectrum antibiotic for several days postoperatively.

If a catheter for the instillation of a cytotoxic drug was inserted into the hepatic artery during the operation, the nurse must make sure that the infusion is maintained and that the catheter is not pulled, tensed, or dislodged.

The skin around the area of the incision must have proper care to prevent infection.

Generally, coughing and moving are resisted by the patient because of discomfort after the abdominothoracic surgery. The nurse will have to help the patient to cough and deep breathe. Tracheal suction apparatus should be kept at the bedside and used if coughing is unproductive. The patient should be turned every two hours and, at these times, careful skin care should be given. On about the third postoperative day the patient is allowed to dangle and, while he is doing this, his vital signs should be closely monitored. Elastic supportive stockings are applied to both legs to enhance circulation and to help prevent phlebitis. The stockings should be removed daily and skin care given before reapplying them. They have been found to be more effective than Ace bandages which often wrinkle and restrict circulation.

During the early postoperative period when the patient is receiving nothing by mouth, he should be given frequent mouth care. Approximately five days postoperatively, bowel sounds return and the patient is placed on a diet which progresses rapidly to normal.

During the entire postoperative period, the patient who has had liver surgery—and his family too—are very dependent on the nurse for emotional as well as psychological and physical support. Whatever surgical procedure the patient has undergone, alert and comprehensive nursing care is of the utmost importance.

LIVER TRANSPLANTATION

The first successful human liver transplant was performed by Dr. Earl T. Starzl on July 23, 1967. By April 1969, 55 orthoptic liver transplantations had been carried out in man. Twenty-two of these patients survived 30 days or longer. Generally, those who did not survive were the victims of technical complications. The survival rate of patients who have had liver transplants at Memorial Hospital has been six weeks to eight months.

At present, there are three liver transplant centers in the world. One is in Denver where Dr. Earl T. Starzl did the first successful orthoptic transplant. Another one, in Cambridge, England is under the direction of Dr. Roy C. Calne who has done the second largest number of liver transplants in the world. The third center is at Memorial Hospital.

The question may be asked, "Why are heart and kidney transplants so much more successful than liver transplants?" Ten or 15 years ago kidney transplantation was undergoing the same difficulties that beset liver transplantation today. However, these difficulties have been largely overcome and kidney transplantation is now usually very successful. In some series, as many as 90 percent of kidney grafts give patients at least two years survival. One difference between liver and kidney transplants is that a living person cannot be a liver donor whereas an identical twin or a sibling may be a kidney donor. Another difference is that there is no machine that can take over for the liver in the way a renal dialysis machine can take over for a kidney in a crisis situation. When a liver is transplanted it must function immediately and must continue to function, so that the demand on the transplant is very great.

The liver is extremely vulnerable to warm ischemia. It must be chilled exactly right in order to preserve it for the length of time it takes to make the transfer. Because of the many vascular anastomoses that have to be done with great precision, the liver is a very difficult organ to transplant. The heart, on the other hand is one of the simplest organs to transplant, but it is one of the hardest to maintain because the slightest imbalance will produce electrical changes and irregularities which can easily cause the patient's death. The liver can accept and recover from a great deal of trauma so, in a way, nature compensates for the other difficulties involved in transplantation.

Coagulation problems can be quite enormous if the donor liver is not properly preserved. The organ is large but, at the same time, it is extremely delicate so must be handled with extreme gentleness.

Candidates for liver transplant include patients with primary hepatoma, those with cancer of the gallbladder or bile ducts, those with metastatic cancer in both lobes of the liver but whose primary cancer was in the colon and had been under control for some years. Other candidates include children with congenital biliary atresia, and patients whose livers have been fatally damaged by acute yellow atrophy of the liver, cirrhosis, chemical or viral hepatitis, or trauma. The patient for liver transplant should have the indicated liver pathology and not be over 50 years of age. Some surgeons feel that the age limit may be extended to 57 years provided the patient is physiologically vigorous. Finally, the operative risk must be acceptable; that is, the prospective recipient must have a healthy heart, good lungs, and good kidneys. And, of course, there must be an acceptable donor-recipient match anatomically, physiologically, and serologically. That is to say, one cannot replace the liver of a young child with that of an adult in most cases, simply because the difference in size of the two livers would make an anatomical fit impossible. The physiological match refers to the fact that the liver being transplanted must be a healthy one. The liver of a person who has cancer cannot be accepted for transplant unless the cancer was primary brain tumor or a small skin cancer, because of the danger of transferring occult cells with the organ. In the two instances mentioned, this danger does not hold. In fact, patients with primary brain tumor are ideal donors. As to the serological match, the important match is between the ABO systems of the donor and recipient; there must be red blood cell compatibility. The direct cross match must be negative in order to rule out preformed antibodies that might act on the liver.

During a year's time, the liver transplant team at Memorial Hospital rejected as donors two patients with a history of cancer; one with encephalitis; one who was an alcoholic; one for age (99 years old); and eight because there was no matching recipient. In addition, three prospective donors experienced sudden circulatory collapse before they could be brought to the hospital.

The pathology of the five patients who had orthoptic liver transplants at Memorial Hospital between February, 1969 and October, 1971 was as follows: hepatoma, two; bile duct cancer, two; biliary atresia, one. Donors for these transplants included patients with brain tumor (primary), intercranial aneurysm, and automobile injury. The sixth liver transplant to be done at this hospital was a heterotrophic or auxiliary transplant, the first of its kind in the world. In this procedure, the patient's liver is left in place and a second liver is inserted. The patient was a 72-year-old woman who was in too poor condition to withstand an orthoptic transplant but who was severely jaundiced and had severe pruritus. She survived for eight months; eventual death was due to a gastric ulcer and an abscess beneath her own liver and behind the obstructed bile ducts. The auxiliary liver functioned well during the survival period, and the cancer did not spread. This could be a particularly helpful procedure to use in children with biliary atresia or in adults with cirrhosis.

The Operation

The diseased liver is removed after the vena cava, portal vein, and hepatic artery have been clamped off and the organ has been freed from the surrounding tissues. While this is being done, the donor is in an adjoining room and his liver is also being removed through a midline incision, after which it is perfused through the aorta, the hepatic artery, and the portal vein so as to chill it and preserve it until there is time to transfer it to the recipient. After the organ has been fitted into the fossa from which the diseased liver has been removed, it is "hooked up" by anastomosing the donor and recipi-

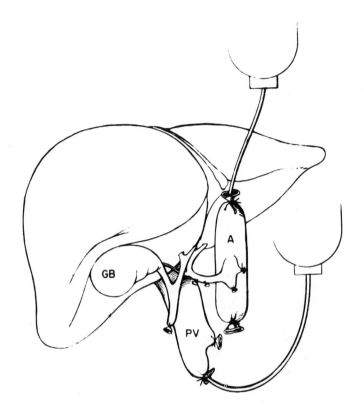

Figure 2. Donor liver has been removed and is being perfused through aortic segment and portal vein. A, aorta; PV, portal vein; and GB, gallbladder

ent suprahepatic vena cavae, portal veins, and hepatic arteries. When the clamps are removed, the liver picks up its functioning, bile begins to form, and the patient awakens promptly from surgery.

Postoperative Care

The nursing care of the patient who has had a liver transplant is similar to that required for any patient who has had abdominal surgery of major proportions, with the addition of some special procedures necessitated because of the nature of a transplant. The patient's room is prepared so that reverse isolation technique can be practiced postoperatively and thus keep to a minimum any contamination from outside sources. It is equipped with its own emergency cart, any medications that might be ordered, and an EKG monitor. Because of the extensive abdominothoracic surgery involved, a tracheostomy is often done and the patient's ventilation is assisted post-operatively. For this purpose, a Bennett MA 1 volume-cycled respirator is used. The sterilized tubing on the respirator is changed daily in order to reduce the danger of respiratory infection.

Daily cultures of urine, sputum, blood, and T tube drainage are done to monitor significant bacterial flora and as a basis for making appropriate changes in antibiotic coverage. Frequent blood gas determinations are made to assess pulmonary function. Coagulation and electrolyte studies are done at least daily and more often if abnormalities present themselves. Daily liver function tests are ordered including SGOT, LDH, total protein and albumin, total and conjugated bilirubin, and alkaline phosphatase. The normal re-action initially to transplantation is an elevation of serum bilirubin, SGOT, and alkaline phosphatase. These elevations are usually the result of ischemic damage to the liver and when this is overcome the levels return to normal. One of the important parameters to be monitored is the concentration of bile salts in the bile; in fact, this is thought to be more important than monitoring the concentration of serum bilirubin when one wants to measure actual liver function.

Complications

The complications that may arise during or following liver transplant in-clude some that are common to all types of surgery and some that are specific to transplantation. Among the metabolic problems encountered in patients who have received liver transplants at Memorial Hospital were acute, but temporary, renal failure and hypophosphatemia.

Coagulation changes that occur during transplantation consist of fibrinol-ysis, thrombocytopenia, and depression of various clotting factors. Several mechanisms apparently account for the sudden decrease in clotting factors during the operation for liver transplant. The most important is probably the consumption of the coagulation factors as a result of intravascular coagulation. The decrease in plasma clotting factors is treated by the use of fresh frozen plasma. Thrombocytopenia, or decreased platelets, is treated by platelet infusion. Although vitamin K therapy is often employed in cer-tain clotting disorders, the nurse should remember that it is never used in an emergency as it takes upwards of 24 to 72 hours for it to reach its peak effect. Coagulation defects and steroid therapy make transplant patients prime candidates for peptic ulcer and gastrointestinal bleeding. Antacids are ordered routinely for all patients as soon as they are able to take fluids by mouth. The stools are checked daily for occult blood.

Most of the bleeding that occurs postoperatively is caused by the residual heparin effect related to the perfusate in which the donor liver is primed for surgery. This is reversed by the use of protamine sulfate, usually given to the patient before he leaves the operating room. Low-dose heparin may also be the physician's treatment of choice for a bleeding patient which sometimes surprises nurses if they do not understand the process of consumption. Consumption coagulopathy, or disseminated intravascular clotting, refers to the process of hypercoagulability within blood vessels, which is accompanied by an increase in the normal mechanism of fibrinolysis which helps dissolve these clots. Eventually all of the clotting factors are depleted and diffused, and generalized hemorrhage occurs. The treatment for this condition, low-dose heparin, helps to slow down the process of fibrinolysis and to restore the clotting mechanism to normal.

The thromboelastograph (TEG), an apparatus that automatically records and produces a writeout of the size and nature of the whole clot within half an hour, is ideal for use in emergency situations. The only technical requirement that must be carefully observed in its use is that blood obtained from an arduous venipuncture should be avoided. All blood samples should be drawn through an 18-guage needle and the first several cc's discarded to rid the sample of IV fluid or tissue thromboplastin. Also, of course, the steel cup that holds the sample should be scrupulously clean.

Rejection is a serious complication that may follow liver transplantation. The body's ability to maintain its integrity as far as foreign tissue is concerned largely depends on the action of lymphocytes. When the lymphocytes come into contact with the antigen from a liver graft, they are stimulated to become lymphoblasts which, in turn, divide and produce more lymphocytes that are sensitized to the foreign tissue. They attack the liver and cause the release of still more antigen. More lymphocytes are thereby sensitized and a vicious circle is set up.

To break this cycle, an *immunosuppressive regimen* is instituted. In health, the body's natural immune system is a multifaceted reaction which in general, protects the body from invasion by such foreign materials as bacteria, viruses, pollen, cancer cells and, of course, transplanted tissues from other individuals. This system does not reach full maturity until the puberty years but it carries on its police functions from early life—even embryonic life. During these years the lymphocytes circulate throughout the body and discover what we are made of. They store this information in their remarkable long-lasting memories so that later when they meet something that does not match up with what they know about our natural makeup, they react to reject the invader. In most instances the outside invader is overcome. For the patient with a newly transplanted liver, this process would result in rejection in every instance unless outside action is taken. This action consists of the administration of immunosuppressive agents. At Memorial Hospital the immunosuppressive regimen consists of Imuran (azathioprine), prednisone, and anti-lymphocyte serum.

Imuran is a purine analogue, a derivative of 6-mercaptopurine. It is cytotoxic in action and thus exerts an anti-proliferating action on newly dividing cells.

The adrenocorticosteroids of the cortisone family, including prednisone, have certain distinctive immunosuppressive properties, the most striking of which is the power to annul a preexisting state of sensitivity if given over a sufficient length of time. In fact, these steroids are now used clinically to maintain rather than institute a state of non-reactivity because as primary immunosuppressants they are rather weak. They have another important property, that is, the ability to prolong the state of non-reactivity engendered by treatment with anti-lymphocyte serum. There is great synergy between these two agents. The acute action of steroids is presumably on the efferent sector of the immune response, that is, they somehow prevent the sensitized lymphocytes from engaging, attacking, and destroying their targets.

The third immunosuppressive agent, anti-lymphocyte serum, is in a class by itself. It is a xenogenous serum that is raised by injecting human lymphoid cells into horses or rabbits. The active principle is an antibody or a complex of antibodies directed against the antigens present. To prevent the harmful effects of prolonged administration of this agent, the gamma fraction of the whole serum is used—anti-lymphocyte globulin (ALG).

Because the liver is sensitive to azathioprine, more dependence is placed on the steroid and the anti-lymphocyte serum. Unfortunately, the steroid may cause gastrointestinal bleeding, so that the dosage must be kept low. Hence the surgeon relies chiefly on ALG to prevent rejection, and the ratio of this agent in the peripheral blood must be closely monitored because it may cause hemolysis in patients who are sensitized to equine globulin. The optimal ratio of ALG in the peripheral blood is about 10 and it is believed that a blood level of about 50 mg% must be maintained to forestall rejection of a transplant. In one of the Memorial series of transplant patients it was impossible to raise the ratio regardless of the amount of globulin administered, because the patient had a sensitivity to horse serum. Thus, one of the mainstays of the immunosuppressive regimen was completely impotent in this particular case.

Immunosuppressive agents are exactly what their name implies; they abolish or weaken the body's immune responses. Strictly speaking, they should abolish only the immune response, but the only one of these agents that fulfills this criterion is the anti-lymphocyte serum. The immunosuppressive action of the other agents in common use is really a by-product of some much more general toxic or inhibitory influence which also happens to affect the cell's immune response. What is known of their action has been gained through experience rather than from a theoretical understanding of how they actually work.

Two major problems may arise during active immunosuppression of the allograft recipient: 1) invasion by such harmful foreigners as bacteria, viruses, and cancer cells; and, 2) an immune reaction to the ALG itself. In the first instance, the problem arises because the immunosuppressive agent suppresses the patient's defenses against infectious organisms at the same time it is suppressing the immune response to the liver graft. In the second instance, ALG provokes immunological responses against itself because it is also a foreign protein that is not much different from the liver graft and therefore the body will try to eradicate it as an invader. Consequently, the physician tries first to induce tolerance toward this agent and, when this is not successful, he treats the patient with such agents as Benadryl and hydrocortisone to reduce the allergic reaction to the ALG and to allow the lymphocyte antibodies to carry out their function. The use of immunosuppression, as it stands today, is less than ideal, but better agents are already being realized and it is possible that soon many patients will be receiving allografts, or even xenografts, and not require any immunosuppressive therapy.

The earlier signs of rejection are associated with anoxic liver damage, elevated bilirubin, SGOT, and alkaline phosphatase. However, the rejection reactions result in cholestasis so that the later signs include T-tube drainage that is colorless, and gray-colored stools.

One of the ways of monitoring rejection is to measure the bile salt concentration in bile. Initially, the patient's bilirubin in the serum may be quite high postoperatively from the ischemic changes that have taken place; later it comes down to normal. Bile salt concentration is then normal, but during a period of rejection the serum bilirubin rises impressively—to 20 or 30 mg%—and the bile salt concentration falls to almost zero levels. With treatment, the serum bilirubin level begins to fall, but preceding that there is a rise in the bile salt concentration indicating recovery of liver function.

This seems to be a better way to monitor liver function than measuring the serum bilirubin levels which may be rendered inaccurate by the fact that hemolysis from the anti-lymphocyte globulin that is being given to the patient raises this level. A second way of monitoring is by measuring the activity of the lymphocytes. A sample of lymphocytes is taken every few days and observed to see whether they undergo blastoid transformation, either by being left alone or by stimulation with phytohemagglutinin. The ratio of cell activity when stimulated is compared to the ratio when the lymphocytes are left alone and a comparison of these rates gives the physician a clue as to whether the patient is suffering from rejection or some other complication.

Special Nursing Needs of the Patient with a Liver Transplant

The nurse who gives postoperative care to the liver transplant patient must be as skillful in coping with his psychological and emotional status as she is in providing for his physical comfort. Preoperatively, too, she is called upon to give an unusual amount of support. She is dealing with a person who is aware of his condition and probably knows the seriousness of the operation that is planned. Almost all hospitalized patients experience an elevated anxiety level, particularly when they must submit to a surgical procedure. Consider, then, the magnitude of the anxiety and fear engendered when the patient must choose between death and undergoing surgery that involves the severe risks inherent in organ transplantation. In addition, he may also experience an unconscious feeling of guilt because another person must die before he is able to have his chance at life.

In *The Magic Mountain,* Thomas Mann expressed the idea that "speech is civilization itself. The word, even the most contradictory word, preserves contact. It is the silence which isolates." During the immediate postoperative period, communication by speech becomes a problem for the liver transplant patient because of his tracheostomy. His feeling of aloneness is further increased by the limitations imposed by the isolation techniques used in caring for him. The nurse needs to anticipate his needs and reduce the demand on him to communicate at a time when it is necessary for him to conserve his energy. His nonverbal communications become very important, and a skillful and perceptive nurse can pick up many clues from them.

Probably because of the pioneering nature of the surgery, these patients demonstrate a tremendous amount of curiosity about everything that is happening to them. They are not satisfied with just being told what is going on— they want to know why. Thus it becomes part of the nurse's role to constantly explain and reinforce information presented by the doctor. This has to be geared to the patient's level of understanding and again points up the need for the nurse to be knowledgeable about the physiological changes that are taking place in the patient. These explanations become much more difficult when complications are present. The nurse will find it advantageous to be present whenever the doctor speaks to the patient, because she can take cues from him about what information to give the patient and can also alert the doctor to some of the fears and problems that are disturbing the patient.

The postoperative reactions of patients who have had liver transplants at Memorial Hospital have followed a typical pattern. They usually arrive from the operating room sleepy but awake, in good spirits, and with a highly optimistic attitude. As the days pass, however, they become increasingly irritable and impatient. They are subjected to so many procedures and tests that they have little time for sleep and rest. As this begins to take its toll, the nurse must set priorities of care so as to allow as much time as possible for uninterrupted sleep. After a time, a certain amount of regression is noticed in the patient's behavior. This sometimes enables him to accept care from others and to look up to the physician as a strong healer. One pertinent consequence of regression is an alteration in one's time sense. A day-to-day orientation offers a refuge that is relatively free from fear, the patient's thinking does not extend months into the future, and he thereby maintains the incentive for limiting his planning and actions. It is important for the nurse to understand how to use the patient's regression in dealing with his helplessness.

Many physiological and psychological disadvantages accompany bed rest, and a regimen that allows freedom and activity compatible with the patient's physical status boosts his morale. The nurse should foster warmth in the often impersonal hospital milieu, and anticipate the patient's needs so that he will feel more comfortable and his fears will be minimized. Helplessness often leads to loss of self-confidence and then coping mechanisms are also lost. Keeping the milieu as constant and unchanging as possible and keeping all channels of communication open are the two most significant contributions of the nurse to the postoperative care of the patient who has undergone a liver transplant.

How Nurses and Nursing Responded to the Establishment of the Transplantation Program at Memorial Hospital

The Board of Manager's approval, in November, 1968, of an allotransplantation program for Memorial Hospital raised many questions for nursing. Who would care for the two patients—the donor and the recipient? To what nursing unit would the recipient be admitted? Would isolation technique be required of the nurses? Would the nurses need special training? How would nursing be involved in the communications network that would be established?

A new special care unit was under construction at that time, so it was decided that the nurses assigned to that unit would be given an intensive four-week training course in the care of transplant patients. During this month many of the nurses who would be involved in caring for the patients experienced quite mixed feelings about organ transplant and the concept of "legal death." They explored and expressed their feelings during discussions and conferences with the physician who would head the program, the chairman of the department of nursing, and the nursing staffs of the recovery room and intensive care unit. The nurses' attitudes toward giving care to the recipient were generally positive. Any anxiety they had was centered on the technical aspects of the care the patient would need and the nursing skills that would be required to give that care. This apprehension was allayed somewhat when it was decided that the patient would receive the care of two nurses around the clock so that no one nurse would be left alone with the patient.

The nurses' attitudes toward caring for the donor patient were generally more negative. Since two teams—a donor team and a recipient team—were to be set up, and since team membership was to be voluntary, it was agreed that those who did not wish to care for donors would not be asked to do so.

One of the most important parts of a transplantation program is an efficient communications center which will function to coordinate all the activities in connection with the transplant. Since the nursing office is the one central office that is in operation 24 hours a day, it was chosen to be the communications center for transplants, and the following system was set up. The surgeon in charge would make the decision whether to accept a donor and would notify the communications center to send out either a "red" alert or a "blue" alert. A red alert would mean that the transplant would take place within an hour, and a blue would mean that it would take place within three hours. If the donor was to be brought from another hospital, an ambulance would be sent for him and the communications center would notify the on-call nurses, anesthetists, resident, and recovery room personnel that a donor was to be admitted. Then the nursing supervisors would man the alert telephones and notify the approximately 40 people who would be concerned—hospital administrator, surgeons, anesthesiologists, pump team members, operating room personnel, medical team support members, admitting office, donor nursing team members, blood bank personnel, the special laboratory technicians, appropriate members of the clergy, hospital security personnel, and public relations personnel.

The next step would be to locate possible recipients and get them to the hospital. The special care unit would be notified so that beds could be prepared for several recipient patients. A file of possible recipients was used to select several on whom a transplant workup had been done and on whom background information was available.

It was expected that potential liver donors would be persons with fatal brain damage, whose liver was intact, and whose blood pressure was at least sustainable—a clinical state that could have resulted from head trauma incurred in an accident or suicide attempt, a ruptured intercranial aneurysm, or a primary brain tumor. As soon as the donor arrived at the hospital, blood was to be drawn for type and cross match (both major and minor blood groups), for leukocyte typing and for SGOT, bilirubin, alkaline phosphatase, prothrombin, serum protein electrophosphoresis, BUN, sugar, cholesterol, and 5-nucelotidase determinations. The donor was to be monitored for vital signs, EKG, EEG, urine output, and central venous pressure. A respirator would be used to maintain adequate respiration. It was expected that most donors would have deficient blood volumes and would require large quantities of blood, plasma, and dextran to maintain their blood pressure. A donor team, independent of the transplant team, would be responsible for seeing that all criteria for death were met. This team would consist of the referring doctor, an internist, and a neurologist or neurosurgeon. When all conditions were met, the neurologist (or neurosurgeon) would certify that death had occurred. The transplant could then be carried out.

On January 10, 1969, the first donor was admitted to Memorial Hospital from another hospital in the city. This man had had a temporal lobe lobectomy for glioblastoma multiforma in December, and had been comatose thereafter. However, he was still responsive to noxious stimuli. On admission, he was treated for bronchial pneumonia and a urinary tract infection. After eight days, his condition became stabilized and remained so until February 14 when a change occurred in his respirations and level of consciousness. His condition deteriorated steadily and he was pronounced legally dead on February 19th. All the criteria for death had been met, despite the fact that the patient had maintained his blood pressure. The recipient selected to receive his liver was a 27-year-old woman with hepatoma. With this transplant, the role and the responsibilities that nurses and nursing would carry in future transplants at Memorial Hospital was established.

QUESTIONS AND ANSWERS

Q. Can a human being get cancer from eating cancerous liver?

A. Probably not.

Q. How does colonic and rectal cancer metastasize to the liver?

A. The cancer cells are carried via the lymphatics through the lymph nodes of the colon and rectum, as well as by the blood drainage system. Metastasis happens when some of the cancer cells have gotten beyond the lymphatic entrapment system or are carried in the portal system to the liver.

Q. How do patients manage the "bowel prep" which sounds exhausting?

A. If the patient is particularly anxious the nurse must do everything she can to reduce this anxiety. Try to give him time to rest between the various activities and help him to verbalize his feelings.

Q. Are patients ever taken directly back to the nursing unit after surgery?

A. No. They are always returned to the special care unit.

Q. What can be done to allay the intense itching that patients with a high bilirubin content often experience?

A. There is really no satisfactory way to relieve itching from extrahepatic obstruction. Benadryl and a variety of other agents are used, but nothing short of surgery is permanently effective.

Q. Are fewer liver transplants being done now than two or three years ago?

A. It may be that publicity about organ transplants is waning—transplantation had quite a flourish of publicity when it first started. However, after several had been done and the excitement over being able to transplant an organ and save someone's life died down somewhat, people began to take a long, hard look and realized that many transplant patients had just as many problems as they had before. Now many surgeons and other interested people are back in their laboratories doing more experimentation before they go ahead with transplants. There will probably be another flourish very soon.

Q. What type of consent is obtained from the family of the donor? How do families react when they are approached about this?

A. The consent is quite specific as to the organs that are to be donated. We try to get as many family members as possible to sign the consent, and each organ that is being donated is listed on the form. Family members' reactions depend almost entirely on how intelligent they are. The less intelligent and the less educated they are, the less chance there is that they will agree to letting the relative be a donor, and vice versa. Most of the donors are accident victims—healthy persons who have suddenly become dead. Generally the family is motivated to make something good come out of this tragedy, and they realize that giving a heart, lung, or liver to someone else so that this person can live will not affect the life after death of their loved one. This is really the most unselfish motivation anyone can have.

Q. Why are patients with primary brain tumor preferred as donors?

A. Patients with primary brain tumors are the preferred donors of livers for transplant because, generally speaking, a brain tumor is not a metastatic lesion. It is a locally aggressive lesion that will not, in any sense, be present in the donor organ, whether it is a liver or a kidney. Therefore, there is no danger of transplanting a cancer along with the liver.

Q. How much preoperative psychological preparation is necessary for the recipient?

A. A great deal. Because transplantation is usually a last resort for a reasonable chance for long-term survival, informed consent is mandatory. The patient should understand what kinds of risks he is facing— and they are considerable—with either type of transplanatation.

Q. On the whole, how does the patient's family cope with the transplant situation?

A. They are moved—as everyone is—by the awesomeness of the procedure. Each family brings to transplant their experiences up to that point. If their emotional bank is sizeable they come to the situation with at least love, understanding, and ability to talk things out, even when the patient is isolated, and they can work with each other and with the attending personnel, among them a social worker whose special skills are in family relationships. If they walk into the situation impoverished emotionally, it goes without saying that this difficult episode is not going to make them much richer. Sometimes a phenomenon may occur in that a family that walks into this experience poor emotionally, walks out of it enriched because of the beautiful nursing and medical care the patient received and because of the support extended to the patient and his family by the whole team.

Q. When the liver is transplanted is the gallbladder transplanted along with it?

A. Yes. It is used in the anastomosis. One of the big problems in liver transplantation, strange as it may seem, is the biliary tract anastomosis which is often the source of leakage. The normal bile duct is very small and difficult to deal with and this has been a problem for all surgeons doing liver transplants.

Q. What does a liver transplant cost?

A. It varies, but the usual hospital cost is about $20,000. No physician's fees have been charged for any transplant that has been done at Memorial Hospital. The hospital cost is for two nurses around the clock, all the medications, and all of the tests, procedures, and equipment that are needed.

Q. What is the most challenging nursing problem in caring for a liver transplant patient?

A. Probably the isolation technique that is required. This is difficult for both the patient and the nurse. Because they are isolated in the room with the patient for so many hours at a time, the nurses feel the same isolation that patients do.

Q. Does the future of treatment of cancer of the liver lie in transplantation or is some other treatment contemplated?

A. Transplantation, obviously, is a less than ideal way to treat cancer. In fact, any surgery is less than ideal for treating this disease. But for patients whose cancer is of such a nature that there is no other way of treating them with any hope of curing them, transplantation is the only treatment presently available.

SUGGESTED READINGS

Books

Alexander, Wesley J. and Robert A. Good. *Immunobiology for Surgeons*. Philadelphia: Saunders, 1970.

Brunner, L. S., Charles P. Emerson, L. K. Fergusen, and D. S. Suddarth. *Textbook of Medical-Surgical Nursing.* Second edition. New York: Lippincott, 1970.

Nealon, T. F. (Ed.). *Management of the Patient with Cancer.* Philadelphia: Saunders, 1965.

Pack, George T. *Tumors of the Liver.* New York: Springer-Verlag, 1970.

Rosenthal, Leonard. *The Application of Radioiodinated Rose Bengal and Colloidal Radiogold in the Detection of Hepato-biliary Disease.* St. Louis: Green Company, 1970.

Russel, Paul S., and Anthony P. Monaco. *The Biology of Tissue Transplantation.* Boston: Little, Brown, 1964.

Scheuer, P. J. *Liver Biopsy Interpretation.* Baltimore: Williams & Wilkins, 1968.

Schwartz, S. I. *Surgical Diseases of the Liver.* New York: McGraw Hill, 1964.

Sherlock, Shiela. *Diseases of the Liver and Biliary System.* Fourth Edition. Oxford: Blackwell, 1968.

Starzl, Thomas E. *Experience with Hepatic Transplantation.* Philadelphia: Saunders, 1969.

Periodicals

Forman, J. V., et al. "Anesthetic and Metabolic Problems of Liver Transplantation," *Anesthesia, 26*:92-93, January, 1971.

Fortner, J. G., M. H. Shiu, W. S. Howland, et al. "A New Concept for Hepatic Lobectomy," *Archives of Surgery, 102*:312-315, April, 1971.

Fortner, J. G., E. J. Beattie, Jr., M. H. Shiu, et al. "Orthotopic and Heterotopic Liver Homographs in Man," *Annals of Surgery, 172*:22-32, July, 1970.

Fortner, J. G., M. H. Shiu, W. S. Howland, et al. "The Donor in Human Liver Transplantation," *American Journal of Surgery, Gynecology and Obstetrics, 130*:988-94, December, 1970.

Fortner, J. G., E. J. Beattie, Jr., R. C. Watson, et al. "Surgery in Liver Tumors," *Current Problems in Surgery,* June, 1972.

Hoyter, Jean. "Impaired Liver Function and Related Nursing Care," *American Journal of Nursing, 68*:2374-77, November, 1968.

Howland, W. S., et al. "Coagulation Abnormalities Associated with Liver Transplantation," *Surgery, 68*:591-6, October, 1970.

Juzwiak, Marijo. "Nursing the Patient with Hepatic Lobectomy," *RN, 31*:43-47, September, 1968.

Molander, D. W. and R. D. Brasfield. "Liver Surgery," *American Journal of Nursing, 61*:72-74, July, 1961.

Taylor, K., N. Commons, and M. S. Jack, "Liver Transplant," *American Journal of Nursing, 68*:1895-99, September, 1968.

Virgadamo, B. T. "Care of the Patient with Liver Surgery," *American Journal of Nursing, 61*:74-76, July, 1961.

Pamphlets

Leevy, Carroll M. "Evaluation of Liver Function in Clinical Practice," Indianapolis, Lilly Research Laboratories, 1965.

Patients with Rectal or Colonic Tumors

Regional Medical Program — Oncology Nursing Seminar

on

**NURSING MANAGEMENT OF PATIENTS WITH
RECTAL OR COLONIC TUMORS**

Seminar Leader

Maus Stearns, Jr., M.D.

Seminar Participants

Martha Atchley, M.S.W., Social Worker

J. Herbert Dietz, Jr., M.D., Consultant, Rehabilitation Program

Frances Gutowski, R.N., B.S., Clinical Nursing Instructor

Clara Horowicz, R.N., Head Nurse

Margaret Lodes, R.N., Head Nurse

Patricia Monk, R.N., Head Nurse

Sheila Reiss, R.N., Public Health Nurse, Visiting Nurse Service
of New York

Guy F. Robbins, M.D., Director, Memorial Hospital Regional
Medical Program

Maus Stearns, Jr., M.D., Chief, Rectal and Colon Service

Cancer of the colon and rectum is one of the most frequently occurring forms of "deep-seated" cancer. In men it ranks second to lung cancer, and in women second to breast cancer. However, it ranks first among both men and women who develop single cancers. It is' a very catholic disease in that no particular type of person is more susceptible than any other. It occurs in people over 12 years of age in all parts of the world, regardless of their race, dietary habits, or manner of living.. The only recognized predisposing factor seems to be a family history of polyposis and long-standing ulcerative colitis. Although even this possibility is debatable, some surgeons make a great effort to search out polyps of the colon and rectum and treat them as premalignant lesions.

Fifty percent of the patients diagnosed as having cancer of the colon or rectum will not only be alive five years after proper treatment, but they will be free of any signs of the disease. Although this may be considered a fairly satisfactory result as far as the treatment of cancer is concerned, it should not lead to complacency but rather to intensified efforts toward earlier diagnosis. Any patient who presents with bleeding from the rectum, excessive flatulence, abdominal distress, or any change in bowel habit or bowel awareness should be examined digitally, by sigmoidoscopy, and possibly gastrointestinal x-ray.

The large bowel, or colon, consists of the terminal five feet of the intestinal tract. Its primary function is to allow for the absorption of water. This occurs chiefly in the right (ascending) colon but is continued in both the transverse and left (descending) colon. Thin watery material from the small intestine enters the cecum and then passes on into the right colon in an almost continuous process. By the time this material reaches the transverse colon, it has become somewhat "pasty" in consistency, but it is still quite thin and moves through the transverse colon at a fairly steady pace. Water is continually being absorbed as the fecal material continues to pass through the colon, so that by the time it reaches the sigmoid (particularly the distal sigmoid) it has become quite solid. These physiological facts explain why irrigation is of little value in controlling evacuation when the patient has a cecostomy but can be of real value in cases of sigmoid colostomy in which case it has the same effect as an enema.

TREATMENT

To date, surgery is the only effective agent for the curative treatment of cancer of the colon or rectum. It is also the most effective means of achieving long-term palliation of the symptoms of the disease.

Preoperative Preparation

Every patient approaches surgery of the rectum or colon with fear and uncertainty, not only about the operation itself but also about what it might disclose and how this will affect his future life. This is true whether the preoperative diagnosis indicates the presence of a simple, benign polyp or a cancerous lesion that will require extensive surgery and the construction of a permanent colostomy.

Most patients approaching surgery have some idea of what their diagnosis is. Those who might have a colostomy usually know that they have some sort of mass or tumor, but they may not know whether it is benign or malignant. Many physicians feel that the patient should be told that although his condition is serious and he may need to have a colostomy, everything that is medically and surgically possible will be done for him.

Upon admission the patient is asked the reason for his coming to the hospital and his answer gives the nurse her cue as to how he perceives his illness and what his expectations are. She tells him how he will be prepared for the operation. She explains the purpose and procedure for each of the diagnostic tests that will be done. In addition to the usual preoperative tests for any type of surgery, an intravenous pyelogram will be done to assess kidney and bladder function. Also, the patient will be given a barium enema followed by x-ray examination to locate lesions that cannot be detected digitally or visually. The laxatives and enemas he will be given to prepare him for these tests may cause considerable distress when the patient is already bleeding, or has soreness, pressure, or sensitivity in the colon or rectum. If a sigmoidoscopy is indicated, doing it on the same morning that the barium enema is given for the x-ray examination will make it unnecessary to repeat the entire preparation.

During the diagnostic period the patient may be distressed and bewildered, especially if this is his first hospitalization. He not only needs emotional support but, after the tests are completed, the diagnosis has been made, and the doctor has told him about the surgery that has been decided upon, he also needs a great deal of explanation. What he is told depends on the type and extent of the surgery to be done. All preoperative explanations are tailored to the patient's questions, and the nurse must answer them in a way that he can understand and accept. She relays queries she cannot answer to appropriate members of the care team.

Often, the patient will have heard the term "colostomy" but he may have misconceptions about what it actually means and implies. If the doctor has told him that he will have a perineal resection and a permanent colostomy, he will probably express anxiety about it to the nurse and ask many questions. Her attitude at this time is extremely important. She can help him overcome much of his fear and apprehension by taking a positive approach and explaining to him how a colostomy is managed. She should stress the idea that a colostomy simply causes a variation in normal bowel function and that control of fecal excretion by irrigation will become a routine, just as showering and shaving are, and then be forgotten as the patient goes about his daily activities. She should tell him that although some people have a few problems managing the irrigations in the beginning, they overcome them and eventually achieve control of their colostomy and are usually able to go back to their jobs or whatever activities they engaged in before the operation. When the patient understands this preoperatively he will be better able to accept responsibility for the care and management of his colostomy. He will appreciate knowing, too, that until he has achieved control of his evacuations, he will be provided with a proper appliance so that he will not be embarrassed by any unexpected discharge of feces.

Female patients in particular are often concerned about the kind of clothing they will wear after the operation. They should be told that at first the stoma may appear large and bulky but that it shrinks as it heals and will not show under ordinary clothing. They will be reassured to know that once they have achieved regulation of evacuation of the colostomy, they will need only a small dressing or shield over the stoma. The patient who has a sigmoid colostomy can wear a panty girdle or athletic supporter.

The physical preparation of the patient for surgery on the colon or rectum includes:

1. *Nutritional buildup.* Supplementary vitamins (vitamin C and multivitamins) are added to the patient's diet. Because the sterilized bowel can no longer synthesize vitamin K, supplemental vitamin K is given. Usually the patient is started on a low residue diet, gradually shifted to a full liquid diet, and finally to a diet of clear liquids and hard candy just prior to the operation.

2. *Sterilization of the bowel.* When an anastomosis is anticipated, partial

sterilization of the bowel is desirable. This is accomplished through the administration of kanamycin or sulfasuxidine for two or three days preoperatively. When an abdomino-perineal resection with colostomy is anticipated, this (bowel sterilization) is usually omitted.

3. *Cleansing of the bowel.* Laxatives and/or enemas or colonic irrigations are given to empty and cleanse the bowel.

4. *Administration of intravenous fluids.* The afternoon before surgery the patient is given intravenous fluids to compensate for the fluid and electrolyte loss that results from the restricted diet and the laxatives. Usually, 1,000 cc of 5 percent dextrose and water with sodium bicarbonate, and 500 cc of 5 percent dextrose and saline are given.

5. *Preparation of the skin.* Bacteriostatic soap and water are used to cleanse the skin and the usual skin "prep" is carried out.

6. *Restriction of food and fluids.* No food or fluids are allowed after midnight immediately preceding the operation.

During the immediate preoperative period, the patient should be taught how to deep breathe and cough effectively and how to do leg exercises, and he should be told why it will be necessary for him to carry out these activities postoperatively. After surgery he will very likely be lethargic and meditative and may not respond to instructions. He is also told that he will return from the operating room with a Levin tube (to prevent distention of the stomach with gas) and a Foley catheter in place, and that he will be fed intravenously for the first few days. The patient who is to have an abdominal perineal resection should know that for the first few postoperative days the perineal wound will be covered with a large dressing which will need frequent changing, and that this is perfectly normal. Otherwise, he may become anxious when he sees the dressing being changed three, four, or even five times a day.

When the family is included in this final preoperative teaching they can be more supportive to the patient afterward and their fears as to what he will look like and be like after the operation are somewhat allayed. A loving, concerned spouse can give a tremendous amount of emotional support which will make it easier for the patient to cope with the many stresses and fears he is experiencing.

The Operation

The two most common operations for cancer of the colon and rectum are based on two very simple principles. Those based on the first principle involve the removal of the bowel that bears the cancer, the theory being that this may preclude local recurrence of the disease. Those based on the second principle involve (in addition to removal of the tumor) removal of the major lymphatics which accompany the major blood vessels that supply areas to which the cancer might metastasize. While it is possible to remove these major lymphatic drainage vessels, there is as yet no surgical procedure for removing all of the possible sites of cancer emboli through blood vessels in this area.

Carcinomas of the cecum, ascending colon, or proximal transverse colon require a right hemicolectomy; those in the distal transverse or descending colon require removal of the left colon. When the cancer is in the sigmoid or upper rectum, surgical treatment consists of a segmental section that is usually spoken of as an anterior resection. By definition, an anterior resection consists simply of an anastomosis in the pelvis below the peritoneal reflection. Cancers located in the mid or distal rectum require a resection that starts with the mobilization of the bowel, followed by a wide resection of the perineum and removal of the entire contents (not the bladder) of the pelvis (abdomino-perineal resection).

Colostomies. In addition to their classification by location in the bowel, colostomies are classified according to whether they are temporary or permanent, and whether they are end or loop colostomies. By and large, a temporary colostomy is performed for one of two reasons: 1) To relieve a complete obstruction in the bowel, a temporary colostomy may be performed in the proximal bowel. After the obstruction is relieved the patient is prepared for a definitive resection and, eventually, the colostomy is closed. 2) Following an anterior resection (anastomosis below the peritoneal reflection) a temporary colostomy serves to divert the fecal stream and thus protects the anastomosis which, in this location, heals poorly because of the lack of peritoneum. Anastomoses within the abdominal cavity heal quite satisfactorily because they have a good serosal surface, but those in the lower rectum are notoriously poor healers and so are subject to fistulas. Rather than have the patient suffer this consequence, a temporary transverse colostomy (or, rarely, a cecostomy) is created. The question is sometimes asked whether all patients who have anterior resections should have temporary colostomies and the answer is "No." In approximately 20 percent of the patients who have this type of operation a temporary colostomy is created because the patient is in the older age group and cannot tolerate a fistula or the peritonitis that may follow the operation otherwise. It is also done occasionally when the patient has had poor preparation for surgery, or when there is some question as to the adequacy of the anastomosis.

The critical area, as far as the need for a temporary or permanent colostomy is concerned, is the two or three inches (6-7 cm) above the anal margin. Tumors below this level can usually be readily felt with an examining finger, and the surgical treatment most often requires the creation of a permanent end colostomy. When the cancer is above this level, many surgeons do a resection and anastomosis with or without a temporary colostomy which may be closed four to six weeks later. Very few patients with a tumor in this location need a permanent end colostomy, provided that the tumor is still operable. However, this is a controversial area, and some surgeons still do an operation leaving a permanent colostomy. When the lesion is below the critical 6-cm level, the bowel and lymphatics of the pelvis, along with the perineal contents are removed and a permanent colostomy is created. This is the most common form of sigmoid colostomy and one that requires extensive rehabilitation effort.

An end colostomy is one in which the end of the resected bowel is brought out as a stoma. It is usually permanent. In a loop colostomy, a loop of bowel (usually transverse or sigmoid colon) is brought out through an abdominal incision and held in place in the abdominal wall by placing a

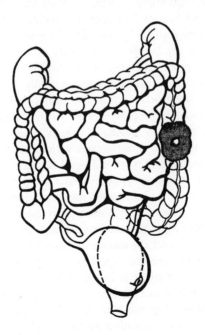

Figure 1. Simple colostomy, descending colon

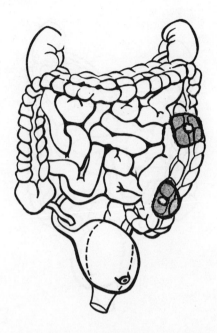

Figure 2. Double barrel colostomy, descending colon

tube or rod under it. It is usually temporary but occasionally may be permanent.

Postoperative Care

After the operation the patient remains in the recovery room until he has reacted from the anesthetic and his vital signs are stabilized. He receives intravenous feedings until an adequate oral intake is maintained. The Levin tube is removed as soon as bowel sounds return. The patient is often uncomfortable with this tube in and he sees its removal as a sign of recovery. Older patients who are intolerant of nasogastric tubes may have a gastrostomy to maintain decompression.

The patient who has had an abdominal perineal resection will have lost a considerable amount of blood and fluid, therefore his fluid balance is carefully watched and his hourly output of urine is monitored. A central venous pressure (CVP) line is usually introduced into the atrium of the heart while the patient is in the operating room so that his CVP can be carefully monitored postoperatively. A low CVP reading indicates hypovolemia or dehydration, and an abnormally high reading indicates possible

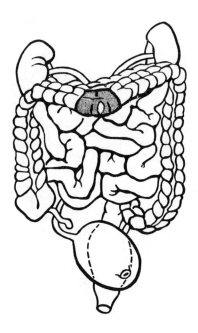

Figure 3. Loop colostomy, transverse colon

congestive heart failure. Blood lost during surgery is replaced either in the operating or recovery room, but sero-sanguineous fluid often seeps from the large perineal wound and this, too, is replaced with blood or plasma. The packing that was placed in the perineal wound during surgery to provide hemostatic action on the open area is removed by the surgeon a little at a time during the first four or five postoperative days. After the packing is all out, the posterior wound is irrigated twice a day with 1:10,000 solution of potassium permanganate or half-strength hydrogen peroxide to remove secretions and tissue debris from the wound and to ensure healing from the inside outward. The doctor determines the direction and depth that the catheter should be inserted for irrigating the perineal defect. If the fluid does not reach the entire cavity, and is not completely returned, an abscess may form in the dead space left by surgery.

When the patient can tolerate it, sitz baths are substituted for the posterior wound irrigations. Since the patient usually leaves the hospital before the perineal wound is healed, arrangements should be made for him to continue the sitz baths at home. The nurse, with the approval of the doctor, routinely initiates referral to a visiting nurse who can be called when necessary to assist the patient when he is carrying out procedures of this kind.

The patient who has had a transverse colostomy is given the same general care as one with an abdominal perineal resection; that is, his fluid and electrolyte balance is carefully monitored, he is fed intravenously, and has a Levin tube until bowel sounds return. On the second postoperative day the doctor opens the colostomy. This is done at the bedside using a cautery machine and it is important that the physician or the nurse prepare the patient very carefully for this so he will not become unduly frightened or anxious.

If a permanent colostomy was created, the clamp that was put on in the operating room is removed on the second postoperative day. Initially, mucus or a small amount of fluid or bile may be expelled and the dressings are changed whenever required.

As peristalsis returns, the patient begins to expel liquid feces through the colostomy. At this time, a temporary appliance is applied if this is feasible and the doctor approves. The appliance is usually readily accepted by the patient who by this time is out of bed and ambulating. He feels more secure with the appliance than with bulky dressings; besides, it helps to control odor and to prevent irritation of the skin and thus gives him a feeling of greater cleanliness and well-being.

The first time the nurse applies the temporary appliance she explains how it is done, step by step, and the patient watches. After that, he assists with the application and soon learns how to do this without help. Most patients, having accomplished this first step in learning to manage a colostomy, approach the second step in self-care—irrigation—with confidence.

Occasionally, however, for psychologic or other reasons, a patient simply will not look at his stoma and, in that case, he cannot learn to care for it himself. This rejection can usually be prevented if the doctor or some other team member explains to the patient immediately postoperatively, if this has not been done preoperatively, just what the stoma will look like eventually and assures him that the early postoperative appearance is not that of a mature colostomy. He should be told that what he sees is the mucosal lining of the intestine and that it has the color of the mucosal lining of the mouth. Hopefully, when the patient knows ahead of time what his stoma will eventually look like, he will not be repulsed when he sees it for the first time. It is important also for the patient's family to show him by their attitudes and expressions that the stoma is not repulsive to them. Often, this alone will help the patient to overcome his feelings of disgust and revulsion so that he can begin to assist in his own care.

Irrigation of the colostomy is started on or about the fifth postoperative day. Precise directions as to how this is to be done should be recorded on the nursing care plan. (See Appendix A, p. 219.) The nurse and the patient together assume responsibility for the first irrigation. At first, the patient is asked to hand things to the nurse or to hold the irrigating bag. Gradually, he takes more responsibility until, eventually, he is able to carry out the procedure unaided.

At Memorial Hospital, the patient with a permanent colostomy is provided with a colostomy accessory kit and irrigator a few days prior to the first irrigation so that he can familiarize himself with the equipment before he uses it. The unit consists of the irrigating bag, a connecting tube with clamp, a No. 16 or 18 French catheter, a plastic stoma cup and an elastic belt, disposable plastic sheaths, rubber bands, and a lubricant.

Eventually, the time and frequency of the patient's bowel movements will very likely be similar to the pattern that he followed preoperatively. From the standpoint of the gastrocolic reflex, the frequency of evacuation and the reaction of the patient to eating will not necessarily change. Therefore, it usually seems best to try to follow the preoperative habit and irrigate at the time of day the patient normally had an evacuation.

Often times the procedure is also taught to a family member when it is believed that they will need to be involved in the irrigation after the patient leaves the hospital.

As soon as the patient is ambulatory, irrigations should be done in a bathroom that is well ventilated and that affords privacy since the procedure can take quite a long time at first, often more than an hour, and the patient is usually self-conscious about it.

Before starting the irrigation, the nurse should review with the patient the following points: 1) how the temperature of the water is checked against the inner aspect of the wrist—it should be lukewarm; 2) how the amount of water needed is measured with an ordinary household measuring cup; 3) how the flow of water is regulated by first using the clamp to release the flow and then placing the bag at a height about 12 inches above the patient's shoulder when he is seated; and, 4) how the well-lubricated catheter is introduced into the colostomy, avoiding any force. (See Appendix A, p. 219.)

Initially, the patient participates in the procedure by holding the plastic irrigating cup over the stoma while the nurse adjusts the belt around his body. After the air has been expelled from the tube by releasing the clamp and allowing the water to run through the tube, the clamp is tightened and the patient is encouraged to thread the tubing through the swing gate of the cup which is then brought forward and lubricated. The nurse then gently guides the patient's hand while he inserts the catheter three to five inches into the colostomy. The patient is instructed to breathe deeply in order to relax his abdominal muscles. After that the cup is brought in place and the nurse releases the clamp thus allowing the water—usually one quart—to flow into the colostomy. With the bottom of the bag at shoulder level the lukewarm water enters the colostomy slowly. The water pressure is controlled by regulating the height of the irrigating bag and can be decreased simply by lowering the level of the bag. Cramping may occur if the bag is held too high or if the water is not comfortably warm. Should this occur, the water inflow may be clamped off for a few minutes. After the fluid is introduced, the clamp is closed, the catheter gently removed, and the swing gate in the stoma cup is closed. The return flow, which drains out through the disposable sheath, can be assisted by gently massaging the abdomen. Sufficient time should be allowed to accomplish satisfactory evacuation. After the procedure has been completed, the area around the stoma is washed and dried, the plastic sheath is discarded, the stoma cup and irrigating bag are washed, dried and returned to the kit. A plastic tote box that can be kept in a closet is ideal for keeping the irrigation equipment together and in order, and for keeping the family bathroom neat.

Until such time as the colostomy has been regulated—usually from one to four weeks—the patient will feel more secure if he is provided with a disposable plastic appliance. The correct size hole is cut in the adhesive backing of the appliance which is then pressed to the skin after a light coating of tincture of benzoin has been applied to the skin around the stoma. If the patient is confined to bed, or if the fecal matter is very liquid, the appliance can be hooked up with a straight drainage system. The appliance should be emptied and cleansed as often as necessary.

After the incision is healed and there is no longer any need to protect it from fecal contamination, the wearing of an appliance is not necessary. A gauze dressing to which vaseline has been applied may be placed over the stoma and secured with paper tape; this will give adequate protection and will help keep the skin in good condition. Once the patient has gained control of his colostomy (and if he is engaged in such heavy work as truck or bus driving) he may guard against trauma to the stoma by wearing a protective shield that is held snugly against the stoma with an elastic belt. Others use a simple dressing held in place by a girdle or abdominal supporter.

Some patients prefer to irrigate daily while others are able to control their evacuations by irrigating at two- or three-day intervals. Patients with transverse colostomies usually will not be able to achieve control through irrigation, but practically all with sigmoid colostomies will.

If possible, the same nurse should assist the patient with his irrigation for several successive days because this provides him with consistent encouragement and reassurance, and he is less embarrassed if he repeats some error or if he forgets something. When this is not possible, a complete and accurate plan of the patient's daily routine should be placed in his chart along with a description of any problems that may have arisen in regard to irrigation. (See Appendix A, p. 219.)

A vital factor in the nursing care of the patient with a colostomy—one that can help make for successful recovery—involves instilling him with optimism and confidence in his ultimate rehabilitation. When achievement of control of the colostomy is possible, the patient should be told frequently that he will be able to carry out his own irrigations and thus regain voluntary control of his stool, that he can do this at any time of day that is convenient for him, and that eventually he will be free of any danger of incontinence for as long as 48 hours at a time. The nurse's attitude has a great effect on the patient's attitude and the rate at which his recovery progresses.

FOLLOW-UP CARE AND REHABILITATION

Ideally, the patient is prepared preoperatively for what will be involved in caring for his colostomy after he leaves the hospital, and he has been learning how to carry out the irrigation procedure from the time of the first irrigation. Occasionally, however, the time comes for him to leave the hospital and he has not learned these things. In such cases, certain arrangements have to be made. Staff nurses initiate visiting nurse referrals for all patients with ostomies. Memorial Hospital patients are also given an instruction card with pointers for the management of their particular stoma. (See Appendix A, B, C, pp. 219–222.) If the patient has no relatives or neighbors who can help with household duties after he gets home, the social worker may arrange for homemaker service through the American Cancer Society or other community agency. As a last resort, the patient may be referred to a nursing home. Every effort is made to avoid this, however, because one objective of aftercare is to help the patient to become independent, and this is usually more easily accomplished if he can remain in his own home. Besides, it is often difficult to secure Medicare or Medicaid funds for nursing home care unless the patient has a very special nursing need.

When the patient has had preoperative and postoperative counseling by the surgeon and nurses as well as other team members, he and his family will be prepared for some of the postoperative and post-hospital problems he will have to face. For example, if the patient can be prepared in advance for the possibility of an unclamped colostomy erupting spontaneously or, better yet, if the precaution has been taken of including a collecting bag in the surgical dressing thus sparing him the humiliation and distress of soiling his bed, he may take a more positive attitude toward learning how to control his evacuations. Pre-discharge counseling will also prepare the patient and his family for what will be needed to give him the necessary care at home. For example, if plans are made ahead of time for accommodating the patient's need for privacy and for adequate time to accomplish his irrigation, many difficulties will be avoided, especially in situations where the entire family must use the same bathroom.

To secure smooth transition from hospital to the patient's home, referral forms are made out several days before the patient is discharged. Practically every colostomy patient can use the services of a visiting nurse after he leaves the hospital. Some patients do very well on their own, but to ensure a successful shift from the dependence of hospital care to the independence of self care at home, referral to the Visiting Nurse Association for at least one visit is a good idea. The only stipulation regarding care is that the patient be under the medical supervision of a doctor or clinic that the nurse can contact should that be necessary. The visiting nurse sees the patient as often as necessary, sometimes every day. As soon as the patient and the family develop confidence in their ability to care for him, and the general home situation is stabilized, the VNA service is discontinued. No patient is refused service even though he may not be able to pay for it.

The first thing the visiting nurse does when she sees the patient at home is to go over the instructions (see Appendix A, B, pp. 219-220) he received while in the hospital and, on the basis of his understanding, helps him set up his irrigation routine. She checks the toilet to make sure the seat is comfortable and the right height for him, and that the items he needs can be placed within easy reach. She discusses with his family his need for privacy and for plenty of time to complete the irrigation without interruption. She may suggest that having a radio in the bathroom, or a clock so that he can check the time occasionally, or a book to read may help him to relax. These are important points because the patient will not feel confident about returning to his job or former activities until he has established an irrigation routine.

The visiting nurse makes sure the patient knows where he can purchase whatever equipment he may need at a reasonable price. She often finds that even though he is allowed a regular diet, the patient is not eating enough because he is afraid of spillage. (See ostomy check list, Appendix A, p. 219.) In that case, she reviews his diet with him and suggests that he eliminate the foods that will cause diarrhea or gas instead of cutting down on his overall intake. Finally, she encourages him to get dressed in street clothes, to see his friends, and get back into society.

Occasionally, a visiting nurse is called to see a patient who has been home from the hospital for a day or two, or even longer, and has refused to have anything to do with his colostomy. The dressings are malodorous and the patient is repulsive to himself and his family. Without showing any signs of rejection, the nurse removes the dressings, disposes of them immediately, irrigates the colostomy, and applies a fresh dressing or a colostomy bag if one is available. She will return daily at the same time to do the irrigation, have the patient assist her with the procedure, and try to find out what his problem is. By not being angry and not showing any revulsion when looking at the stoma, the nurse gives the patient a chance to express his feelings openly. It may be some time before he is willing and able to take the complete responsibility for his irrigations, but most patients do this sooner or later. If the nurse finds that he cannot or will not learn to care for his colostomy himself, she may suggest that he use a medication that will keep the stool soft enough to allow evacuation to occur spontaneously and teach him how to properly apply an appropriate ostomy appliance.

Poor communication is probably responsible for the fact that many private physicians and their nurses and secretaries do not know what the Visiting Nurse Service can do for the patient after he leaves the hospital. Programs for informing them about this service—seminars or wider distribution of the literature, for example, would help these people to feel that they are as much a part of the care team as the hospital and visiting nurses are. Also, the working relationship that might result from such programs would help provide more patients with needed home services.

Social Service Follow-up

Many patients can benefit from counseling by a social worker both while they are hospitalized and after they go home. Often, both the family and the patient need to know how and where to secure financial assistance.

They also frequently need emotional support and this takes different forms depending on the individuals involved. By reading the patient's chart, talking with nurses and doctors about the patient, and by listening to the patient the social worker can find out a great deal about the impact of the colostomy on the individual and what his expectations are. The patient will often express feelings to the social worker that he would hesitate to mention to anyone else. She needs to know when to listen and evaluate what he says, when to offer information or advice, and when to refer him to his physician. Remarks the patient may make often point the way to alternate solutions of particular problems. For example, one woman told the social worker, "I never liked to play in the sand when I was a child, and I never wanted to have babies because I could not stand the thought of having to change diapers." One patient's daughter, in speaking of her father's colostomy, said, "I never could look at sores."

One case report will serve to illustrate the value of the social worker's contact with the colostomy patient and his family:

> Mr. Samuels, a 57-year-old truck driver, had an anterior resection for cancer. Several postoperative complications developed. He was referred to a social worker when his wife asked for assistance in caring for him at home. She had been taught how to irrigate the wound (there was no colostomy) but found that doing this sickened her. She spoke emotionally of her own problems— diabetes, arthritis, and a heart condition—but refused visiting nurse assistance in caring for her husband because she was afraid she would have to pay for it. Later, Mr. Samuels was re-admitted to the hospital and, at this time, had a colostomy. He was very distressed about this recurrence, about having to have a colostomy, and about the fact that he thought his wife was beginning to keep things from him. Although his anger and fear were less explicit than hers, both people came across as hostile and bitter, and they managed to frequently antagonize the doctors and nurses.

> During the following months, Mr. Samuels was in and out of the hospital several times. The social worker persuaded his wife to use a part-time homemaker from the American Cancer Society, but she was so torn between her wish to take complete care of her husband and her need to be relieved of some of this burden that she could not admit that having the help was a good idea.

> Throughout her husband's final hospitalization, Mrs. Samuels continued to fight for his life in the only way she knew. She de-

manded more of the nurses, blamed the hospital for her husband's condition, complained that relatives were neglectful. After sessions in which she would unload her anger on the social worker who assured her that she had done everything a wife could for her husband, Mrs. Samuels would relax and even admit affection for the worker.

Two weeks after Mr. Samuel's death, his widow came to the hospital to pick up his belongings and, after reviewing his entire medical history with the social worker, remarked, "You must have found me an awful pest!" Opportunity for the deceased person's relatives to review the entire experience helps them to handle the situation and to close the chapter, even though the mourning period continues.

Vocational Counseling

If the patient plans to return to work after his colostomy, he may need vocational guidance. Some jobs require physical effort or exposure that a person with a colostomy cannot undertake. For example, a man's stoma may be at exactly the level of the work bench against which he must lean, and this means that something will have to be done about the level of the bench or about finding a different job for the man. It is possible that had the surgeon known about this possibility, he could have altered the placement of the colostomy and thus this problem could have been avoided.

Long-Term Follow-up

The colostomy patient's first visit to the outpatient department, clinic, or doctor's office usually occurs about a week after he has left the protective environment of the hospital, and often one or more problems have developed by that time. The discipline that was started in the hospital is carried out during the entire recovery period and, indeed, throughout the remainder of the patient's life.

Patients sometimes complain about cramping during the irrigation. This may be due to the fact that the procedure is not being accomplished quickly enough. In that case, the patient is advised to use a little less water each time until a good evacuation can be secured with just one quart. The nurse also explains that massaging the abdomen will stimulate peristalsis and evacuation. If the patient reports back-flow from the stoma, the nurse explains that the water is probably entering the colon too rapidly, and that keeping the bag at a lower level while the water is flowing in will solve this problem. He should also be told that sometimes back-flow can be prevented by threading the catheter through a nipple which can be held against the stoma, and in some situations a Laird tip is used for this purpose. An extra catheter with a nipple threaded through it is given to all colostomy patients and is kept with the other equipment in the patient's colostomy accessory kit.

If the patient has diarrhea following some dietary indiscretion, he may be advised to take an antidiarrhetic agent such as Kaopectate. He is also advised to wear a temporary colostomy appliance, to always carry an extra one with him, to take good care of the skin around the stoma, and to call his physician should the diarrhea persist.

Occasionally, the patient will complain about offensive odor of the stool. Such foods as garlic, onions, certain cheeses, or asparagus may cause this. Charcoal, chlorophyll, or bismuth subcarbonate tablets are helpful in preventing odor from developing within the body and can be purchased without a doctor's prescription. Frequently, the patient will be psychologically upset by the embarrassment he feels when odorous gas is expelled through the stoma. He can help prevent this by avoiding gas-producing foods such as beans, cabbage, and asparagus. Usually, the patient can tolerate and enjoy most of the foods he enjoyed before his operation, and he is encouraged to take a well balanced general diet. Sometimes the doctor orders yogurt or buttermilk which will help repopulate the intestinal flora.

The patient should report to the clinic or outpatient nurse any skin irritation that may develop. This is usually due to improper cleansing. The regular use of bacteriostatic soap and water is recommended and, when the skin is excoriated, Karaya powder or a piece of Karaya seal or Collyseel may be used. (Compound tincture of benzoin is to be avoided as it causes skin irritation.)

The patient who has an ascending colostomy can never hope to establish control of it and will always need to wear a permanent appliance. The stools will be loose and will contain irritating digestive enzymes that cause excoriation, so good skin care is absolutely necessary. A rare skin infection, pyoderma, may develop. It is characterized by small pustules on the skin around the stoma and should be called to the doctor's attention at once. Other conditions that must be treated by the physician include ulcers on the stoma or the skin around it, or herniation about the stoma.

Patients sometimes complain to the office or clinic nurse that they feel rejected because their doctor never looks at their stoma, and if even the doctor finds it repulsive it must be rather dreadful to look at. The nurse should explain that the doctor is primarily concerned with the patient's general condition and that he cannot learn much by looking at the stoma. If she will look at it and assure him that it appears normal, she can let him know that his having a colostomy does not make him repulsive to her. However, his feelings about his stoma are greatly influenced by the doctor's attitude. If the doctor will look at it while chatting with the patient about his diet, irrigations, work, and social activities, the patient will begin to feel more acceptable. Eventually, most patients accept their colostomy and the stoma and are able to pursue a normal life without paying very much attention to their colostomy once they have achieved control of it. A very few, however, need long-continuing assistance in managing their colostomy. In New York City a stoma clinic has been established for the purpose of helping these patients.

Prior to 1970, (New York) patients who were having problems managing their stomas would call the American Cancer Society for help in securing supplies and equipment as well as in the management of the colostomy. (A list of these patients revealed that 55 of them had had abdominal perineal resections and had received assistance from the ACS for over 20 years. One woman who had had her surgery five years previously was still receiving help because she became nauseated whenever she looked at her stoma.) When such a call for help was received, the ACS sent a visiting nurse to the home to assess the situation. Often she found that the patient had never received any instruction at all from his doctors or nurses about how to care for his colostomy, so she would teach him the basic facts. But in many cases the problems were so deep-seated that a practical nurse would be sent to visit him four days a week, sometimes every day, for as long as six to eight weeks. Recently, the demand for this kind of service has abated somewhat because patients now seem to be getting more instruction while still in the hospital. But the problem still exists as far as the private physician and his patients are concerned. Often the surgeon and the hospital discharge the patient to his private physician, communication has not been established, and the patient does not have any follow-up care or advice. Consequently he flounders, with no psychological or emotional support and no help in solving such practical problems as where and how to obtain supplies and equipment. The ACS can act as intermediary between the visiting nurse (or other interested person) and the stoma clinic to obtain referrals for such patients. The Society is currently working with members of the New York medical community to develop a program that will improve communication among the private doctors, their patients, and the various agencies so that more and better follow-up care can be provided for private patients.

Impotence is a sequela that sometimes follows an anterior resection or abdominal perineal resection. More men commonly complain of this than women; in fact about 50 percent of males report sex loss and another 50 percent have varying impairment of sexual potency, such as lack of ejaculation. However, in one group of men who were queried, 64 percent stated that they had the same amount of sexual desire as before the operation, and 32 percent said they had less. In terms of actual sexual activity, 25 percent said they experienced no change postoperatively, and 41 percent reported that they were less active sexually. Only 45 percent indicated that they were still having sexual relations, but since it was not known whether they were sexually active before the operation, this figure probably should be accepted with some reservation.

Female patients do not complain of change in sexual activity as much as male patients do. Of those who were questioned in the study mentioned in the preceding paragraph, 38 percent indicated the same sexual desire as before the operation, 28 percent said they had less, and 21 percent reported pain or lack of sensation during intercourse; only one said that her husband was "afraid" and kept away from her. All of the women indicated that their husbands were understanding and considerate.

Changes in sexual desire and activity are often psychological and have nothing to do with the operation per se. In fact, telling a patient that he may be impotent afterwards may actually cause this to happen when it might not have occurred otherwise. Occasionally, it is reported that, although a man is not impotent after an abdominal perineal resection, he no longer produces any sperm. This is probably due to the nature of the operation, as is true physical impotence, either of which may result from mechanical interference with the nerve supply to the genital organs, severance of the presacral nerves, or actual organ destruction.

When there is no true impotency, all the male patient usually needs is reassurance that his loss of sexual desire or potency was, indeed, caused by the operation and does not in any way reflect failure on his part as a man. Much of the adjustment during the follow-up and rehabilitation periods depends on the kind of understanding that exists between the sexual partners.

From the foregoing discussion it becomes clear that the chief role of the office, clinic, or outpatient nurse is to reinforce the teaching that was begun while the patient was in the hospital and to provide constant support and encouragement that will help him develop a sense of security and independence. It is imperative that the nurse be skillful and confident in her ability to guide the patient in learning to control his colostomy and to solve the problems that arise in connection with it. As these problems decrease in magnitude, so do the patient's psychological problems. Recovery of the colostomy patient is a gradual process and the clinic nurse needs to be empathetic and willing to spend time with him.

REHABILITATION

Rehabilitation of the colostomate involves every member of the care team and extends from the preoperative period through the patient's hospitalization, the follow-up period and, indeed, throughout his life. It involves pointing out ways in which the patient can live with his family and in the community, and how he can make use of the various services that the community provides. Rehabilitation also involves prevention—that is, prevention of any degree of disability that can be foreseen. Further, it includes the instruction of the patient by team members in how to circumvent disabilities, how to recognize them, how to appropriately care for oneself in the event that a disability develops, and how to compensate for any disability that may occur.

The impact of a clostomy on the patient varies from mild concern to deep depression which may be manifested by complete withdrawal and which, in its extreme form, may be a prelude to suicide. Depression of this depth is rare, but it does occur—for several reasons. Some patients have an exaggerated idea of how badly they were mutilated or maimed by the surgery; they feel they have lost irreplaceable structures; and that they will never recover from the damage that was done. In such cases, the patient should be told exactly what was done and how little change there has been, and will be, in his body economy.

Another important reason for some patients' difficulty in accepting a colostomy has to do with a basic concept of social acceptability. Perhaps one of the first evidences of parental discipline is associated with toilet training, when it is impressed on the child that fecal incontinence will not be tolerated. Some parents place a high degree of emphasis on this, try to train the child at an early age, and become angry when the child is incontinent. These early experiences undoubtedly create a lasting impression on the individual. Other parents are more permissive in regard to toilet training, and perhaps patients who had such parents are the ones who have less difficulty in adjusting to a colostomy.

Sometimes a patient has an unexpressed fear of the cancer that made the colostomy necessary and may confuse the colostomy with the disease. Often he will have had an experience or close contact with someone who had a colostomy but whose cancer was incurable and who lived, or is living, a miserable life. He identifies with this person and this leads to even more confusion in his thinking about his own colostomy.

All of these problems and attitudes must be taken into consideration when trying to reassure and rehabilitate the patient. He needs to be told, over and over again, that very little real damage was done to his body, and that eventually he will learn to control his evacuations. When the outlook is positive, the patient should be given as much reassurance as possible that there is no evidence to indicate that he will have any further trouble with the disease.

In every instance, rehabilitation can be expected to provide the greatest possible restoration of the patient's ability to live a full and unrestricted life. When there is no hope for the patient except ongoing disability, rehabilitation procedures can provide palliation and survival with the least possible restriction and handicap. For the in-between patient—one who can look forward to some degree of continuing disability and perhaps a series of operations that will curtail his personal and community life, but who will also probably have a relatively long survival—rehabilitation can provide support through the services of such team members as the visiting nurse, the social worker, and the vocational counselor.

The nurse also has an important place in the rehabilitation program. She can be very helpful in assisting the patient to cope with the anxiety and depression that often affects the patient with a colostomy. She can discuss with him the problems he may be having with loss of control of his evacuations, leakage, soiling, or the noisy expulsion of gas. An explanation of the causes of these problems and assurance that proper diet and training will eliminate some of them can help dispel the patient's fears about his acceptability, and may even prevent his going into a period of social withdrawal.

Problems that may develop later in the patient's rehabilitation are many and varied. The stoma may become constricted or an angulation may develop in the colostomy loop that may interfere with adequate evacuation following irrigation. A patient who has achieved control of his colostomy may experience some unusual personal or professional change—an advancement, perhaps, that involves increased responsibility—and the emotional impact of this will cause him to lose control of his colostomy. Perhaps all this person needs is advice regarding the time, method, or procedure of irrigating. He may have been taught to irrigate his colostomy at night. But fecal matter collects during the night and, when the patient is under stress during the day, it becomes difficult for him to control his evacuation. Simply having him change to morning irrigation may solve that problem. When the difficulty is due to a stricture, a dilatation may be recommended. Sometimes surgical revisions are required. And, for a long time, many patients need continued instruction about how to manage their work and vocational rehabilitation, how to control odor, and how to plan their meals.

Most patients respond to rehabilitative measures and learn to manage their colostomies independently. However, some patients do not seem to be able to accomplish this. They never become rehabilitated to the extent that they can go back to work in a situation where it would be necessary for them to have control of their colostomy. They return again and again to the doctor or the clinic complaining of the same problems although there does not appear to be anything wrong with them organically. Regardless of how much teaching and supervision they get, they will always need constant assistance. Rehabiliation doctors and nurses sometimes encourage these patients to look back on their preoperative life and then they have to admit that their bowel function never was very reliable. Some of them may have had parents who were rigid about bowel control and, even though the particulars of their toilet training are forgotten, the ingrained problem is still there. Also, many of these patients are very intelligent; they analyze their problems and often make completely impractical suggestions, and thus the problem is a continuing one. Fortunately, these patients are in the minority for, although it may take some patients considerable time to develop a healthy attitude toward their colostomy, most of them are able to return to their former occupations and find that they are in no way inhibited from again leading useful lives.

Physicians, and patients too, differ in their opinions about whether it is a good idea for a person who has had a colostomy to become a member of a colostomy club. On one hand, belonging to such a club may be helpful in giving the patient an opportunity to associate with a group of people who all have the same problems and who can discuss their common concerns with some degree of mutual understanding. Particularly, it may be helpful to the patient whose perception of himself has been so altered that he now sees himself as repulsive and unacceptable socially. But, on the other hand, the fact that many of the members of such clubs will not be cured of their disease could mean that membership might not be conducive to building a healthy outlook and that the patient would do better to look to professionals for help.

Some of these clubs have been organized by individuals who did not know where else to find help and who, therefore, organized as a group of mutually supporting people. Unfortunately, many of them have not had the advantage of medical advice and have tried to help members solve their problems without being aware of the specific needs of the individuals involved. If such clubs were directed by professional personnel who could channel the club's efforts into appropriate, honest, and medically sound approaches, there would be more value in membership in a club. Also, the American Cancer Society might make better use of club volunteers as it has done with those from the Reach to Recovery group. But when a club exists simply as a default organization, it could conceivably do the patient more harm than good. Patients who go to meetings seeking help are apt to be exposed to people whose disease is not cured or curable, and identifying with them could be a negative experience.

Many professionals who work with colostomy patients during the rehabilitation period believe that the patient should return to an active, normal life as soon as possible and not focus all his thinking on his colostomy. At colostomy club meetings the focus is all on the members' stomas and their problems. At Memorial Hospital the aim is to get the patient *not* to focus on these things but to care for his colostomy once a day and then forget about it and go on living a normal life the rest of the time. All colostomy patients at this hospital are visited by a carefully selected, well rehabilitated volunteer. These volunteers are former Memorial patients who have expressed a desire to help other colostomates by demonstrating personally that living with a colostomy need not be a catastrophe and that a normal, satisfying life is still possible.

CARE OF THE PATIENT WITH ADVANCED, INCURABLE CANCER OF THE COLON OR RECTUM

To give support and encouragement to the patient with incurable cancer is difficult for the physician and the team members alike. Sometimes the patient has not been told that he has cancer. In such a case, the physician can do little more than to say that things are not going quite as well as had been hoped; that, however, everything possible will be done for the patient; that it takes time to recover and that he will do all he can to keep the patient comfortable. This, of course, leaves many of the patient's questions unanswered.

Most physicians feel that they do not have the right to remove all hope from a patient, regardless of his condition. Oliver Wendell Holmes once said, "Be careful about how you take away hope from any patient." The doctor's attitude as well as that of all team members, the way they face the situation, and the way they convey to the patient that he is not being deserted are all-important. Even a small child can sense that he is being deserted unless those caring for him maintain a cheerful attitude and do little things that give him moral support. Many patients can accept knowing that they have cancer and that they will probably die of it, but no patient wants to have all hope taken away from him.

QUESTIONS AND ANSWERS

Q. Who does the preoperative teaching of the patient before he has a colostomy?

A. The doctor is the one who tells the patient that he will have a colostomy, but it is usually up to the bedside staff who are caring for him to re-explain and reinforce what the doctor has said and to answer most of the questions the patient will ask. If there are questions the nurse cannot answer, she refers the patient back to the doctor or to another appropriate team member.

Physicians differ considerably in what they tell patients beforehand regarding the possibility of a colostomy. Some do not mention this possibility even though they are reasonably sure that the patient will have a colostomy. Others mention that it might be necessary to do a colostomy, but do not make an issue of it. They feel that going into too much detail creates a lot of emotional problems for the patient and has a direct influence on his rehabilitation and his ability to get along with his colostomy.

Q. What special steps are taken to prevent and treat excoriation of the skin around a stoma?

A. First, it is necessary to find out what kind of colostomy a patient has. If it is a right side (ascending) colostomy, there will be constant spillage of fecal matter that contains enzymes which are very irritating to the skin. The use of a temporary ostomy bag with a Karaya washer, or a Hollister bag with a belt that holds it close to the body, will help prevent skin irritation.

When the stoma has shrunk to its permanent size, the patient will be fitted by the stoma therapist with a permanent type of appliance.

For all patients, cleanliness is of the utmost importance because the presence of feces on the skin can be very irritating. The skin around the stoma should be washed with mild soap and water whenever necessary. Maalox or some other antacid substance can be used on the skin when the colostomy is in such a location that the drainage contains digestive juices. If the skin is extremely sore, Karaya powder may be dusted on the area around the stoma and several coats of tincture (not the compound tincture) of benzoin applied before applying the rubber cement. This gives good adherence and helps to hold the appliance in place in addition to protecting the skin. Karaya powder and tincture of benzoin may also be used when a dressing is to be applied.

If the skin is extremely irritated, the doctor may give permission to expose the entire area to a heat lamp after covering the stoma with gauze that has been soaked in normal saline solution. Also, sometimes the application of Maalox, A & D ointment, or zinc oxide directly on the skin, and then covering it with a dressing, help dry up and heal the excoriated area.

Q. Does the colostomy bag for a loop colostomy have to be removed for the irrigation procedure?

A. No. If the bag is adhering it is pointless to traumatize the skin by removing the bag and applying another one. It is better to cut a hole just large enough to admit the lubricated catheter in the part of the bag that is directly over the stoma. The irrigation is done with the bag hanging down between the patient's legs as he sits on the toilet. While waiting for the evacuation, the hole is sealed with a piece of adhesive tape. At the completion of the precedure the bag is flushed out using an Asepto syringe and normal saline solution. In this way the bag does not have to be removed and changed until leakage around the stoma occurs. Never patch a leaky bag; change it.

Q. Is it necessary to change the colostomy bag after every evacuation?

A. No. The disposable type of bag can be opened at the bottom and then flushed out using an Asepto syringe and normal saline solution which removes any feces or mucous shreds. The bottom of the bag is then folded over and closed with a double rubber band.

Q. How long does it take to establish regulation through the irrigation technique?

A. Usually regulation can be achieved in about two to four weeks. However, it is difficult to say how long it will take an individual patient because people normally differ as to bowel habits. For example, before their surgery, some people habitually had one movement a day and some two; others had a movement every second or third day. This fact influences the time it takes to establish regularity after surgery. A few patients never do achieve it.

Q. How long does it take a colostomy patient to learn to regulate his movements through diet alone?

A. This is not a method commonly followed in the United States, although some New England physicians employ it for certain patients. Two American physicians spent several months in Great Britain studying the non-irrigating method as it is carried out there and concluded that it should be restricted to patients who are so debilitated that they cannot manage their colostomy, or who are physically handicapped in some way (by a stroke or hand amputation, for example) that makes it impossible for them to care for themselves, or who refuse to do so.

Q. Are alcoholic drinks and beer contraindicated for the colostomy patient?

A. There is no contraindication for alcohol other than its use in excess. Alcohol may, in fact, be a digestive aid and thus be useful to the colostomy patient. Beer may cause over-production of gas in some patients and is contraindicated when this is the case.

Q. How do aspirin tablets placed in the ostomy appliance help control odor?

A. Probably the reason is that aspirin is an acid—acetylsalicylic acid—and, since in most people the bowel content at the end colostomy level is alkaline, it acts to neutralize the feces and so perhaps reduces odor. Also, aspirin will form a salicylate when in combination with any salt and may therefore alter the chemical composition of the stool in the appliance, thus changing or eliminating odor.

Q. Are tub baths or swimming contraindicated for colostomy patients?

A. No. If the patient is going to swim in a private pool or where others are also swimming, he should put on a temporary appliance and cover the edges with waterproof tape which keeps water from getting under the shield of the appliance.

APPENDIX A

MEMORIAL SLOAN-KETTERING CANCER CENTER
DEPARTMENT OF NURSING
INSERVICE EDUCATION

(front)

Colostomy Accessory Kit

Equipment*   Keep equipment in
tote box
Irrigating set—doctor's choice
Accessory kit:
    Blue Handi*Tote box
    Lubricating jelly
    Antibacterial skin cleanser
    Paper tape
    Tincture of benzoin
    Nilodor deodorant drops
    Alcohol swabs
    4 x 4 unsterile sponges
    Bongart bags* emergency use

Care of Equipment

1. Wash reusable equipment with
   mild soap and warm water. Never
   boil or autoclave equipment.
2. Rinse equipment with warm water.
   Use one-quarter cup of white vinegar or bleach to one quart of
   warm water in final rinse as a
   deodorizer.
3. Dry equipment and return to tote
   box.
4. Wash colostomy belt when soiled
   using mild soap and water. Rinse
   well and dry away from heat.

KEEP THIS CARD IN BLUE ACCESSORY KIT

(reverse)

Important Points in Irrigating a Colostomy

1. *Measure the water* —Never any more than two quarts. Try using a little less water each time you irrigate.
2. *Check temperature* —Test temperature on your wrist. Water should be warm, never hot or cold (about 105° F.)
3. *Remove air from tubing* —Let water run through tubing to dispel air.
4. *Check height of bag* —The bottom of the bag should be at shoulder level.
5. *Insert catheter with care—use no force* —Insert catheter 4-5 inches into stoma. Take deep breath when inserting catheter.
6. *Irrigate the same time each day* —This will help establish control and prevent soilage between irrigations.
7. *Keep lubricated gauze over the stoma* —This will prevent sticking of gauze to stoma and will help absorb mucus.
8. *Skin care* —Clean skin around stoma with an antibacterial soap and water.
9. *Odor control* —Use one drop of Nilodor on the dressing or bag.

APPENDIX B

MEMORIAL SLOAN-KETTERING CANCER CENTER
DEPARTMENT OF NURSING
INSERVICE EDUCATION

Care of the Loop Colostomy or Double Barrel Colostomy

General Information:
1. Obtain blue ostomy accessory kit from pharmacy. Keep all stoma equipment in kit.
2. Add bulb syringe set for emptying and rinsing appliance. Add large Bongart bags.
3. Most temporary colostomies are not irrigated. If there is an order to irrigate, order a temporary irrigation set from pharmacy and follow doctor's orders.
4. The patient will have a rod on for several days to keep the colostomy exteriorized.
5. The patient will need to wear an appliance constantly since the loose stool will cause skin excoriation. Meticulous skin care is essential.
6. Daily unnecessary changes of the appliance will cause skin problems. Change the appliance only when necessary, *e.g.,* if the bag leaks.

Prepare the Appliance:
1. Cut a round hole in a large Bongart bag to keep the stoma exposed while protecting as much skin as possible. Leave about ⅛ inch of skin exposed.
2. Remove protective backing and lay appliance aside.

Prepare the skin:
1. Wash skin with warm water and Non-Hex or Phisohex, rinse well and pat dry. (Have patient or family member hold gauze over stoma while you work.)
2. Apply 2 coats tincture benzoin or similar skin preparation to skin surrounding stoma, fan dry the skin.

Apply Appliance:
1. Place prepared appliance carefully by inserting hand into appliance and centering the hole over the stoma. Keep gauze over the stoma while you are doing this. Be careful not to cap or rim the stoma.
2. Apply firm pressure for a minute to assure a good bond.
3. Remove protective gauze through bottom of bag and secure bag with Acco fastener or two rubber bands.
4. Reinforce appliance at top with tape for extra security. Never put pinpricks into the bag for release of gas. Empty gas from bottom of appliance by releasing clamp or rubber bands.
5. Empty bag from below and flush appliance with lukewarm water as often as necessary.

APPENDIX C

MEMORIAL SLOAN-KETTERING CANCER CENTER
DEPARTMENT OF NURSING
INSERVICE EDUCATION

Return to Enterostomal Therapist   *Keep in Nursing Care Kardex*
(upon discharge)
Name_____   Unit_____

COLOSTOMY CHECK LIST

Dressing Change:		*Colostomy Irrigation:*	
Date	Nurse	Date	Nurse
Patient observed		Irrig. set explained	
Patient performed		Patient observed	
Family performed		Family observed	
		Patient performed	
Stoma Care:		Family performed	
Patient observed			
Patient performed		*Miscellaneous:*	
		Procur. supplies	
Posterior Wound Care:		Colostomy kit	
Irrigations		Ostomy hygiene	
Sitz baths		Follow up care	
Patient performed		V.N.S. referral	
Family performed			
		Diet:	
Appliance:		Discuss with patient	
(if indicated)		Discuss with family	
Patient applied		Seen by volunteer	
Family applied			

—over—

Discussion Pointers

1. Prepare a travel irrigation kit. Discuss travel.
2. Discuss skin problems and their management (redness, excoriation, etc.).
3. Discuss appliance and measurement of stoma if patient needs to wear an appliance.
4. Discuss sports activities permitted or prohibited.
5. Discuss underwear and wardrobe.
6. Discuss resumption of social activities (sexual if applicable).
7. Discuss management of emergency situations.
8. Discuss with patient his thoughts and feelings about his changed body image.
9. Discuss return to work and what to tell family and friends.
10. Discuss need for privacy and time for irrigation.

11. Discuss the ostomy procedure generally.
12. Discuss the care of the posterior wound at home.
13. Discuss management of constipation and diarrhea.
14. Availability of hospital personnel to help with problems which may occur following discharge from hospital (emergencies).

N.B. Discussion is best done with a family member, volunteer, enterostomal therapist, patients and nurse in attendance.

REVIEW COLOSTOMY IRRIGATION TECHNIQUE

SUGGESTED READINGS

Books

Bacon, Harry E. *Cancer of the Colon and Anal Canal.* Philadelphia: Lippincott, 1964.

Beland, Irene L. *Clinical Nursing,* 2nd ed. New York: The Macmillan Company, 1970.

Bouchard, Rosemary. *Nursing Care of the Cancer Patient.* St. Louis: Mosby, 1967.

Happenie, Sylvene Dillon. *Colostomy—A Second Chance.* Springfield, Ill.: Charles C Thomas, 1968.

Jackman, Raymond J., and Oliver H. Beahrs. *Tumors of the Large Bowel.* Philadelphia: Saunders, 1968.

Shafer, Kathleen Newton, et al. *Medical-Surgical Nursing,* 4th ed. St. Louis: Mosby, 1967.

Periodicals

American Cancer Society. *1970 Facts and Figures.* New York: American Cancer Society, Inc., 1969.

Cihlar, Jean, Nancy Newhouse, and Charlayne Lenz. "Courage with a Colostomy," *American Journal of Nursing,* 5:1050-51, May, 1967.

Dericks, Virginia C. "Rehabilitation of Patients with an Ileostomy," *American Journal of Nursing,* 61:48-51, May, 1961.

Devlin, H. B. "Abdomino-Perineal Resection of the Rectum," *Nursing Times,* 64:1364-68, October, 1968.

Devlin, H. B. et al. "Colostomy and Its Management," *Nursing Times,* 65:231-4, February, 1969.

Dyk, Ruth, and Arthur Sutherland. "Adaptation of the Spouse and Other Family Members to the Colostomy Patient," *Cancer,* 9:123, 1956.

Eisenberg, Samuel W., Rita P. Napoli, and Beatrice Redding. "Proctosigmoidoscopy," *American Journal of Nursing,* 65:113-115, January, 1965.

Gutowski, Frances. "Ostomy Procedure: Nursing Care," *American Journal of Nursing,* 72:262-267, February, 1972.

Katona, Elizabeth A. "Learning Colostomy Control," *American Journal of Nursing,* 67:534-541, March, 1967.

Lenneberg, E. et al. "Colostomies—A Guide for the Patient," *Diseases of the Colon and Rectum,* 12:201-17, May-June, 1969.

Levine, S. M. et al. "Intestinal Bacterial Flora After Total and Partial Colon Resection," *American Journal of Digestive Diseases,* 15:23-28, June, 1970.

Mendelssohn, A. N. "Management of the Colonic Stoma," *Surgery, Gynecology, and Obstetrics,* 129:1046, November, 1969.

McKittrick, J. B., and Jane H. Shotkin. "Ulcerative Colitis," *American Journal of Nursing, 62*:60-64, August, 1962.

Rowbotham, J. L. "The Stoma Rehabilitation Clinic," *Diseases of the Colon and Rectum, 13*:59-61, January-February, 1970.

Sill, A. R. "Bulb Syringe Technique for Colonic Stoma Irrigation," *American Journal of Nursing, 70*:536-7, March, 1970.

Sterling, W. A. et al. "A Normal Life with a Colostomy or Ileostomy," *Postgraduate Medicine, 47*:80-85, February, 1970.

Turrel, Robert et al. "Symposium on New Perspectives in Colorectoanal Surgery," *Surgical Clinics of North America, 45*:1067-1329, October, 1965.

United Ostomy Association and Quarterly, Vol. 7, No. 4, Fall, 1970.

White, Dorothy Ruth. "I Have an Ileostomy," *American Journal of Nursing, 61*:51-52, May, 1961.

Wolfman, Earl F. Jr., C. Thomas Flotte, and Jeanne C. Hallburg. "Carcinoma of the Colon and Rectum," and "The Patient with Surgery of the Colon," *American Journal of Nursing, 61*:60-66, March, 1961.

Problems Associated with Gynecologic Cancer

Regional Medical Program — Oncology Nursing Seminar

on

PROBLEMS ASSOCIATED WITH GYNECOLOGIC CANCER

Seminar Leader

John L. Lewis, Jr., M.D.

Seminar Participants

Martha Atchley, M.S.W., Social Worker

Donald L. Clark, M.D.

Dorothy Donahue, R.N., Clinical Nursing Instructor

Marilyn Hafner, R.N., B.S.N., Head Nurse

Walter B. Jones, M.D., Assistant Attending Surgeon, Gynecology
Service

John L. Lewis, Jr., M.D., Chief, Gynecology Service

Susan Sargent, R.N., Clinical Nursing Coordinator, Operating
Room

Shirley Weatherly, R.N., Nursing Supervisor

The first of three interesting and unique facts about gynecologic malignancies is that this field furnished the first instance of human malignancy that could be totally eradicated if a routine, non-painful, inexpensive test were done every year on every female in the world population. Proper screening of all females could literally eliminate mortality from cancer of the cervix which, for generations, has been one of the great killers of women. Unfortunately, almost one-half of the women—in the United States, at least—who should have this test annually, or oftener, have never had one. This is the Papanicolaou cytologic examination (Pap test) that was developed by Dr. George Papanicolaou while he was associated with the department of anatomy at Cornell University. The only problems that exist in connection with the examination are concerned with its utilization; that is, education about it and motivation to use it are in great need of strengthening.

The Papanicolaou cytologic examination usually allows the physician to detect invasive cancer of the cervix but, more importantly, it enables the detection of two conditions of the cervix that precede carcinoma—carcinoma in situ, and even before that, dysplasia—both of which can be treated simply and are totally curable. The test is most useful for picking up atypical cells when the patient presents with no apparent disease of the vagina, cervix, or uterus; everything appears to be perfectly normal on general examination.

One Papanicolaou examination will pick up perhaps 80 percent of the lesions that are, or that may become malignant. But three consecutive examinations will pick up more than 95 percent of them. Consequently, the secret is not to have just one test and then five or six years later have another test, but to have it done regularly at least annually. This holds for all women, regardless of age. Along with the Papanicolaou examination, the routine examination should include a thorough pelvic and breast examination by a competent physician. This triad, if carried out regularly, would greatly help in getting treatment for cancer or precancerous conditions of the female reproductive organs before a malignancy reaches a stage that makes heroic measures necessary and cure doubtful.

The second interesting fact about gynecologic malignancies is that one of these diseases, choriocarcinoma, was the first malignancy shown to be curable by chemotherapy after it has become metastatic. Choriocarcinoma is a disease that starts in the placenta, during pregnancy, metastasizes rapidly and, historically, has almost always killed the patient within one year. Since 1968, 21 patients who had not been treated elsewhere have been admitted to Memorial Hospital with some form of malignancy that began during pregnancy; that is, gestational choricarcinoma or hydatidiform mole. All 21 patients were admitted for chemotherapy and all are now well, even though 14 of them had metastatic cancer. In 50 similar patients originally treated at the National Institutes of Health, there have now been 88 successful pregnancies, consequently these patients are also considered cured.

In 1955, Dr. M. C. Li of Memorial Hospital and Dr. Roy Hertz of the National Institutes of Health showed that methotrexate could be used effectively in treating choriocarcinoma, and in the 1960's they found that actinomycin D could also be used for this purpose. When this tumor grows, it always produces chorionic gonadotropin and, therefore, the accurate measurement of levels of this substance in the urine allows the physician to determine the patient's response to therapy.

The third unique fact about gynecologic malignancies is that about one-third of the patients with endometrial carcinoma will respond with prolonged regression to treatment with progestational hormones, even after the disease has become metastatic.

THE PHYSICIAN'S ANSWER TO "SHOULD THE PATIENT BE TOLD?"

Sometimes, even before she enters the hospital, the patient will ask the doctor outright, "Do I have cancer?" Physicians' attitudes differ as to how this question should be answered and often the response is a reflection of the man's own personality. Some physicians will answer the question positively if absolutely sure of the diagnosis, and will tell her all she needs to know about her disease for her comfort, while reassuring her that she will be properly cared for. On the other hand, some physicians rarely tell a patient she has cancer, since they honestly think that most patients don't really want to know and that even those who are quite sure of their diagnoses do not want to be told because, psychologically, they want to continue to deny it to themselves.

A patient may be inquisitive enough to demand a definite answer but in such a case the person is usually also intelligent enough to know that a direct question may bring a direct answer. Then, all the physician can do is tell her that she has a malignancy, and that means cancer, and that this is a threat to her life unless it is properly treated.

Some physicians find that most of their patients know they have a malignant disease—if not before their first visit to the doctor's office, at least after they are admitted to the hospital for surgery. But their fears really relate to whether they are going to die. Sometimes the patient will ask the question on two different days, but in perhaps different ways. If they are told "Yes," the next question will be "Can you do something about it?" What they really are asking is "Can you do something about it so that I won't die?"

The preoperative discussion with a patient scheduled for possible radical pelvic surgery, associated with the necessary urinary stoma or colostomy, must anticipate the possibility that such diversions may not be feasible or necessary. The patient should understand that there may be alternative means of treatment, both in terms of extent of surgery or radiation, and that the proposed operation has two purposes, namely, to evaluate the precise nature of her problem and, if indicated, to treat it. After the surgery, time must be taken to explain the course adopted in her particular case.

It may be easier for the patient to accept the situation if she is told that she has a "malignancy" instead of using the word "cancer." She should know that the reason it is imperative that this tumor be removed is because it is a threat to her life. Then, if the tumor is in an early stage, the doctor might quote statistics, if accurate statistics are available and favorable. For example, a patient who has a definite diagnosis of cancer of the cervix can be told that she has a malignancy at the mouth of the uterus, but that it is in an early stage and she has an 80 percent chance of being alive, well, and without any evidence of this disease five years from now, provided she accepts the proper treatment.

If it is easier to talk to a patient about unusual or "abnormal" cells that will shorten her life if they are not removed, then that may be the best way for the doctor to handle her questions. But if a patient is told a direct lie when she really wants to know her diagnosis, and she finds out that the doctor lied, she will not trust him again, and the faith that must exist between doctor and patient is lost. His answer must always allow for the contingency that the patient will not respond favorably to therapy; then, if this happens, and the patient learns that her condition is hopeless, the trusting relationship will still be there.

It is difficult to keep a patient from finding out that she has cancer when she is under some kind of therapy. When this happens, the nurse's most difficult job is to take care of the patient's anxiety, and one of the best ways of doing this is to see that she receives the best possible care by concerned, informed personnel. It is important for the oncologic nurse's attitude to be based on the philosophy that there is always hope—always one more thing that can be done—and to project this philosophy in all her contacts with the cancer patient.

TREATMENT

The treatment of gynecologic cancer today is a multidisciplinary phenomenon. It consists of more than just operating on people, radiating them, or putting them on a chemotherapy regimen. Of course, certain diseases can be treated with just one of these modalities of treatment and some of them get well. But in all cases of gynecologic cancer, the best knowledge of qualified personnel in each of these fields should be considered when the decision as to treatment for a particular patient is made. Each case has to be judged on its individual characteristics and the treatment tailored to the state of the patient and the state of the lesion.

Although the final management of the patient is the responsibility of the attending physician, all of the nursing staff who come into contact with her— the resident staff, the social worker, the radiotherapist, the chemotherapist, and any one else who works with the patient in any capacity—bear part of the responsibility.

Gynecologic cancer is an all-inclusive term that covers cancer of the vulva, vagina, cervix, endometrium, body of the uterus, ovary, fallopian tube, and placenta. Breast tumor is also sometimes included in this category. Obviously, some patients will be faced with massive operations, but many will be cured by a simple conization of the cervix or a simple hysterectomy. Some will be found, at surgery, to have a benign condition although the signs and symptoms may have suggested a malignancy. Some are treated with radiotherapy which has serious local consequences during the course of treatment. Others may be treated with chemotherapy and these patients, too, require special care and observation because some of the drugs used are highly toxic. And, happily, some of the patients who enter the hospital for possible treatment of cancer will be found not to have this disease. Families often try to protect the patient from knowing she has cancer because for people the world over, the word "cancer" is synonymous with hopelessness and ultimate death. This is not the attitude that prevails at Memorial Hospital where, as far as gynecologic cancer is concerned, the overall cure rate for invasive cervical carcinoma is between 57 and 60 percent; for vulvar carcinoma, 70 to 80 percent; and for endometrial carcinoma, 70 to 80 percent. So it is evident that the majority of the patients with a gynecologic malignancy who are admitted to this hospital for primary therapy get well.

The female reproductive organs are, to a certain degree, much more accessible for physical examination than many others. The vulva can be seen in its entirety if the patient is in the proper position and the light is good. The vagina can be inspected thoroughly when a speculum is used, and the cervix can also be visualized. Usually, the uterus can be felt by the physician doing a bimanual examination and, in some cases, the adnexa (the tubes, ligaments, and ovaries) can also be felt; if the patient is tense and apprehensive about this examination, giving her a light anesthetic will relax her enough to permit the surgeon to do a more thorough examination.

CANCER OF THE VULVA

Cancer of the vulva is most common in older women—those in their sixties, seventies, and even eighties. This malignancy is often preceded by a premalignant leukoplakia of many years' standing. This condition is curable by removal of the plaque-like or ulcerous leukoplakic lesion. However, once cancer has developed, it is necessary to remove the entire vulva and regional lymph nodes because of the frequency of spread to these areas.

The cause of vulvar cancer is not known. It is assumed that the causative agent has a slow induction time or is one that happens to be present later in life. But since there is no definite knowledge about what causes cancer of the vulva, it is not possible to try to intercept its action in producing the disease. The suggestion has been made that, when the hormonal balance changes after the ovaries cease to function, women start secreting different substances in their urine, and these may cause cancer of the vulva. However, there is no evidence so far to verify this theory. Any lesion on the vulva should be regarded as possibly malignant and, if it does not respond promptly to local measures, should be biopsied. The overall cure rate for all stages and sizes of vulvar cancer is between 70 and 80 percent.

It is not unusual for the first signs of cancer of the vulva to be itching and burning. These discomforts may take the woman to her physician who will elicit a general history, give the patient a clinical examination, take a Papanicolaou smear or a biopsy, or possibly both, do a bimanual pelvic examination, and inspect the vagina and cervix. Later signs are pain and perhaps bleeding. Although the disease is usually recognizable on sight with the patient in the lithotomy position, when these signs have appeared, a biopsy will confirm the diagnosis.

The treatment for vulvar cancer must be tailored to the individual patient and the stage of the lesion. The physician will consider the size first; then whether it has apparently spread from the original site; and then whether this patient can be subjected to radical surgery or whether she should be treated by radiotherapy. If the disease has progressed to a stage that is not treatable by either surgery or radiotherapy, he will consider the use of chemotherapy which is more time-consuming but less traumatic than either of the other two possibilities.

Generally, however, the preferred treatment for cancer of the vulva consists of a complete removal of the vulva and a bilateral, superficial dissection of the lymph nodes in the femoral triangle below the inguinal canal and down to Hunter's canal. If any of these nodes are found to be positive for cancer, on one side or both, a deep dissection is done. This includes removal of the lymph nodes along the abdominal vessels from the external iliacs up to the common iliac and including the obturator nodes. (This operation was first described by Antoine Bassett at the University of Paris. It has been adopted by surgeons the world over as the standard treatment for cancer of the vulva.) The sartorius muscle which, with its parallel fibers, is about two inches wide in the upper thigh, is transplanted from its origin so that it lies over the denuded femoral vessels that would otherwise be covered only with skin; this also provides a flatter bed for the skin to drop back on, so that healing is probably enhanced. These wounds frequently break down and it is helpful then to have this muscle tissue covering the vessels and acting as a protective layer between them and the open air.

Hemovac catheters are inserted into the retroperitoneal space on both sides to provide proper drainage, because most of the lymph channels on both sides have been cut, and this results in the collection of fluid under the skin. The wound across the groin is closed, and the skin of the thigh is approximated to the vaginal mucosa. The procedure appears more traumatic than it actually is. Since no major cavity of the body is entered, the patients do remarkably well after operation. The chief problem is that most of them are elderly, and the immobilization necessary to obtain satisfactory healing leads to such complications as pneumonia which, in the past, has been the principal cause of death following radical vulvectomy. Today, antibiotics are used to combat pneumonia, but some bacteria are resistant to antibiotics and good nursing is still necessary to prevent pneumonia as well as sepsis, both of which continue to kill some of these patients.

Treatment of cancer of the vulva by radiation is slower than in cancer of the cervix because it is difficult to secure the radiation source in the proper location for an adequate length of time. Also tissues low in the vulva and around the vaginal orifice are quite sensitive to radiation and discomfort becomes an important factor. Finally, it is not the treatment of choice because the cure rate is much lower than that achieved with surgery.

Postoperatively, turning the patient frequently and positioning her with pillows will lessen tension on the suture line which, in these cases, is quite taut. Sometimes, even with good nursing care, wound breakdown occurs. When this happens, frequent irrigations with sterile saline solution, the heat lamp, and sitz baths are employed. Occasionally, butterfly flaps are applied, in the hope that this will encourage granulation. Sepsis is another serious complication that sometimes follows this operation.

By starting the patient on deep breathing, coughing, and leg exercises immediately after the surgery, the nurse can often save her from unnecessary endotracheal aspiration or the complication of atelectasis.

CANCER OF THE VAGINA

Cancer of the vagina is relatively uncommon, but when it does occur it is usually epidermoid in origin. Occasionally, this disease may arise in glandular remnants in the vaginal wall or in glands near the orifice. Rarely, a melanoma will arise in the vagina; this is a very aggressive cancer that is difficult and usually unsatisfactory to treat either by surgery or radiotherapy. Even a combination of these two modalities has not given good results.

Cancerous lesions in the vagina are often discovered during a routine pelvic examination. They also can be diagnosed from a Papanicolaou smear. Cancers in the lowermost part of the vagina are similar to vulvar malignancies in type, in manner of spread, and in problems associated with their treatment. Those in the middle and upper third of the vagina very closely resemble epidermoid carcinoma of the cervix in type and manner of spread. These are treated either by surgery similar to that employed for treatment of cancer of the vulva or by radiation.

CANCER OF THE CERVIX

The incidence of cervical cancer is second only to that of cancer of the breast. It occurs mostly in young women, women who married at an early age, women who have had children, and women from the lower socio-economic groups. The disease is rare in Jewish women and virginal women. The process may be present for as long as five to ten years before frank invasive cancer develops and, in this early stage, is often referred to as cancer in situ. Non-invasive cancer of the cervix is potentially 100 percent curable.

Cancer of the cervix, and the premalignant conditions that lead to it if left untreated, are most frequently diagnosed by the Papanicolaou cytologic examination. However, it is well known that frank invasive cancer of the cervix may not show up in this examination. This is due to the fact that often the superficial cells that are picked up in the smear are necrotic, and the picture is confused by an overlying infection. Therefore, whenever a lesion on the cervix is visible to the naked eye, it is best for the pathologist to look at a biopsied specimen under the microscope.

The initial symptom is almost always bleeding at times other than the menstrual period; that is, intermenstrually, postmenopausally, or following sexual intercourse.

Treatment for cancer of the cervix depends on the conditions present in any individual case and on the extent of the disease. Actually, the clinical stage of the tumor is the principal factor in determining the particular treatment that will be instituted. The following general classification of cancers of the cervix is used by most surgeons:

Stage I = the neoplastic growth is confined strictly to the cervix.

Stage II = the growth has spread to the upper part of the vagina, or into the surrounding tissues, but has not reached the pelvic wall.

Stage III = the growth has spread to the lower third of the vagina, or has reached the pelvic wall at some point.

Stage IV = the growth has spread to the bladder or rectum, or both, or to some organ beyond the pelvis.

The so-called dysplasias of the cervix—early changes in the cells that are considered potentially dangerous—can be treated quite simply and effectively by conization. This involves removing the affected part of the cervix, primarily the area at the squamo-columnar junction, around the os. The pathologist thus has an adequate piece of tissue for cytological examination and confirmation of the diagnosis of dysplasia. If a patient has neither cancer in situ nor invasive cancer, the amount of tissue removed for the biopsy is often adequate to effect a cure.

The same procedure is often used when the patient has cancer in situ in which the cells are indeed malignant, but have not begun to grow through the basement membrane into the surrounding tissue. Often patients with cancer in situ are quite young; it can occur in teenagers and is fairly common in women in their early twenties who have not yet had children. Therefore, if the biopsy shows the lesion to be carcinoma in situ, if the disease is confined to this lesion, and if resection at the margins is clear, conization may be all that is needed to effect a cure. If a patient can be carefully and competently followed up, she may then proceed to have children.

Invasive cancer of the cervix presents different problems for the gynecologist. This disease usually appears first as an ulcerating lesion on the surface of the cervix. It tends to spread by direct extension to the vaginal wall and out to the pelvic wall, as well as to the rectum and bladder. It often metastasizes to the pelvic lymph nodes but not often to distant organs. When the disease is diagnosed early in young women, or in women who are in good physical condition, the usual treatment consists of radical hysterectomy and pelvic lymphadenectomy. In various adaptations of the so-called Wertheim operation, the body and cervix of the uterus are removed and also the tissue around it—the parametrium; that is, the paracervical and paravaginal tissues on each side of the cervix extending out to the pelvic wall. This technique, described about 60 years ago by Dr. Ernst Wertheim, of Vienna, was the primary treatment for cancer of the cervix before the advent of radium, and it still has a place in the management of some forms of cancer in some patients. However, it fell into disuse for several years because of the high morbidity and mortality that attended it at a time when less was known about the operation and about postoperative care. In the years following World War II, the development of modern techniques of anesthesia, blood replacement, maintenance of electrolyte balance, and improved postoperative care prompted Dr. Joe Meigs, of Boston, to utilize the Wertheim principle in the development of an operation he called a "radical hysterectomy with pelvic node dissection." Basically, it consisted of Wertheim's operation plus dissection of all the lymph node-bearing areas around the external iliac and common iliac vessels on both sides, the hypogastric vessels, obturator spaces, and tissues around the bladder. This operation is now the standard surgical procedure.

At about the same time that Wertheim was developing his radical hysterectomy, Dr. Friedrich Schauta, also of Vienna, began doing a similar operation via the vaginal route. His procedure was much less traumatic and produced equally good results. There were fewer problems with anesthesia and fluid loss, and the operating morbidity and mortality were lower. This operation is still being done, especially in Austria where it is the primary means of treating cancer of the cervix.

At Memorial Hospital three types of operations are done for invasive cancer of the cervix and uterus which has extended beyond the tissue removed in a radical hysterectomy and pelvic node dissection: 1) the anterior pelvic exenteration; 2) the posterior pelvic exenteration; and, 3) the total pelvic exenteration. These operations are all variations of the radical hysterectomy and pelvic lymphadenectomy, plus excision of the bladder and or rectum, with diversion of the urinary and/or fecal streams. They are all massive procedures and an immense amount of tissue is removed. Serious problems often develop in regard to fluid and electrolyte loss, the formation of fistulae from the ureter which comes down beside the cervix and sometimes has to be dissected out, and impaired blood supply to the parts. The advantages are that the tumor can be removed in its entirety and the outlook is generally good, with about one-fourth of the patients being cured. The anterior or total exenteration involves transplantation of the ureters into an isolated loop of bowel (sigmoid, ileum, or jejunum), which may or may not be brought out to the abdominal surface with the creation of a stoma. This is essentially a conduit and does not serve as a storage bladder. The posterior pelvic exenteration combines the radical hysterectomy and pelvic lymphadenectomy with an abdominal perineal resection of the rectum, and necessitates the construction of a colostomy. The total pelvic exenteration consists of a radical hysterectomy, pelvic lymphadenectomy, excision of the bladder, transplantation of the ureters into the bowel, abdominal resection of the rectum, and the creation of a colostomy. For this operation, the patient must be prepared in terms of cleaning out the bowel completely so that the surgeon has a clean field to work in and contamination can be kept to a minimum.

The particular operation used depends on the location and extent of the tumor. Among the factors taken into consideration by the doctor when he is evaluating the patient for an exenteration are age, stage of the disease, whether the patient has received radiotherapy, and very importantly, whether he thinks the patient can cope with the conditions that follow exenteration. The exenterations are done mostly on patients who have recurrent cancer after radiation; patients in which the disease remains confined to the tissues that can be removed by this operation. Fortunately, this is often the case in cancer of the cervix which, biologically, tends to remain in the pelvis for a long period of time before it metastasizes to areas that cannot be reached by surgery.

How is a woman who is to have a pelvic exenteration told of this possibility, and how are her various questions about it answered? This is a difficult question, because what and how a woman is told about the proposed operation depends almost entirely on the individual patient and the particular doctor involved. Physicians vary in their basic concepts about how much to tell the patient. Of course, it is impossible for a woman who is going to receive 30 cobalt treatments after surgery to think she is being operated on for some minor ailment. Most of them know when they are admitted to the hospital that they have cancer. They know, too, that they are desperately ill, and that their disease is life-threatening. They are seeking and are willing to accept almost any help that is available, and the possibility of an exenteration provides a very real hope that there is at least some chance for life.

These patients should be told what an exenteration involves in terms of a colostomy and an ileal conduit, and how these are managed postoperatively. They should also be assured that, although they give operative consent for these things to be done, no more will be done than is absolutely necessary to save this person's life.

Pyelonephritis is the most common, and certainly the most serious, complication that follows pelvic exenteration. When the patient has an ileal conduit and the urinary stream is separated from the fecal stream, the problem is not so great. Most of the cases of pyelonephritis with kidney loss result from chronic infection that develops when the ureters are transplanted into the colon as in a wet colostomy, or when urine and stool are evacuated together through the rectum. Only recurrent cancer exceeds kidney disease as the cause of death after this surgery.

Although the pelvic exenteration operations would appear to be so drastic as to be incompatible with social adjustment postoperatively, many patients with both a colostomy and a urinary conduit manage to live quite normal social and professional lives. Among the patients who have been treated by pelvic exenteration at Memorial Hospital, the one who has survived the longest was operated on in 1947 by Dr. Alexander Brunschwig, who originally devised the operation. The overall survival rate for patients treated at this hospital (approximately one thousand in the last 20 years) is about 20 percent, including cases that received the treatment early in this surgical program as a purely desperation measure, with the sole purpose of providing palliation. After it began to be done only for curative purposes, the survival rate has improved to about 30 to 35 percent, with many of the patients having a fairly high quality of survival. Patients are expected to recover from the operation quite rapidly and to be at home taking care of their families within a reasonably short period of time. Follow-up is simplified because the tumor has been removed and the organs, too, so it is easier for the physician to determine whether or not a recurrence has taken place.

Radiotherapy is often the modality that is used for cervical cancer that involves the parametrium and for early cancers that occur in women who are not good operative risks. The radical hysterectomy is a major procedure that can take as long as six or seven hours, and women who are grossly over-weight, diabetic, or who have had a myocardial infarction are not good surgical risks. The radiotherapy used usually consists of an intrauterine and an intravaginal applicator of a radioactive source, followed by external high-voltage radiation.

CANCER OF THE ENDOMETRIUM

Cancer of the endometrium occurs chiefly in older women, but not always. Bleeding is the primary symptom of this disease. It has been estimated that 30 to 40 percent of postmenopausal bleeding is caused by endometrial cancer. Intermenstrual bleeding in younger women is also indicative of endometrial cancer in some cases. In these younger women with endometrial cancer, there is usually a history of anovulatory flow.

Endometrial cancer is sometimes discovered through a routine Papanic-olaou examination, but this is not as reliable in these cases as in cancer of the cervix. This is because cells shed from the uterus are not as easily picked up in the top of the vagina as are those from the cervix. (This is one of the shortcomings of the self-administered "Pap test.") However, if the smear is taken by a competent examiner, and includes two specimens—one from the mouth of the uterus that picks up cells that may show changes taking place in the cervix, and one from the posterior vaginal fornix (the so-called vaginal pool) that may pick up cells shed from the inside of the uterus—the chances of obtaining a positive result are greatly increased. Because of the possible unreliability of the Papanicolaou examination in diagnosing this particular gynecologic malignancy, the surgeon often relies for his diagnosis on the pathologic examination of curettings or an endometrial biopsy.

Cancer of the endometrium is treated by surgical procedures similar to but simpler than those outlined for cancer of the cervix. Because the disease, in general, is up in the fundus of the uterus, it can be removed with little more than a simple hysterectomy. At Memorial Hospital, the surgeons tend to do an operation that is not nearly as radical as the one done for cancer of the cervix, because it has not been shown that the super-radical procedure results in any better cure rate for this particular disease than a simple total hysterectomy. Actually, the cure rate for endometrial cancer is about 70 percent. Preoperative radiation therapy is now being used in most of these patients.

One of the common sites for recurrence of cancer of the endometrium is the vault of the vagina, or the remnant left after the uterus has been removed and, for this reason, the patients are further treated by radiation after their surgery.

In the later stages of cancer of the endometrium, when the disease has infiltrated down into the cervix or has spread beyond it, treatment is primarily by radiotherapy.

CANCER OF THE OVARY

Cancer of the ovary is not as common a disease as cancer of the cervix, but, unfortunately, it is the disease that kills most of the women who die of a gynecologic cancer. In 1970, about five New York state women died of cancer of the ovary for every three who died of cancer of the cervix. This particular statistic is fairly representative of the mortality rate in the United States generally. The reason for this high rate is that cancer of the ovary is the gynecologic malignancy most difficult to diagnose by our present techniques. Unfortunately, in its early stages the disease is asymptomatic. Often, by the time the patient sees a doctor, the symptoms have become those of advanced ovarian cancer. Ovarian cancer is associated with massive ascites and spread of the disease throughout the abdomen, or with a big mass that has grown rapidly and can be felt by external examination of the abdomen. By this time the patient may have lost considerable weight, increased in girth, and have such symptoms as abdominal pain, dysuria, urinary frequency, constipation, and sometimes, vaginal bleeding.

Several suggestions as to how ovarian cancer might be diagnosed earlier than it is at present have been advanced. One recommendation is that Papanicolaou smears be taken from the cul-de-sac that lies between the uterus and the rectum. This has been done by some diagnosticians. It has also been recommended that whenever cancer of the ovary is suspected, the doctor perform a laparoscopy; that is, an examination with a cystoscope-like instrument that is passed into the abdominal cavity so that one can take a look at the ovaries. Any abnormality in the pelvis should be regarded with suspicion until it is proven not to be a cancer of the ovary. Furthermore, less strict criteria for laparotomy for the removal of ovarian lumps or ad-nexal masses should be employed than has been the case in the past; that is, a mass had to persist over a certain number of cycles; had to be of a certain size; and had to be solid rather than cystic before the surgeon would con-sider doing a laparotomy. The concensus now seems to be that the diag-nostician ought to rule out the idea that perhaps these masses might just be simple cyclic physiologic phenomena; that after they are followed for a month at various times in the menstrual cycle to see if they disappear, they should be regarded in much the same light as a lump in the breast is re-garded, that is, potentially lethal until proven not to be. Hopefully, a blood test or serological test for this disease will one day be developed. But until it is, aggressiveness in the exploration and evaluation of any unexplained mass in a woman's abdomen is the only acceptable course.

The cure rate for cancer of the ovary is very low. The reason for this is that these cancers are usually far advanced by the time the patient seeks help. Only about 25 percent of patients with ovarian cancer survive for five years or longer.

Patients with cancer of the ovary challenge the ingenuity of the patient, the surgeon, the radiologist, and the chemotherapist. Also, surgery is some-times required to relieve an intestinal obstruction which is a dreaded com-plication because these patients often then develop fistulas, and they tend to have reobstructions.

Every now and then, even in advanced cases, patients do very well on radiotherapy. Chemotherapy, too, offers some significant palliation in one-quarter to one-third of patients; it makes them more comfortable and pro-longs their lives. Women have not only been cured of their primary tumor with chemotherapy alone, but of metastatic disease as well. Many have lived for significantly long periods of time—well over five years. On the relatively rare occasions when the diagnosis is made early, and the primary tumor is confined to the ovary (or ovaries) (Stage I), treatment by hysterectomy and bilateral salpingo-oophorectomy (at Memorial Hospital) has resulted in about 65 percent survival rate. The addition of radiotherapy to the pelvic area has not seemed to make any difference in the five-year survival rate or in the length of time the patients have lived. About two-thirds of these patients have lived several years without any evidence of the disease.

Cancer of the ovary is a rather odd tumor which does not generally recur locally or persist locally as cancer of the cervix sometimes does. This disease spreads by early seeding from the ovaries into the peritoneal cavity, and it implants itself on the serosa of the bowel, the parietal peritoneum and omentum, and over the liver and diaphragm. Some years ago, it was thought that perhaps the best way to handle this kind of dissemination would be to give a good dose of radiation to the entire peritoneal cavity. Now this has become possible since the introduction of radioactive isotopes. Initially, radioactive zinc, then radioactive gold and, finally radioactive phosphorus were tried and a technique was achieved whereby the peritoneal surfaces of the abdomen could receive radiation without radiating the entire abdomen from an external machine—not an easy thing to do. Patients at Memorial Hospital are given about 10 or 15 millicuries of phosphorus-32 into the peritoneal cavity after abdominal surgery is completed and, as a result, the five-year survival rate has risen from about 65 percent to about 90 percent in patients with stage I ovarian cancer. It is unfortunate that only a small percentage of patients with cancer of the ovary are in this early stage when first seen by a physician and can be treated in this manner. The procedure is rather simple. When the operation is finished, two polyethylene sprinkler tubes that look like tiny garden hoses and give off a fine spray from the end of one to the end of the other, are placed through a large needle puncture in the abdominal wall. One of them is placed across the upper abdomen and the other across the lower abdomen. The abdominal wall is closed tightly and no drain is placed either at the place the tubes are inserted or in the pelvis. The radiotherapist accompanies the patient to the recovery room and pumps phosphorus-32 into these tubes. The radioactive substance spreads through the abdomen, the tubes are withdrawn, and that is the only treatment given.

The question often comes up as to when and why the ovaries are sometimes removed and sometimes left behind when a hysterectomy is done. This is usually decided after considering the patient's age and the disease for which the surgery is being done. The incidence of ovarian cancer is not as high as cancer of the cervix, but its cure rate is low unless the disease is diagnosed early. If the uterus is being removed for a benign tumor and the woman is in the menopausal age group, the surgeon is likely to remove the ovaries as a preventive measure. If the woman is young, and the tumor for which the surgery is being done is benign, or if it is a stage I cancer of the cervix, the ovaries are not usually removed.

CANCER OF THE FALLOPIAN TUBE

In many ways, cancer of the fallopian tubes resembles cancer of the ovary, although it is a far less common disease. The tube is thin-walled, and the disease perforates it and then spreads rapidly. But patients can be cured of this disease. Here, too, as in cancer of the ovary, there is an adnexal mass that is difficult, sometimes impossible, to define. The Papanicolaou smear can occasionally be of diagnostic value because cancerous cells may come down through the tube, through the uterus, and into the vagina where they can be picked up in a Papanicolaou smear.

Treatment for cancer of the fallopian tube is essentially the same as for ovarian cancer. Frequently cancer of the ovary involves cancer of the tube also and, in these instances, it may be that the cancer arose in the tube and then involved the ovary, so this kind of tumor may be more common than the statistics indicate. Although there are clear-cut criteria for making an accurate diagnosis of cancer of the fallopian tube, a differential diagnosis is not very important because the treatment is the same as for ovarian cancer. Also because of this similarity, the disease has a poor prognosis.

COMPREHENSIVE CARE FOR THE PATIENT WITH A GYNECOLOGIC MALIGNANCY

The Nurse-Patient Interview

The nurse is usually the first professional person to see the patient after she enters the hospital. The initial nurse-patient interview can set the mood for the patient's entire hospitalization. It can be the basis for establishing short- and long-term nursing goals, and for the nursing care plan. If this is the patient's first admission to the hospital, she should be given information about the various routines, and an explanation of the functions of the staff members who will be seeing her frequently.

During her early interviews with the patient, the nurse can help dispel some of the "old wives' tales" that the woman may have heard regarding her female organs, and help her distinguish between fact and fiction. Many women think that after they have a hysterectomy they are not really women any more and that they will not be able to function sexually as they did before. It is up to the nurse to tell the patient that this is entirely untrue and why it is untrue. The nurse should plan to make rounds with the doctor so that she can be completely aware of what the doctor has told the patient and can reenforce this information later on when she is alone with her.

The newly admitted patient may have many worries. She has had some symptoms that may have been alarming and, because gynecological disorders involve such an intimate part of the anatomy, it may have been difficult for her to seek medical advice. Then when she is told that she must enter the hospital for surgery or whatever seems appropriate, she is often in a very disturbed emotional state, because she has had to leave her husband and children, and step out of the role that she has functioned in most successfully in the past. As the nurse gets to know the patient, she can pick up specific clues that might relate to such problems as the fact that there may be no one at home to care for the children. In such a case, the social worker can often be helpful in solving this particularly worrisome problem. Sometimes just making arrangements to have the children cared for will make it possible for the patient to remain in the hospital for her much-needed treatment.

One important fact the patient should understand early in her hospital stay is that while several members of the team will be doing things for and to her, everyone works collaboratively according to the medical plan of care. The concept of flow of care needs to be emphasized.

Preparation for Surgery

The preoperative care of the patient who will have gynecologic surgery includes many tests and procedures not included in the preoperative preparation of patients for other types of surgery. The nurse should explain these to the patient in terms she can understand.

The physical examination will include a pelvic examination, and often Papanicolaou smears will be repeated several times. The patient's body weight, the fluid and electrolyte determinations, and the laboratory reports on blood tests that are ordered, furnish the base line for the doctor's management of the patient preoperatively and allow him to make any needed replacement prior to surgery. Along with these tests, an EKG and a urinalysis add to the base line for treatment during and after surgery.

An intravenous pyelogram (IVP) is often ordered. To the gynecologic surgeon it can show displacement of pelvic organs as well as hydronephrosis caused by a pelvic mass pressing against the kidney. It can also serve as an indicator for the kind of management the patient will require during the time of surgery for the urinary diversion.

Cystometric studies are also done. Cystometry is a very simple procedure in which saline is instilled into the bladder to determine its capacity and also to demonstrate its muscle tone.

It may come as a shock to the patient to know that she must undergo all of these tests, when she thinks she has come to the hospital just to get a little vaginal bleeding taken care of. She may say, "There's nothing wrong with my heart. Why do I have to have an electrocardiogram?" Many things the care team takes for granted on admission of all patients may cause anxiety in the gynecologic patient. This is important for the nurse to realize because she may have to spend most of the short preoperative time with the patient just answering questions. But if the nurse can answer the questions in a meaningful way, it may help the patient to approach her surgery in a more positive mood. She may fear any number of things—disfigurement, cancer or the spread of cancer, or the consequences of radiation—many of which she may not mention except, perhaps, her immediate fear about what will happen to her in the operating room. The nurse can do much to allay this particular fear by explaining to the patient that she will be well sedated before she goes to the operating room, and that she will be well cared for by nurse specialists in the recovery room.

For the patient who is to have radical pelvic surgery, certain preventive nursing measures will help to make the postoperative course smoother and less complicated. The preparation of the vagina for surgery involves the use of sulfonamides, antibiotics, suppositories, and douches. Sometimes the doctor will agree that the patient be allowed to take care of the douching herself, but not all patients are knowledgeable about how to perform this task. In fact, the nurse often has to teach them the rudiments of female anatomy. This preparation is also required for the insertion of uterine or vaginal applicators for a radiation source. Any draining lesions must be cleared up before the patient is scheduled for surgery. Enemas and laxatives are often ordered, along with sulfa and antibiotic therapy, to prepare the bowel for surgical manipulation and/or dissection. The patient is usually placed on a low residue diet at least two days prior to surgery, and on the day just before the operation she receives only clear liquids. During the preoperative period, the patient's intake and output should be strictly recorded because this record, along with fluid and electrolyte determinations, can serve as a guide for fluid replacement which may be required to correct the dehydration that can occur rapidly when the patient reacts to the bowel preparation with violent diarrhea.

Because gynecologic surgery interferes with circulation in the extremities, elastic bandages are applied postoperatively and, when the patient has a history of thrombophlebitis, they are applied for several days before surgery. The bandages should be applied, with even pressure throughout, to the entire area from the toes to the mid-thigh, and should include the heel and knee. Careful palpation of pulses at the ankle should always be done prior to putting on these bandages to be sure there is no arterial insufficiency.

If the patient will be returned to an environment that is different in any way from her preoperative environment, she should be prepared for this change. All patients should be told that they will go from the operating room to a recovery room. In addition, if the patient is going to return from the operating room with vaginal or uterine applicators for insertion of a radiation source, she should be told that she will be placed in a single room to reduce the radiation hazard to people who will be having contact with her. She may be relieved to know that her family and friends will still be able to visit her even though they will remain outside of the area of radiation exposure. She should know that she will receive adequate nursing care and attention but that the nurse will perform the essential tasks as quickly as possible and then leave the room. It would also be well to tell her that when she returns from the recovery room she will be placed on bed rest, and will have a Foley catheter inserted. Knowing these things before going to the operating room often makes it possible for the patient to be more relaxed and cooperative during the postoperative period.

Routine preoperative preparation, of course, includes a bath with germicidal soap. The patient must void immediately before going to surgery to make sure that the bladder is empty, and to avoid trauma to it during surgery. The "prep" includes a vaginal "prep" and is usually done by the nurses on the unit. The nurse who does the "prepping" should know the patient's history, and especially whether any previous treatment has included radiation. The disease may extend down into the vagina and, if radiation therapy has been used, the tissues may be extremely friable.

It is essential that all preoperative procedures be done efficiently and that all reports that may be abnormal are relayed to the doctor as quickly as possible.

Care in the Operating Room

The operating room nurse plays a vital role on the team that cares for the patient having surgery for a gynecologic malignancy. The nature of the surgery in these conditions causes considerable emotional stress and, during the time immediately preceding the operation, the nurse can communicate either security or fear. During the actual surgery, her responsibility for the patient's physical needs continues. The judgment, skill, and quiet efficiency required in caring for the patient in the operating room make the presence of a professional nurse necessary. She knows how to function expertly in such emergencies as hemorrhage or cardiac failure. The surgeon too is often dependent on her for assistance. Whether a patient is going to be cured by her surgery is often determined in a relatively short period of time in the operating room.

The high point of the patient's hospitalization is her operation, and probably the most psychologically stressful experience she has is actually going to the operating room. Consequently, she needs assurance and reassurance, either verbal or nonverbal, when she arrives there. The nurse confirms the identity of the patient by calling her by name or by checking her Identaband. She checks the chart to see that the various required forms are there and are in order. The operative consent, in particular, must be filled out completely and, if it is not, and if the patient has been premedicated, there are medicolegal aspects to be considered.

The operating room nurse has to prepare herself for each operation, whether it is a dilatation and curettage or a pelvic exenteration, and must learn the different procedures that are performed. She also needs to know the preferences of each individual surgeon. Preoperative communication with the resident or surgeon may pave the way for a very smooth operation, and the nurse must be flexible in adapting to a change in plans. Positioning the patient for surgery is of great importance; the nurse should concern herself with the patient's safety and comfort and call upon other members of the team for assistance if necessary. At Memorial Hospital, draping is also done by the nurse, sometimes with the assistance of the surgeon. Blood loss, operating time, and even the final outcome of the operation may be directly related to the nurse's efficiency, so she must develop a total awareness of all that is happening around her and act accordingly. Standardization of procedures, instrument setups, and drapes are essential. However, patient care cannot be standardized; therefore, flexibility, dexterity, and technical confidence are all desirable skills in the operating room nurse whose patients include those having gynecologic surgery. The end result of adequate preparation on the part of the nurses within and outside of the sterile field should be a successful operation for the patient and a satisfied surgeon.

Postoperative Care of the Patient with a Pelvic Exenteration

The postoperative care required by gynecologic patients often puts them in the intensive care unit. Not all of them go to the ICU, however, although all require detailed attention because their condition may be unstable. The nurse must be able to recognize and evaluate their needs in order to understand what has to be done for them.

Seventy percent of patients who have pelvic exenterations have some kind of major complication postoperatively. Thus, they require nursing care of the highest order. Many of the problems that arise are concerned with the care of the ileal conduit stoma, because the urine drains out onto the skin and causes irritation. Because of this factor, the nursing focus is on this area. The patient returns from the operating room with a temporary appliance in place over the stoma. Since the stoma is often quite edematous immediately after surgery, the hole in the bag must be fairly large. Consequently, the nurse must be very attentive from the start, and deal with the problem competently in order to prevent widespread excoriation of the skin around the stoma.

The skin must be kept as clean and dry as possible, and the bag securely in place, if this condition is to be prevented. After routine cleansing of the skin, the application of tincture of benzoin and Karaya powder helps to protect the skin and to keep the bag attached. If the skin is excoriated, the Karaya powder is used before the benzoin is applied. It is important that there be no leakage, because accurate monitoring of the patient's urinary output is essential, in addition to the need to protect the skin by keeping it dry. The nurse must be very conscientious about this; continuity of care around the clock is of the utmost importance. The bag is held in place only by adhesive during the early postoperative period and is inclined to come off when the patient moves about in bed, so constant observation is important.

As soon as the edema of the stoma has subsided and the patient is able to tolerate a diet, she is fitted with a permanent appliance after consideration of her size, weight, and the bag most suitable for her. This cannot be done unless the skin has been kept in good condition by meticulous skin care and avoidance of unnecessary appliance changes. The patient is taught from the start to care for her ileal conduit stoma.

The nurse must make the patient feel that she is being given really good nursing care because, although she may have been told exactly what would happen during and after the operation and that she would be eliminating urine through a stoma on the abdominal wall, the patient never seems to be fully prepared for the actual situation. Therefore the nurse's attitude at this stage is as important as her nursing skill. She must take a positive approach to the care of the stoma, of the skin, and of the patient in general, in order to help her and her family adjust to the patient's postoperative requirements, for this is the foundation of her recovery and her rehabilitation.

Patients with an ileal conduit often complain of odor from the bag, but this is not likely to occur if the appliance is changed every five to six days and carefully washed with soap and water. It is usually the alkaline content of the urine that causes the odor. Adding cranberry juice to the diet is effective in reducing the alkaline nature of the urine and hence in preventing the bag from becoming "smelly." Unpleasant odors that persist after the bag has been washed and aired may sometimes be overcome by soaking the appliance in a urinary appliance deodorant solution or a solution of ½ cup of vinegar and ¼ cup of Clorox in a quart of water. The appliance should then be rinsed and allowed to dry thoroughly prior to reuse.

If the skin around the stoma becomes excoriated, a Colly-seel or Karaya seal appliance is recommended. Also, the application of heat, using an ordinary goose-neck lamp, will hasten epithelialization. The permanent appliance should never be used until the skin is healed. In the meantime, the nurse continues to carry out the measures to protect the skin that have been described above.

The skin around a colostomy stoma is also protected by a temporary drainage bag which is applied in the operating room. The same care that is prescribed for the ileal stoma is utilized, and is very satisfactory. At first, there is only minimal drainage from the colostomy. It may be mucus-like or it may be a watery stool, so it is important to have a bag always in place.

Severe excoriation can also occur around a colostomy stoma. The pH of the fecal drainage depends on the level of the bowel from which it comes. If it is from the upper part of the small intestine it will be acid in reaction, and if from the lower part it will generally be alkaline. A buffering agent such as Amphogel or Maalox can be used, but the real secret in preventing skin problems is to keep the fecal drainage from coming into contact with the skin. This is accomplished by close fitting of the bag and its proper application to the skin so that it will adhere and not leak.

Patients who have a colostomy in addition to their ileal conduit are taught to take care of that stoma also. As soon as bowel sounds return, which is usually about five or six days postoperatively, routine colostomy irrigations are started. The equipment and procedure are explained fully and the first irrigation is done while the patient is still in bed. She will probably be rather weak, but she can participate in the procedure by holding some of the equipment or lubricating the tube, perhaps. If the nurse takes the attitude that the procedure will not create any problems, the patient is likely to start out feeling the same way. The next irrigation is done in the bathroom and, at this point, the patient can be instructed in how to judge the amount of fluid she can tolerate and how long it will take to complete the irrigation. As the teaching program progresses, the patient learns that her colostomy may be regulated by irrigation and that eventually she will not need to wear a colostomy appliance. A small gauze square is all that will be necessary to protect the stoma. It is helpful if the same nurse can be assigned to teach the patient and help with the irrigation for several consecutive days so there will be continuity and consistency in the instruction.

Follow-up Care

The follow-up program for a patient who has had therapy for a gynecologic malignancy should continue throughout her life. Regular examinations by a gynecologist should include rectal and breast examinations. If radiation therapy was used in her treatment, she should also be seen by a radiologist regularly.

The transfer from hospital to home is more smoothly accomplished when the nurses have prepared the patient for it by their accepting, understanding and hopeful attitude. Many times the gynecologic cancer patient has abdominal or vaginal fistulas that drain constantly and require several hours of nursing care daily. Nurses spend time making her comfortable physically by utilizing nursing techniques that are directed toward preventing drainage from excoriating her skin. They also focus on the patient's feelings and her reactions in coping with her body alteration. But the patient's entire progress depends, to a great extent, on the nurses' attitudes while caring for her. Her feelings about whether she will be acceptable socially are often based on clues she gets from them. When nurses accept her as a complete woman whose condition is not revolting or repulsive, the patient is more apt to return home in a hopeful mood and to enter the rehabilitative phase of her illness in a positive frame of mind.

Many patients are apprehensive about whether they will be able to care for their stoma or stomas after they leave the protective environment of the hospital where they can always call for help if a problem arises. Because of this fact, the nursing department makes a routine referral to the Visiting Nurse Association when the patient who has had an exenteration is about to be discharged. This should be done early enough so that plans can be made for a visiting nurse to see the patient the first day she is at home. Even though the foundations of self care have been well established during the patient's hospitalization, she finds things very different at home where she must use the family bathroom and set up her own equipment. She tends to become nervous and insecure about whether she can ever learn to manage her own irrigations. The visiting nurse can be very supportive and helpful at this time. She can also evaluate whether the patient needs additional help from some other agency and, if this is the case, she can refer the patient to a social worker.

When the patient returns to the clinic or outpatient department for follow-up care, she frequently has complaints about her appliance. Often, double adhesive rings are used with tincture of benzoin to protect the skin, and a cement is used for adherence, but sometimes the technique of applying the bag has to be changed or altered so as to make the bag secure enough to prevent leakage.

Most doctors recommend that the bag be changed every three or four days after the patient goes home, if only to check the skin underneath for irritation or excoriation, and to observe the stoma. Some people who have worn an appliance for a longer time say that they do not change the bag oftener than every six or seven days, and that they learn, after a while, just how often they must do this. As to the appliance itself, it is fitted to the particular patient, and she should have two, preferably three, so that she can rotate them. The stoma may continue to shrink for some time after the patient leaves the hospital and, in this case, the patient will be re-fitted with an appliance to suit the size of the stoma and protect the skin around it.

Although it is often the visiting nurse who brings the social worker into the care group for the patient at home, in many instances the patient has seen a social worker while in the hospital, and this same person visits her at home. While the patient was still in the hospital, the worker may have ascertained whether she had relatives or neighbors who could be depended on to help her with her personal care or with household duties. She may also have determined whether the patient should be referred to The American Cancer Society, Cancer Care, or some other agency. Often, too, the patient needs to talk to someone outside the family in regard to her feelings as a woman and mother following her radical surgery, and the social worker can be helpful just by listening. Sometimes the patient will test the worker's reactions by showing her the wound, scar, or whatever; probably because she is trying to find out how acceptable, or unacceptable, her disfigurement is.

Many of these patients are eligible for public assistance, but securing it is often a tedious and frustrating process for the patient, and the social worker can work with the patient to secure the help she needs. Very often the family has been getting along on a minimal budget without welfare assistance but, when the time comes for the patient to be cared for at home, extra help is needed in terms of a homemaker, housekeeper, or perhaps just someone to come in and clean every week or two, and this cannot be managed on the family's limited income. In such cases, the worker can help to process an application to the department of social services and funds will be provided to meet this extra expense of the patient's illness.

QUESTIONS AND ANSWERS

Q. How do nurses usually relate to patients who are anticipating radical gynecologic surgery, and do they draw parallels with themselves?

A. Of course the nurse may draw parallels with herself if the patient is young, or if she reminds her of her mother or some other older relative. The nurse-patient relationship in these situations is often difficult to deal with, because the patient may have many distressing fears. As far as the surgery is concerned, most patients expect to return from the operating room alive and, hopefully, cured. Their most disturbing preoperative thoughts are usually concerned with what the operation will do to their role as wife, mother, and homemaker. The nurse needs to understand their normal life styles before she can answer some of their questions. She needs to know how they have adjusted to previous stressful situations in order to help them.

Q. When a hysterectomy is to be performed, is the possible effect on their future sexual relations discussed with both the husband and wife?

A. Often the physician sees the patient first in his private office and her husband accompanies her. This gives the physician an ideal opportunity to discuss the nature of the operation proposed and the changes it will have, if any, on the sexual relationship between the husband and wife. In the clinic situation, the patient is often from out of town and the husband is not present when she is first seen by a resident. But after she is admitted to the hospital, and before the operation is carried out, the resident tells her what the operation consists of, what the anatomical defect will be, and what effects this will have on her sex life.

Q. What are some possible ways for nurses to handle the patient's questions about what her sexual feelings, sexual adequacy, and body image will be after extensive gynecologic surgery?

A. Much of what the nurse says will depend on what the doctor has told the patient.

If the nurse has had good communication with the patient preoperatively, she knows how the patient has adapted to serious problems in the past, and so has some idea of how she might accept her present situation. These questions are important to the nurse, because they give her an idea of how the patient might accept her present situation. Her answers will give the patient an idea of what her social acceptability will be, and this general help is sometimes more useful than specific answers. One of the ways the nurse can help the post-surgical patient is to help her to feel socially acceptable.

Q. At what age should routine Papanicolaou examinations be started?

A. "Pap" tests should be started at whatever age the woman begins to have sexual intercourse, since every study that has been made of the etiology of cervical cancer has shown that its incidence correlates with sexual activity. The virginal female should start having the tests at about 20 or 21 years of age.

Q. Are any statistics available concerning the findings when fluid from the cul-de-sac have been subjected to the Papanicolaou examination?

A. Whether cancer cells are picked up when fluid from the cul-de-sac is examined by a "Pap" test depends on whether there is ovarian carcinoma in situ. This test is not done for Memorial Hospital patients with ovarian cancer because studies that have been repeated several times have shown that only in about 26 of 1,000 cases will the cells found be abnormal and, of these, very few turn out to be cancer. Most pathologists think that a rather peculiar layer seen on the ovaries of these women is simply a layer of serosal cells that are not at all malignant or premalignant. Two other studies, carried out elsewhere, were also discouraging because no cancer cells were found when over 1,000 women were given the cul-de-sac test, but many known cases of ovarian cancer were missed.

Q. Should a woman continue having Papanicolaou examinations after having a total abdominal hysterectomy?

A. Yes, because there is still a possibility that the patient will develop carcinoma of the vagina. Also, a number of women who have hysterectomies because of dysplasia or cervical cancer in situ may develop cancer of the vagina, so they too should have the "Pap" test, along with a general and a pelvic examination, at regular intervals after recovery from surgery.

Q. Has there been an increase of cancer of the cervix or endometrium since IUD's have come into common use?

A. There does not appear to be any evidence at present that would implicate the intrauterine devices in carcinogenesis. However, the IUD may not be as effective as the contraceptive pill in controlling conception for the following reasons: 1) about 15 to 20 percent of women reject the IUD; that is, they expel it; 2) some women react to it with very heavy bleeding and it has to be removed; and 3) it is sometimes the source of erosion or infection, and, again, has to be removed. For many women, it is an adequate method of contraception.

Q. When a woman has an IUD and becomes pregnant, is the IUD removed or left in to be expelled during delivery?

A. It is left in until delivery because the physician tries not to do anything to the uterus that contains a normally implanted pregnancy.

Q. Is there any real evidence that contraceptive pills cause cancer?

A. There does not appear to be any concrete evidence that contraceptive pills cause cancer. However, a study done under the auspices of Planned Parenthood reported that a comparison of "Pap" tests done on women who chose the contraceptive pill and those who chose the diaphragm or condom showed a higher incidence of carcinoma in situ in women who used the pill than in those who used either of the other two methods of contraception. This has been widely interpreted as implying that contraceptive pills cause cervical cancer. But it is equally possible that the diaphragm or the condom protects the woman from a causative agent such as a virus or, more importantly, that women taking oral contraceptives have intercourse more frequently.

Because contraceptive pills are the most effective method of birth control outside of surgery, they came into wide general use before many controls or studies were set up. By the time studies were set up, the subjects were usually women who had had multiple pregnancies or who had some gynecologic condition that correlates with a high incidence of cancer in situ, dysplasia, or invasive cancer. Consequently, there is no way to find out which women might be likely to develop cancer from the use of contraceptive pills.

An important fact about the use of birth control pills is that the woman who takes them is not the same endocrinologically as she would be otherwise. This is because, to be effective, the pill must contain a pro-gestational agent. Some physicians have expressed concern about the long-term effects of suppression of pituitary gonadotropin. Others are concerned about the long-term effects on the breast in regard to the development of breast cancer.

All that can be said now is that if there is an effect, it is not very great.

Q. Do monilial or trichomonal vaginal infections with constant chronic irritation predispose a woman to cancer of the vulva?

A. There is no evidence to indicate monilial or trichomonal infections are implicated in the causation of vulvar cancer. Some granulomatous dis-eases, condylomata, and perhaps viruses may be implicated in the causation of cancer elsewhere.

It is important to note that there is a high incidence of venereal disease among women with cancer of the vulva.

Q. Is pregnancy and delivery possible after vulvectomy?

A. There is no reason why a patient who has had a vulvectomy cannot become pregnant. Delivery might be difficult, however, and a cesarean section would probably be done. Since most of the patients who require vulvectomy are in the older age group, this problem does not often arise.

Q. Is sexual intercourse possible after vulvectomy? If so, is it enjoyable for the woman?

A. Yes, intercourse is still possible after vulvectomy, because the vagina is still present. Reasonably satisfactory sexual intercourse is possible after many radical pelvic procedures. It may involve some change in position or in technique. In some situations, the only change needed is for the woman to keep her thighs close together; this lengthens the distance from the vaginal vault so that, although the penetration is not so deep, it can be satisfying to both partners.

Sexual compatibility depends not only on the physical organs that are connected during intercourse, but it also involves a great deal of psychological coordination. The most important factor in relation to in-tercourse after pelvic surgery is whether the partners care enough for each other that they are willing to make adaptations to techniques that will give both of them sexual satisfaction. Some women have reported enjoying intercourse more after having radical pelvic surgery than they did before.

Q. Is plastic surgery ever employed in the reconstruction of the vaginal orifice and canal?

A. Yes. However, one of the problems in the treatment of gynecologic cancer is that regardless of the modality employed, be it radiation or surgery, deformity does occur in many cases. The physician who treats these patients tries first to cure the disease, and second to reconstruct the remaining functioning organs to whatever degree is possible.

In the past, the surgeon tended to proceed without considering reconstruction, because it was believed that a better result could be obtained that way. Currently, the tendency is to attempt some reconstructive measures. For example, an artificial vagina has been constructed by making a cavity and lining it with a skin graft or an intestinal transplant, and this has been fairly satisfactory. Whether it functions is really decided by the relationship between a woman and her sex partner. A woman may ask to have an artifical vagina constructed because she wants to feel that she has all the facilities for intercourse to offer her husband, but many women who have radical pelvic surgery have managed to maintain reasonably adequate sexual relations, even though the vagina may be considerably smaller or shorter after the surgery. If both partners care enough, a satisfactory solution can usually be reached. Nevertheless, reconstructive surgery certainly has a place in gynecologic surgery.

Q. What is the significance of erosion of the cervix?

A. An erosion is a visible lesion, a raw area, not necessarily pathologic. It can be a simple inflammation or it can be a malignancy. A "Pap" test may disclose the presence of malignant cells but it is often negative when there is actually a gross abnormality present; therefore it is not, in itself, considered an adequate basis for diagnosis. The physician depends on the pathologist's report of a biopsy of the affected part for his diagnosis.

Q. How accurate is Schiller's test in diagnosing cervical cancer?

A. The Schiller test consists simply of applying Lugol's solution to an area that is suspected of containing malignant cells which do not ordinarily take the brown stain. So if part of the area to which the solution is applied fails to take up the stain a biopsy can be taken from that area.

This will not necessarily result in a positive biopsy for cancer, because there are several other pathologic conditions in which the cells will not take this stain. Thus, it is not a very accurate test, but sometimes is of help in locating an area where one would be more apt to get a positive biopsy for cancer, if a malignancy were present.

Q. Should the patient who has had gynecologic surgery receive hormones for the rest of her life and, if so, what hormones?

A. Whether a post-hysterectomy patient receives hormones depends on why the operation was done. The only malignancy in the female reproductive tract that is thought to be stimulated by hormones is endometrial carcinoma, so estrogen is almost never given to a woman who has been treated for this disease. Similarly, it is considered risky to use hormonal therapy in patients who have had carcinoma of the breast.

The decision as to whether it is safe for a woman to take hormones for the rest of her life relates to the question of whether estrogens can cause cancer in an organ where it would not develop otherwise, and all that can be said about this is that the danger probably exists in a small number of women. The best evidence for this latter statement is that, over the last 20 years, most menopausal women who have gone to a private gynecologist have been given some form of hormonal therapy, that is, estrogen, and there has not been an overwhelming increase in the incidence of breast or endometrial cancer in the United States during that time. This fact has also been interpreted as indicating that estrogens can cause gynecologic malignancies because, with the improvement in health care over the past 20 years, the incidence rate should be going down, and it isn't.

Most women go through menopause without hot flashes and the vagina does not necessarily dry out, because the adrenal gland continues to produce estrogen.

Many patients develop breast or endometrial carcinoma while on the estrogens and, on the other hand, many more do not. Any woman on estrogen therapy should be under the care of a physician who takes the responsibility for doing regular breast and pelvic examinations. She should also be on a regimen in which the dosage is suspended for a prescribed length of time during the month so as to give the structures that are being stimulated by the estrogens some time to rest.

Q. Can phosphorus-32 be used more than once in a patient with cancer of the ovary?

A. It has been used as often as three times in patients at Memorial Hospital.

Q. What criteria are utilized in selecting candidates for pelvic perfusion?

A. The problem with pelvic perfusion in cases of gynecologic cancer, particularly the type that is likely to remain localized in the pelvis (cervical cancer), is that we do not, at present, have an effective chemotherapeutic agent to use for this purpose. It was tried in a few cases at Memorial Hospital some years ago but abandoned because it did not offer any particular advantage and, in fact, was moderately hazardous.

Q. What can be done to aid the patient who has continued incontinence after discharge from the hospital?

A. The answer to this question depends on what one means by incontinence, since there are many kinds of incontinence. In a medical sense, the word really means a loss of control over the evacuation of body wastes such as feces or urine. This can result from a number of causes in addition to surgery; neurological disease, for instance. In gynecologic patients, incontinence usually has to do with fistulae that cause the contents of the bowel or the bladder to leak out uncontrolled by a normal sphincter. These situations are usually corrected by repair or by diversion. How it is handled depends on the exact nature of the involvement.

Q. How should the nurse answer the patient who asks if she will receive any nursing care when she returns to the nursing unit after having a radium or cobalt insert?

A. The patient should be told that she definitely will receive all the care she needs, but that the nurses will work much faster because of the possibility of radiation exposure. She should also know that her family and friends can visit her, but that they will be required to remain outside of the area of exposure. She needs to be told, in addition, that she will be on certain physical limitations such as bed rest, that she will have a Foley catheter inserted, and will be on a low residue diet. Knowing all these things ahead of time will affect the patient's acceptance of the necessary conditions after the radioactive substance is inserted. And, of course, immediately after the applicator or source of radiation is removed, all restrictions are lifted. Sometimes patients worry about being a hazard to their children and others after they have had external radiation, and need assurance that no one in the environment can be affected, and that they can see their family and friends as often and for as long as they wish. The only exception to this is that physicians tend to limit visitations by pregnant women.

Q. Is it ever advisable to tell a patient with gynecologic cancer that she is going to die?

A. If the patient asks, "Am I going to die?" the physician might answer by saying, "Yes, you are going to die. We are all going to die. The question you are really asking me is *'When* am I going to die?' and I cannot answer that." If the patient is very ill, the doctor may say, "You are very sick, but we are doing everything in our power to make you live as long and as comfortably as you can. Beyond that, I cannot give you a definite answer."

As far as the nurse is concerned, there is no one recipe or direct route that can be recommended when she is faced with giving an answer to the patient's questions about her possible death. However, it will be helpful for her to be aware of, and to keep in mind: 1) what the doctor has told the patient; 2) her own attitude toward cancer; and 3) her own limitations and response to the stress this question creates. It is a very difficult question to answer and one the nurse is often asked.

Q. How can the nurse best support the patient who is afraid she will die as a result of her surgery?

A. Any cancer patient who goes to surgery thinks of this possibility. If she is fully aware of what is going to be done, she needs to be assured that all of the nursing personnel will be available to take care of her both during and after the operation, and that she can rely on their care and expertise. The nurse who can convey to the patient that she expects her to survive her surgery can provide a great deal of comfort for the patient who fears dying in the operating room.

Q. Should a woman who has gynecologic cancer and whose prognosis is fatal, be revived if she has a coronary attack?

A. The general concensus seems to be that the patient who is terminally ill with cancer should not be resuscitated. On the other hand, the patient who may survive for three or four years, or more, with treatment— even though she is not curable—is resuscitated. If the nurse is new on the shift or on the nursing unit and does not know all the facts about the patient, or what the doctor's order is in this regard, the answer is "Yes," resuscitate her.

The diagnosis of cancer does not mean that a patient would not be resuscitated; many patients live for a comparatively long time in reasonably good symbiosis with cancer.

SUGGESTED READINGS

Books

Ball, T. L. *Gynecological Surgery and Urology,* 2nd ed. St. Louis: Mosby, 1964.

Bouchard, Rosemary. *Nursing Care of the Cancer Patient.* St. Louis: Mosby, 1967.

Brewer, J. I., D. M. Molbo, and A. B. Gerbie. *Gynecologic Nursing.* St. Louis: Mosby, 1966.

Brunner, Lillian S. et al. *Textbook of Medical-Surgical Nursing,* 2nd ed. Philadelphia: Lippincott, 1970.

Fitzpatrick, G. M. *Gynecologic Nursing.* New York: Macmillan, 1965.

Hawkins, J. *Shaw's Textbook of Operative Gynecology,* 3rd ed. Baltimore: Williams & Wilkins, 1968.

MacLeod, D., and J. Hawkins. *Bonney's Gynecological Surgery,* 7th ed. New York: Harper and Row, 1964.

Miller, N. F., and H. Avery. *Gynecology and Gynecologic Nursing.* Philadelphia: Saunders, 1965.

Nealon, T. F. (Ed.). *Management of the Patient with Cancer.* Philadelphia: Saunders, 1966.

Nelson, James H. *Atlas of Radical Pelvic Surgery.* New York: Appleton-Century-Crofts, 1969.

Novak, E. R. and G. I. Jones. *Novak's Textbook of Gynecology,* 6th ed. Baltimore: Williams & Wilkins, 1961.

Shafer, K. N. et al. *Medical-Surgical Nursing,* 4th ed. St. Louis: Mosby, 1967.

Smith, D. W., and C. D. Gips. *Care of the Adult Patient, Medical-Surgical Nursing.* Philadelphia: Lippincott, 1963.

TeLinde, R. W. *Operative Gynecology,* 3rd ed. Philadelphia: Lippincott, 1962.

Urquhart, Audrey L. *A Study of Nursing Care of the Vulvectomy Patient, A. N. A. Regional Clinical Conferences, 1967.* New York: Appleton-Century-Crofts, 1968.

Periodicals

Alpenfels, E. J. "Cancer in Situ of the Cervix—Cultural Clues to Reactions," *American Journal of Nursing,* 64:83-86, April, 1964.

Anderson, N. J. "Vulvectomy—Nursing Care," *American Journal of Nursing,* 60:668-670, May, 1960.

Barber, H. R. "Septic Shock in Obstetrics and Gynecology," *Minnesota Medicine,* 53:393-7, April, 1970.

Barber, H. R. "Relative Prognostic Significance of Pre-Operative and Operative Findings in Pelvic Exenteration," *Surgical Clinics of North America,* 49:431-47, April, 1969.

Chalfant, R. L. "Diagnosis and Treatment of Cancer of the Uterus," *Nursing Forum, 4*:67-75, No. 3, 1965.

Dillon, H. B. "The Woman Patient," *Nursing Clinics of North America, 3*:253-261, June, 1968.

Durbin, M. S. Jr. "Geriatric Gynecology," *Nursing Clinics of North America, 3*:253-261, June, 1968.

Funnell, Joseph W., and Betsy Roof. "Before and After Hysterectomy," *American Journal of Nursing, 64*:120-122, October, 1964.

Gray, M. J. "The Use of Radiation Therapy in Gynecologic Malignancy," *Hospital Topics, 45*:103-7, September, 1967.

Gusberg, S. B. "Cancer in Situ of the Cervix—Treatment as Preventive Medicine," *American Journal of Nursing, 64*:76-79, April, 1964.

Harris, R. E. "The Role of a Nurse Clinician in the Gynecological Cancer Detection Clinic," *Medical Times, 98*:157-60, July, 1970.

Hilkemeyer, R. "Nursing Care in Radium Therapy (Uterine Cancer)" *Nursing Clinics of North America, 2*:83-95, March, 1967.

Hofmeister, Frederick J., Robert R. Reick, and Nancy Jane Anderson. "Vulvectomy—Surgical Treatment and Nursing Care," *American Journal of Nursing, 60*: 666-668, May, 1970.

Hresachyshyn, M. M. "A Critical Review of Chemotherapy in the Treatment of Ovarian Carcinoma," *Clinical Obstetrics and Gynecology, 4*:885-890, September, 1961.

Lewis, G. C. Jr. "Cancer in Situ of the Cervix—Screening and Diagnosis," *American Journal of Nursing, 64*:72-75, April, 1964.

Lewis, J. L. Jr. "Chemotherapy and Surgery in the Treatment of Gestational Trophoblastic Neoplasms," *Surgical Clinics of North America, 49*:371-80, April, 1969.

Mayo, P. and N. L. Wilkey. "Prevention of Cancer of the Breast and Cervix," *Nursing Clinics of North America, 3*:229-241, June, 1968.

McCulley, L. B. "Health Counseling of Women," *Nursing Clinics of North America, 3*:263-273, June, 1968.

McGowan, Larry. "New Ideas About Patient Care Before and After Vaginal Surgery," *American Journal of Nursing, 64*:73-75, February, 1964.

McFayden, Iain R. "Choreocarcinoma," *Nursing Times, 64*:793-94, June 14, 1968.

Robbins, L. C. and E. Walker. "Cancer in Situ of the Cervix—Problems of Control," *American Journal of Nursing, 64*:80-83, April, 1964.

Stone, Martin L. and Allan B. Weingold. "Cancer of the Ovary," *Hospital Medicine, 1*:33-38, September, 1965.

Symmonds, R. E. "Where Gynecologic Cancer Should Be Treated," *Obstetrics and Gynecology, 35*:144-8, January, 1970.

Volk, William L. and John D. Foret. "The Problem of Vesico-Vaginal and Uretero-Vaginal Fistulas," *Medical Clinics of North America, 43*:1769-1777, November, 1959.

Weed, J. C. "Gynecologic Malignant Disease in Geriatric Patients," *Geriatrics, 22*:126-31, December, 1967.

Patients with Urologic Tumors

Regional Medical Program — Oncology Nursing Seminar

on

NURSING MANAGEMENT OF PATIENTS WITH
UROLOGIC TUMORS

Seminar Leader

Willet F. Whitmore, Jr., M.D.

Seminar Participants

Jacqueline Clare, R.N., Professional Nurse Practitioner

Mary McCormack, R.N., B.S.N., Head Nurse

Kathleen O'Horo, R.N., Head Nurse

Carl J. Schmidlapp, M.D., Assistant Attending Surgeon, Urology
Service

Mary Wall, M.S.W., Social Worker

Malcom Wells, R.N., Stoma Therapist

Willet F. Whitmore, Jr., M.D., Chief, Urology Service

Although urology is sometimes regarded as one of the less glamorous of the surgical specialties, both physicians and nurses, once they have learned something about it, find it very interesting. There are three reasons for this interest when studying urologic malignancies. First, urology treats of a variety of diseases in a variety of organs. Second, this specialty is unique in the relatively high degree of accuracy that is associated with diagnostic investigations. And third, the frequent effectiveness of therapy is gratifying to both physicians and their patients.

Cancer of the kidney, bladder, prostate, and testis make up the bulk of the urologic neoplasms that occur in people in the United States.

RENAL CANCER

Renal cancer alone accounts for approximately eleven thousand cases annually in this country, and about six thousand of these are fatal. The disease occurs most often in people who are in their late fifties and early sixties, and the incidence is almost twice as high in the male as in the female, the ratio being 1.7 to 1. It ranks third among genitourinary malignancies. In one-third to one-fifth of the patients, the disease has already become metastatic by the time the patient first sees a physician and the diagnosis is made. Sixty percent of the metastases are to the lung and 33 percent are to the liver and bone.

The several types of renal cancer are classified according to the specific tissue of origin. Tumors that develop in the connective tissue are sarcomas. Papillary carcinomas develop in the epithelial tissue of the renal pelvis. Then there are embryonal tumors, such as Wilms' tumor in children, as well as metastatic tumors from other organs. However, 85 percent of malignant renal tumors are renal cell carcinomas or parenchymal tumors—often misnamed hypernephromas. There are two types of renal cell carcinoma, the clear cell type which has a relatively good prognosis, and the granular cell type which has a relatively poor prognosis.

Diagnosis

The three classic symptoms of renal cancer are bloody urine, pain, and a palpable mass. The first and primary symptom that the patient notices is hematuria, but he will probably not experience any pain when voiding unless he happens to pass a blood clot. Blood in the urine does not always mean that the patient has renal cancer, but its presence is a mandate for a thorough investigation. Some, but not all patients may have pain in the renal area. In others, a mass may be palpated, generally not by the patient but by the physician. However, these tumors are rather slow growing and sometimes the patient can feel the mass himself. Other symptoms which also occur in other diseases and thus are not of specific significance diagnostically are malaise, anorexia, loss of weight, and sometimes gastrointestinal disturbances, peripheral neuropathy, and congestive heart failure. Fever of undetermined origin is an important sign if it accompanies the three classic symptoms and should suggest the possible presence of renal tumor. The patient with metastatic renal cancer may have pain in the long bones, especially the upper end of the humerus, and in the spine or skull. Varicocele is an important sign in the male, particularly if it occurs on the right side because this suggests obstruction of the right spermatic vein by possible tumor.

Abnormalities in the blood count, and blood chemical aberrations are not especially helpful in making the diagnosis of renal cancer. Neither is cytologic urinalysis, because in renal cell carcinoma the cancer cells are rarely sloughed off into the urine; in fact, the urinalysis may be normal.

The intravenous pyelogram is an important diagnostic tool, however. The findings in pyelographic studies often contain important diagnostic signs that lead the physician to suspect the presence of a tumor and then angiograms can be performed which will show abnormalities in the vessel architecture if a renal tumor is indeed present.

After excretory urography is performed, sometimes nephrotomography is done to determine whether the tumor is solid or cystic. Arteriography will also give some clue as to whether it is benign or malignant if there is "puddling" of the contrast medium. The venacavagram is important in determining whether the disease has involved the venous system. Lymphangiography may delineate metastasis to lymph nodes in the renal area but is relatively unimportant as far as "staging" of renal tumors is concerned. The chest x-ray is certainly important because the prognosis is extremely poor when metastasis to the chest has occurred. A skeletal survey plus a bone scan will show lesions in the bones and are important procedures because, in these instances, cryosurgery or radiation can be used as palliative measures.

Treatment

Radical nephrectomy is the treatment of choice for renal cancer. At Memorial Hospital, the surgeons who perform this operation often remove a rib or use an abdominal incision and remove all of Gerota's fascia and the kidney within it. The adrenal gland is also removed as well as pericaval or periaortic lymph nodes.

Radiation is not of established value in treating renal tumors because they are very radioresistant, but it is sometimes used as a palliative measure for pain in metastatic disease and is under investigation as a therapeutic adjunct in early stages of the disease as well.

Progestational agents such as Provera have been widely used in this country, and may be considered in the treatment of tumors that cannot be removed or cured.

The overall five-year cure rate for resectable renal cell cancer is 40 to 50 percent.

Papillary cell tumors of the renal pelvis are treated by nephroureterectomy. This is usually done through two incisions and a cuff of the bladder is removed in the process. If tumor develops in the opposite kidney after one kidney has been removed, it is sometimes possible to treat it by open fulguration, possibly leaving a nephrostomy tube in, and using Thio-Tepa instillations postoperatively.

The five-year cure rate in papillary tumors of the renal pelvis varies from 5 to 50 percent. Staging of papillary tumors shows that in stages I and II, the five-year survival rate is about 70 percent; in stage III, 30 percent; and in stage IV, 6 percent.

For squamous cell carcinoma the cure rate is almost zero.

Comprehensive Nursing Care of the Patient with Renal Cancer

All patients who are under study for a possible diagnosis of cancer, or who are about to undergo surgery for a malignancy, are very anxious. In this respect, patients with urologic malignancies need the same kind of understanding and awareness of their fears and anxieties as patients with any other type of malignancy. The nurse's awareness of these feelings, from the day of his admission onward, will make the experience much easier for him and his family to accept and to tolerate.

Preparation for the various diagnostic tests is an important aspect of the nurse's role in caring for patients with urologic malignancies. Patients should be kept well hydrated, but fluids and food must be withheld after midnight before most tests, including x-ray examinations. A simple explanation of why these tests are being done, and why fluids and food must be restricted, will help to gain the patient's cooperation and confidence, but this should be given well in advance of the tests and not at the last moment. The patient's questions should be answered in a friendly manner, of course, but his family's questions should also be answered in the same way because their understanding of the situation will help alleviate uncertainties and anxieties that might otherwise be transferred to the patient. Many of these patients are in the older age group and have become malnourished, partly as a result of their disease; therefore, a good dietary regimen must be instituted. On the other hand, some are obese and must be put on a strictly calculated, low-calorie diet.

Cardiovascular and/or pulmonary disease is often present in the patient with urologic cancer and, when this is the case, a complete medical workup and clearance is necessary before any surgical treatment is carried out. If the patient is on digitalis before surgery, this will be continued postoperatively. Patients who receive antihypertensive medication preoperatively may become hypotensive during or after surgery. Intermittent positive pressure breathing is sometimes utilized preoperatively for patients with pulmonary disease, along with mucolytic agents that aid in the dissolution and expectoration of thick secretions.

It is also imperative that any patient being considered for surgery be taught how to deep breathe and cough effectively, and that he practice these exercises at regular intervals without fail. Changing the patient's position from side to side helps loosen secretions and increases the effectiveness of coughing. With the patient in the upright position the nurse instructs him to take a deep breath and then coaxes him, during exhalation, to breathe out as slowly and for as long as he can. He is also given an explanation of any machine that may be used postoperatively to induce coughing and has a chance to try it out before he goes to surgery. Being familiar with the mouthpiece or mask will help alleviate any fear he may have of not being able to breathe during postoperative treatments.

Leg exercises, such as rotation, flexion, and extension of the ankle are also taught and practiced preoperatively.

All patients are weighed on admission, preoperatively, and every day after surgery unless otherwise ordered. The important point of the weighing procedure is that it be carried out at the same time and in the same manner on each day.

Nephrectomy is the usual surgical procedure carried out when the patient has renal cancer. Although hemorrhage is not a frequent complication of nephrectomy, its occurrence must be watched for carefully. Hemorrhage is indicated by profuse red, thick drainage, clots, and perhaps distention at the suture line. Massive hemorrhage will be reflected in a drop in blood pressure and a rise in pulse rate, but excessive slow oozing may not be reflected in these signs for several hours. Therefore, the patient should be turned slightly to the side when dressing observations are made.

During the first 24 postoperative hours, the patient should be turned at least every two to three hours. Positioning him on the operated side will allow the pressure of the other organs to help fill in the dead space at the operative site and improve dependent drainage. Deep breathing and coughing is carried out each time the patient is turned, or more often if necessary.

Unless contraindicated, ambulation is begun within 24 hours. Sitting up for inhalation treatments will facilitate coughing and make it easier for the patient to deep breathe and expectorate. Supporting the incision with both hands during the coughing and deep breathing exercise, and the use of narcotics during the early recovery period, will help to ease or eliminate the pain that occurs with coughing.

When the thoracic approach has been used, the patient will return from the operating room with a chest tube in place. The nurse must make sure the tube is kept properly positioned and free of kinks so that it will provide for good drainage. A liberal use of pillows makes proper positioning easier and contributes to the patient's comfort. In these patients, the possibility always exists that the pleura will be perforated. Therefore, the nurse should watch for signs of pneumothorax—sudden, sharp chest pain, dyspnea, anxiety, and increased pulse rate. The patient should be maintained in high Fowler's position, and oxygen and a thoracotomy set kept at hand for emergency use.

On the second or third postoperative day, or as soon as the gastrointestinal function has returned, the patient is started on a liquid diet of 30 cc's per hour, although he may still have a nasogastric tube in place. Accurate recording of intake and output cannot be over-stressed. If an indwelling catheter is in place, hourly monitoring of the urine is done; the volume should be 30 cc's per hour, or more. When the patient does not have a catheter, and has not voided within eight to ten hours postoperatively, a catheterization is done to determine the volume of urine present in the bladder and to relieve discomfort.

Throughout the postoperative period, words of encouragement about their progress, and reassurance that the discomforts they have are transitory, allays apprehension and gives comfort to most patients.

Guidelines for the patient's follow-up care begin to be formulated as soon as he is hospitalized, but they need to be expanded and reinforced as the time for his discharge approaches. The importance of maintaining good health habits, of taking in an adequate amount of fluids, and of securing immediate treatment for any respiratory infection are pointed out. Reassurance that life with one kidney can be normal should be stressed, beginning early in the postoperative period. Follow-up appointments are made with the outpatient department and the patient is urged to make further appointments whenever he feels the need of some attention or advice.

CANCER OF THE BLADDER

Cancer of the bladder is the second most frequently occurring genitourinary malignancy. About twenty thousand new cases develop each year and there are about nine thousand deaths from this disease annually in this country. It accounts for about 3 percent of all deaths from cancer and, again, it occurs more often in males than females—three times as often, in fact.

The primary symptom of cancer of the bladder is hematuria which may be described as "gross total," meaning that it occurs throughout the act of micturition, although it can occur at the beginning or at the end of the act. It can also be painless, but generally pain or some other symptoms are associated with it. Hematuria is not necessarily a continuous symptom; it may come and go. But every time blood is found in a patient's urine, a complete investigation is merited. Vesicular irritation, with frequency and urgency, even without hematuria, also deserves investigation, especially when it occurs in people fifty years of age or over.

Infection is often a concomitant of bladder carcinoma that has been present for a period of time. Ureter obstruction may occur in stage C and D tumors and the involvement of the ureteral orifices causes hydronephrosis and back pain that may or may not be accompanied by infection. Metastasis can occur, of course, just as it does in many other types of cancer.

Diagnosis

Urinalysis is an important diagnostic tool, even without gross total hematuria. A urinalysis will reveal the presence of red blood cells, and more than one or two cells per high-powered field is reason for further investigation. Whereas urinary cytology is not very helpful in the diagnosis of the clear cell carcinoma of the kidney, it is quite important in diagnosing bladder carcinoma. Papanicolaou tests done on the urine are very often positive. A negative report does not mean that there is no tumor present, but if the test is repeated, the chances are that a good pathologist will pick up tumor cells if cancer is present.

An intravenous pyelogram is an important tool for delineating any problems that may be concerned with function in the upper urinary tract and the degree of hydronephrosis. The cystogram and the angiogram are seldom of any diagnostic value. However, cystoscopy is a procedure that must be employed at the time hematuria first appears, and the physician should not wait for a second attack before doing this. A cystoscopic examination may be done in the doctor's office, but it is better to have the patient in the hospital where it can be done under anesthesia, where a good bimanual examination can also be done, and where generous biopsies can be taken. The cystoscopist may well stage the tumor in 80 percent of the cases, and the biopsy will reveal the grade and extent of the tumor present. In vesical cancer it is very important to know the grade and stage of the tumor because this will determine the therapy that will be carried out.

Jewett's classification, which has been used for some years for staging cancer of the bladder, stages the lesions as follows: Stage O cancer is an in situ carcinoma and involves only the mucosa of the bladder. In stage A, the lesion extends down into the submucosa. In stage B, it extends into the muscle of the bladder. In stage B_2, it extends through the muscle of the bladder, but does not involve the perivesicular fat. In stage C, the tumor involves the entire thickness of the bladder and extends into the perivesicular fat. Stage D represents metastatic disease. Stage D_1 represents a lesion that involves the lymph nodes in the pelvis (such as the obturator nodes). In stage D_2, there are distant metastases in nodes above the pelvis, or higher up in the torso, or in the chest.

Treatment

Endoscopic destruction by fulguration is the therapy used in the low-grade and low-stage vesicular tumors. The morbidity is almost zero. How-

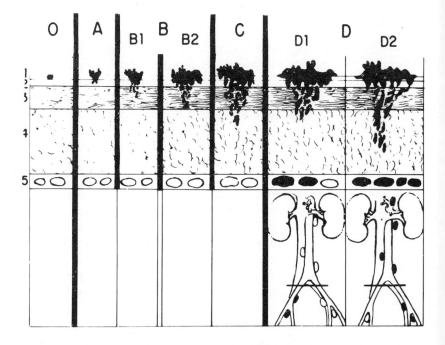

Figure 1. Stages of vesical neoplasms

O—limited to mucosa;
A—not beyond submucosa;
B1—not more than halfway through muscle layer;
B2—beyond the halfway level of the muscle layer, but not into fat;
C—beyond the muscle layer, but not metastatic, or invading the
    substance of adjacent organs;
D1—metastatic to the pelvic lymph nodes and/or invading the sub-
    stance of adjacent organs;
D2—metastatic beyond the pelvis.

ever, it is possible for dissemination or implantation to occur during the procedure. Also, the bladder is left intact so that whatever caused the tumor to
develop in the first place may produce other bladder tumors later. Consequently, even though all the tumor is cleared out, this procedure is repeated every three months thereafter.

Suprapubic destruction is employed only for huge tumors that cannot
be treated endoscopically, and of course the morbidity is slightly higher be-

cause this is an open operation. Again, recurrence is possible because implantation may occur when the bladder is opened and tumor cells are spilled. The bladder is left in place as in the endoscopic procedure.

Segmental resection is a somewhat more extensive operation than the suprapubic one and it also has higher morbidity and mortality rates. It entails removing a full-thickness section of the bladder with a margin of at least 2 centimeters. In this operation, too, the bladder is maintained. Curability statistics are about the same for this operation as for cystectomy, but segmental resection cannot be done when the tumor is near the bladder neck or ureteral orifices where appropriate margins cannot be obtained.

Simple cystectomy is no longer commonly employed except for patients who are given radiation treatment for a tumor and who later develop radiation cystitis with intractable bleeding; then a cystectomy may be mandatory as an emergency procedure.

Radical cystectomy is the procedure used at Memorial Hospital for most high-grade, high-stage tumors. In this operation, all of the bladder, the perivesical fat, the lymph nodes on both sides of the pelvis and, in males, the prostate, seminal vesicles, and occasionally the urethra are removed. The reason for removing the urethra is that it may be the site of recurrence of the disease. In female patients the uterus and adnexa, as well as the urethra, are removed at the time the cystectomy is performed. This operation carries a mortality rate of about 10 to 15 percent. The morbidity is high. The intravesical recurrence rate, however, is zero because the bladder has been removed. However, tumors may develop in the ureters that are implanted in the ileum or the sigmoid, or brought out to the skin. Radical cystectomy is a drastic procedure. The problem, of course, is that it creates a major change in the patient's body and his urine drains out onto the abdominal wall. Also, an occasional patient requires a colostomy along with the ileal conduit and this complicates his care. The male is completely impotent after the operation. In the female, the vagina is foreshortened but, although this does not cause any great problem as far as sexual relations are concerned, she still has urine draining out through a stoma in the abdominal wall.

With all these reasons for not doing a radical cystectomy, why is it done? One reason is that sometimes even low-grade and low-stage tumors recur so frequently and become so extensive that, after a period of years, the surgeon finds he cannot keep ahead of this disease and is really forced to do something drastic. Another reason is provided when patients have infiltrating lesions that are unsuitable for segmental resection.

Radiation therapy may be used to treat the patient who refuses to undergo cystectomy. Several modalities are available. External radiation with supervoltage up to six thousand rads will cure some patients but it may produce a contracted bladder and, occasionally, intractable bleeding from radiation cystitis. Intracavity irradiation is accomplished by putting a radium bomb within a Foley catheter, and can be used for treating lesions near the bladder neck. Interstitial radiation can be given either through an instrument or through the open operation in which seeds are implanted in the bladder itself. Radiation may also be used as an adjunct to other therapy. Some years ago, a protocol was developed in which a dose of 4000 rads was given over a period of about four weeks prior to cystectomy. Recently, the dosage has been changed to 2000 rads given over about seven days immediately prior to surgery, and the results seem to indicate that this protective radiation apparently does not increase the morbidity of the operation or the difficulty of it and that it may improve survival prospects.

Chemotherapy is employed for patients who have metastatic disease and who are inoperable, but no effective programs of treatment have yet been developed. Thio-Tepa can be used in the treatment of multiple recurrences of papilloma of the bladder, mainly in the hope of producing a bladder that the surgeon can do an endoscopic resection on later. Generally, the response to the Thio-Tepa is erratic and, if absorption of the drug is excessive, hematologic toxicity may occur; therefore, blood counts should be done frequently if the drug is given over a period of time.

In summary, a study of the five-year survival rate following various modalities of therapy show that excision and fulguration have a high cure rate and a low morbidity rate. There is also a good chance for a patient to survive segmental resection—the mortality rate is between 4 and 5 percent. However, it must be remembered that segmental resection is reserved for highly selected tumors that are not located at the base or neck of the bladder. The mortality rate for patients who have radical cystectomies is between 10 and 15 percent; the cure rate for those with stage C tumors is from 8 to 26 percent, and for patients with stage D tumors only 3 percent.

Comprehensive Nursing Care of the Patient with Cancer of the Urinary Bladder

In addition to the preoperative laboratory studies, tests, and treatments that are performed for patients undergoing renal surgery (see page 268), a urine for culture and a sensitivity determination are obtained. Procedures employed to confirm a diagnosis or to plan treatment include direct visualization by endoscopy or cystoscopy, transurethral resection, or segmental resection of the bladder.

Post-cystoscopy discomfort is relatively mild. The patient may complain of frequent, burning urination and the urine may be slightly blood-tinged. Increased fluid intake and warm sitz baths will often take care of these discomforts.

When the patient returns to the unit following a transurethral resection of the bladder, an indwelling catheter is in place. This catheter is not irrigated unless it is not draining well, and then gentle irrigation with normal saline is ordered. Often this dislodges a small plug in the catheter and this is all that is needed; sometimes a slight squeeze of the tubing will suffice. Frequency and burning are to be expected, and the patient is told that there may be some gross hematuria off and on for up to four weeks after the operation. This is secondary to the sloughing off of coagulated areas in the bladder. If hematuria persists, or is associated with the passage of clots, the doctor should be notified.

Multiple lesions and infiltrating growths are often treated by radical surgery. After medical and surgical clearance for surgery is complete, and a proper pulmonary toilet has been carried out, the patient is ready for a radical cystectomy and ileal conduit operation. The anticipation of such radical surgery may have an overwhelming impact on the patient and his family, and the nurse can be very helpful to him when he is faced with making the decision to undergo such surgery—just by being there and listening when he wants to talk about it. Preoperatively, the patient is placed on a regimen designed to prepare the bowel by lowering the bacteria count of the intestinal flora and reducing the volume of formed feces. This is accomplished through the administration of antibiotics, cathartics and enemas, and placing the patient first on a low residue diet, then a clear liquid diet 24 hours previous to surgery. The nurse carries the major responsibility for making certain that the prescribed regimen is followed. During this preoperative period, most patients are physically uncomfortable and this serves to heighten their anxiety. Therefore, the nurse should be liberal in dispensing

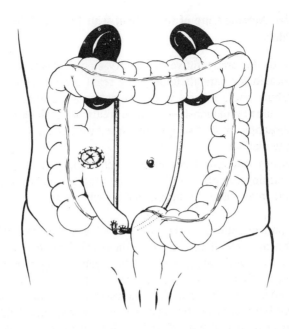

Figure 2. Ileal conduit

explanations, encouragement, and understanding. In addition, Ace bandages are applied from the toes to the groin area on the morning of surgery.

Postoperatively, meticulous measurement and accurate recording of intake and output are of the utmost importance. Intake will be solely by parenteral fluid until gastrointestinal function returns and oral feedings are resumed. Output will consist of gastric juice, urine, and wound drainage. Measurement of these fluids determines, in part, the fluid and electrolyte replacement needed. Some degree of paralytic ileus will be present. Drainage from the nasogastric tube may be high in volume, causing a significant loss of electrolytes. The tube is irrigated several times a day to facilitate drainage and to prevent intestinal distention which could cause tension at the intestinal anastomosis of an ileal conduit.

Using the patient's preoperative weight as a base line, daily postoperative weights are plotted against it to determine whether there is any retention of fluid and to serve as a guideline for fluid replacement. Because of the significant loss of body fluids, it is important that the patient receive the total volume of fluid ordered, at the time prescribed. The intravenous drip as well as the urine output should be checked hourly. Blood is drawn daily to determine electrolyte levels, and intravenous corrections are determined by these results. Because the anesthesia time may be anywhere from five to eight hours, the possibility of pulmonary congestion and pneumonia is increased. Frequent turning and coughing, and early ambulation are necessary to prevent respiratory and circulatory complications. These activities also improve urinary evacuation and help to elevate the patient's morale. In the early postoperative period, narcotics are administered as frequently as the order permits, unless there are signs of hypotension, shallow slow respirations, or stupor.

Wound edema and abdominal distention often cause severe incisional pain during the first postoperative week. After construction of an ileal conduit, the patient returns from the operating room with a temporary appliance which is connected to a straight drainage system. Skin irritation is a problem that is sometimes encountered when caring for a patient who has an ileal conduit. A common cause is the too frequent changing or lack of gentleness when changing the temporary appliance. A solvent that is specifically made to remove any residue adhesive should be used, since it will be less irritating to the skin. Mild irritation subsides quickly when the area is cleansed gently with soap and water, dried thoroughly but not vigorously, and exposed frequently to a heat lamp. The skin around the stoma must be perfectly dry for a watertight seal to be achieved. A layer of tincture of benzoin just before securing the temporary appliance in place improves adhesion to the skin and also coats and protects it. The temporary appliance should be left in place as long as there is no leakage; signs of skin or stoma irritation can be clearly seen through the plastic bag. Each time the skin is cared for, the patient is encouraged to participate and is shown how to change the appliance. Then, when a permanent appliance can be used—that is, after abdominal distention and edema of the stoma subside—he knows how to handle the equipment and how to give himself proper skin care. An ileal conduit accessory kit and instruction card will help the patient to master the principles of stoma and skin care. (See Appendix A, p. 301.)

Because of the alteration in the patient's self-image, a member of his family—usually his wife—is included in the early instruction concerning the care of the stoma so that his acceptance of this lifetime alteration can be shared with someone close to him.

The patient who has had a uterosigmoidostomy has a rectal tube with a large lumen inserted to take care of both urine and fecal drainage. If this

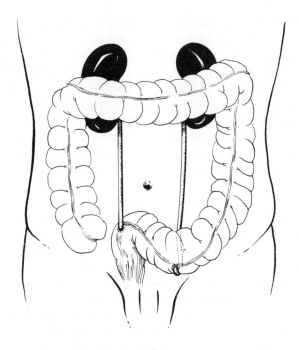

Figure 3. Ureterosigmoidostomy

tube becomes dislodged at any time it must be reinserted (no more than four inches). One complication of this operation is that there may be a reflux of fecal material and infection may develop as a result. Enemas and rectal temperatures are contraindicated. Perineal exercises in which the anal sphincter is strengthened by alternately contracting and relaxing it, and emptying the bladder at timed intervals, will help the patient to gain control of urination per rectum.

When the patient has had a cutaneous ureterostomy, special stoma care is needed to prevent sloughing and stricture. The stoma is kept moist for from five to ten days using a sterile 4 x 4 moistened with normal saline. A splinting catheter is usually placed in the ureterostomy in the operating room and is not removed until satisfactory healing occurs.

Once the urine output is adequate, plans are made for the patient's discharge and he is fitted with a permanent appliance. He must be made aware of the importance of good hydration and early treatment of any infection. He should be told that the urine may be cloudy and have mucous shreds in it, but that he should report to the doctor immediately should there be any other alteration in the urine, such as an increase in volume or the presence of blood or clots. Follow-up appointments are made for the patient and continuity of care continues to be closely and carefully supervised until his health and strength are regained.

CANCER OF THE PROSTATE GLAND

Prostatic cancer is the most common urologic cancer in men over 50 years of age. For purposes of classification, four stages of prostatic cancer are recognized: stage A, latent cancer; stage B, clinically early cancer; stage C, locally extensive cancer that has not metastasized; stage D, cancer that has metastasized. On digital examination, the patient with stage A carcinoma of the prostate presents nothing to make one suspect the presence of a neoplasm. Indeed, this cancer, by definition, is found only by the pathologist. It is not recognized by the clinician, but if an operation is performed in which some prostatic tissue is removed, the pathologist will find the cancer when he examines the tissue. This is, by all odds, the most common cancer that is recognized in our population.

Diagnosis

Stage B prostatic cancer characteristically produces a nodule of induration that is relatively sharply defined from the rest of the prostate. Patients with these lesions, too, have no symptoms that indicate the presence of cancer, the lesion characteristically being found in the examination for some other complaint. At Memorial Hospital, the single most common source of patients with such cancers is patients who present at the head and neck clinic with some type of head or neck lesion. During the routine medical evaluation, a digital examination reveals the presence of a prostatic nodule. (All men past the age of 50 are advised to have periodic digital rectal examinations as a means of detecting these cancers early.) Acid and alkaline phosphatase levels are apt to be within normal limits. As in all cases of malignancy, the final diagnosis rests with the pathologist.

Patients with stage C prostatic cancer characteristically have an area of induration in the prostate that involves not only that gland but also the contiguous structures—frequently the bases of the seminal vesicles. The patient will have some symptoms of prostatic obstruction because the tumor is large enough to obstruct the urinary outlet. The patient with a benign prostatic tumor may also have symptoms of prostatic obstruction but, on digital rectal examination, the extensive induration characteristic of stage C cancer cannot be felt. An intravenous pyelogram may show that the tumor has invaded the bladder base and has reached high enough toward the apex of the seminal vesicle to also obstruct the ureter. In about 30 percent of these patients the serum acid phosphatase level will be elevated.

The prostatic cancer with which the physician is most commonly presented is the stage D type. When a patient consults a physician because of bilateral or unilateral sciatica, the physician thinks instantly of prostatic cancer, particularly if the patient is elderly. In stage D prostatic carcinoma, the lesion in the prostate is usually very extensive. The patient may or may not have urinary symptoms. He may or may not have bone pain, depending on whether his bones are involved, but he often has sciatica because of nerve root involvement. He may present with lymphedema in one or both lower extremities as a consequence of massive involvement of lymph nodes in the pelvis. The serum acid phosphatase is elevated in about 75 percent of the patients, and the alkaline phosphatase is almost invariably elevated if there is bone involvement. Thus the serum acid phosphatase elevation is a useful diagnostic criterion, but lack of elevation should not exclude the diagnosis of cancer.

Treatment

Two features of prostatic cancer make it difficult for one to be dogmatic about the proper treatment for this disease. One is the uncertain natural history of the host and the other is the uncertain natural history of the disease. As far as the host is concerned, the uncertain natural history is evidenced by the fact that between one-third and one-half of the patients with prostatic cancer will die of some other cause before they die of prostatic cancer. Furthermore, even in patients who are destined to die of prostatic cancer, the growth rate of these tumors is extremely unpredictable. Some patients with untreated disease may live for many years without much evidence of progression of the cancer, while others may have an aggressively growing tumor that kills them in a few months.

Urologists have accumulated various preferences in the treatment of this disease and, from the several therapies available, it is often possible to select a regimen that will have an impact on the course of the disease. First of all, it is possible to treat the patient with no treatment; the reason for this is that 90 percent of patients with stage A prostatic cancer have a normal five-year life expectancy if nothing is done and, of course, treatment itself does have some ill effects. The alternative for patients with this type of carcinoma is excision of the tumor.

The alternatives in the treatment of stage B cancer of the prostate are no treatment, excision, or irradiation. In these cases, the usual procedure at Memorial Hospital is to advise no treatment until there is evidence of local growth of the tumor on serial digital rectal examination. At that point, irradiation is utilized because excision results in impotence and possibly incontinence. With radiation there is some risk of impotence, but appreciably less than with excision, and no risk of incontinence. With either of these modalities, however, the degree to which the cancer can be controlled is uncertain. There is no reliable data on this point. It is known that at least 60 percent of patients treated with surgery or irradiation will live for five years, but it is not known whether they live because they were treated or because they would have lived five years without any treatment.

Stage C prostatic cancer is usually treated surgically with a transurethral resection. Whether or not anything further is done depends upon the rate at which obstruction occurs following the resection. If it occurs rapidly, the physician is usually inclined to advise irradiation by means of a cobalt unit.

The surgeon may remove the prostate in any one of several possible ways. The perineal route involves an incision that begins in front of the anus, goes through the perineum to the prostatic capsule posteriorly and involves removing the entire prostate and the seminal vesicles. When the transurethral route is used, an instrument is inserted through the urethra and the adenomatous or central portion of the gland is removed, most often for urinary obstruction or for biopsy. The suprapubic route involves opening the bladder and enucleating the prostate from within the bladder, but it is not used for known prostatic cancer. The retropubic route involves going behind the symphysis distal to the bladder neck, excising the prostate and removing also the seminal vesicles and pelvic lymph nodes. Many cancers of the prostate begin in the part of the gland that is left behind after a conventional prostatectomy for benign disease. Enucleation of the prostate in the treatment of benign prostatic obstruction by any of the conventional routes leaves the patient with a digitally palpable prostate, and with the same risk of developing carcinoma in the gland that was present before the operation.

Endocrine therapy is certainly justified in the treatment of the patient with disseminated disease; that is, stage D prostatic cancer. Recently, endocrine therapy has come under attack as a means of treatment of prostatic cancer, the claim being that it does not produce the high percentage of remissions that was once thought and, furthermore, some of the agents have undesirable side-effects. Certainly the latter seems to be true, but the former is not; there is good reason to believe that endocrine therapy has a profound and favorable effect in about 80 percent of patients with metastatic, prostatic cancer.

Comprehensive Care of the Patient with Prostatic Cancer

Because patients with prostatic cancer experience so few distressing symptoms, many do not seek medical advice until after the disease has advanced and prostatic obstruction has occurred. Therefore, by the time the patient enters the hospital he may have developed pain, difficulty in voiding, and sometimes hematuria. He may also complain of sciatica, which is caused by nerve root involvement. Sometimes he presents with severe urinary retention. In this instance, bladder drainage by an indwelling catheter is instituted or, if the obstruction is severe, a suprapubic cystotomy may be performed. When a catheter is inserted, the nurse must be sure to see that it is patent and, if urine is not draining, she should check the tubing to see whether the patient may be lying on it or whether it has become kinked. Frequently, changing the patient's position will reinstitute drainage. There should be no loops of tubing below the level of the drainage bag. The tubing should be clipped to the lower bed sheet and the excess length coiled on the bed, and the rest of it should go straight down to the collection bag or bottle.

Since hematuria is frequently a problem, clotting and plugging of the tube must be prevented. This can be accomplished by *gently* irrigating the tube as frequently as ordered or required. Vigorous irrigation tends to irritate the bladder and increase bleeding. From 20 to 30 cc's of the irrigating solution is instilled and allowed to drain out by gravity. The purpose of irrigation is to maintain the patency of the tube, not to lavage the organ. The doctor should be notified if the irrigation appears to be unsuccessful. Should the catheter seem to be plugged with a clot or with mucus, it may be "milked."

The closed drainage system is a precaution against infection. Even when the patient is up and walking, gravity may be maintained by coiling the excess tubing and clipping it above the collection bag. A leg bag can be used when necessary, but careful measures should be used to prevent contamination when changing from one system to another. The drainage system itself should be changed every week; the catheter is changed only by order of the physician. The catheter acts like any foreign body in that prolonged use of it causes irritation and infection. For this reason, good hygiene including cleansing the skin around the meatus, is necessary, and a high fluid intake should be maintained.

Preoperatively the patient who is to undergo curative prostatectomy is given such tests as chest x-ray and EKG. A blood chemistry and complete blood count will also be done. In addition, the workup will include a skeletal survey, bone scan, and intravenous pyelogram (IVP). The IVP will delineate the amount of obstruction present, while the skeletal survey will demonstrate the presence of any bony metastases. The bone scan will discover anything missed by the skeletal survey. Routine Papanicolaou tests will be done on the urine and a urine culture will be taken to ascertain whether the obstruction has induced stasis and infection. Coagulation studies are necessary to determine the fibrinolysin levels, since fibrinolysin is a particular enzyme of the prostate gland and high levels of it in the blood may lead to uncontrollable hemorrhage from dissolution of the blood clots. The nurse must be aware of any unusual medical problems for which medical clearance must be obtained preoperatively. As in most operative cases, the patient is taught the necessity for breathing and coughing exercises, as well as the leg exercises, and how to do them. The emotional implications of this kind of surgery involve both the patient and his family and the nurse must be understanding of their anxieties.

The preoperative preparation for retropubic prostatectomy is the same as for any abdominal surgery. When the perineal procedure is used, an incision is made anterior to the anus and, for this reason, it is necessary to place the patient on a "bowel prep" which consists of cathartics, enemas, and a low residue diet.

Postoperatively, the initial consideration for the patient who has had prostatic surgery is careful monitoring of the vital signs. Because of the average age of the prostatectomy patient, hypertension may be present preoperatively and any drop in blood pressure will be significant. Close observation and accurate measurement of the urinary drainage are also of prime importance. An indwelling catheter is attached to straight drainage and hourly urine measurements are taken.

Since there may be some bleeding, the nurse should make frequent observations of the amount and color of the drainage; and she must be able to distinguish between arterial and venous bleeding. Bright red drainage,

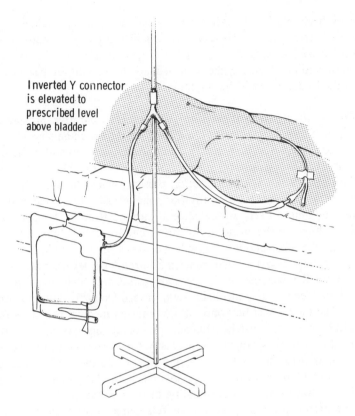

Figure 4. Bladder decompression

when associated with increased viscosity and bright red clots in the tubing, demonstrates a significant loss of blood and the physician should be notified immediately. Hypotension and pallor indicate that an emergency situation exists. Serious bright red bleeding without clots is indicative of a blood dyscrasia or possibly hemolysis. Reports of the preoperative coagulation studies will help to identify the dyscrasia. Irrigating the wound with an isotonic solution will counteract hemolysis.

Venous bleeding is characterized by a dark burgundy discoloration of the urinary drainage. In excessive amounts, the viscosity of the drainage may increase and black clots will form. This can be controlled either by decompression or by intermittent irrigation. Decompression prevents the bladder from emptying rapidly and the small amounts of urine that always remain in the bladder act as a tamponade. This is accomplished by having the urine that drains from the catheter go uphill through a prescribed length of tubing before it goes into the collection bag. The tubing from the catheter is attached to an inverted Y connector taped to an IV pole at a prescribed height. Since it is necessary for the urine to travel uphill, against gravity, a certain amount will always remain in the bladder. The inverted end of the Y is kept open to provide a safety exit in the event the pressure in the system gets too high. The vent also prevents the siphon from falling, thereby draining all the urine from the bladder. It is important to note that the bladder may be full of clots, yet the system seems to be working freely. Persistent complaints of suprapubic pressure and discomfort may indicate this, and palpation of the bladder suprapubically for distention can confirm it. Again, the doctor should be notified. Venous bleeding will gradually subside until the urine is amber in color, or slightly pink tinged, by about the fourth postoperative day.

Intake and output measurements are necessary but of no value unless accurate. The importance of subtracting irrigating solutions from the urinary drainage and of distinguishing routes of intake and output cannot be over-stressed. Blood, plasma, and fluid replacement, as well as accurate electrolyte balancing depend upon these records. Any apparent decrease in urinary function should be immediately reported, but not until the patency and positioning of the tubing are checked.

Wound care following suprapubic or retropubic prostatectomy is similar to that following any abdominal operation. The dressing should be changed as often as necessary and a dry, sterile dressing applied. Initially, the drainage tube is sutured to the wound, but the sutures are cut when the drain is advanced and a sterile safety pin is run through the drain to prevent it from slipping back into the wound. When a suprapubic cystotomy tube is used, even though it is connected to a straight drainage system, there may be drainage around the tube. If this is copious, the position of the tube must be checked frequently for patency or dislodgement.

After a perineal prostatectomy, perineal care is instituted on or about the second postoperative day, or after the first change of dressing. Washing with a cleansing agent and exposure to a heat lamp will promote healing. Sitz baths are begun after removal of the drain.

Early ambulation and good pulmonary hygiene are of importance in preventing pulmonary and cardiovascular complications. Antiembolic stockings or elastic bandages should be applied, especially if the patient is elderly.

Intravenous therapy is continued for 24 to 48 hours after surgery, depending on the patient's ability to tolerate fluids. Fluids are started slowly and the diet is increased gradually. Perineal prostatectomy patients are kept on fluids or a low residue diet to minimize bowel activity, since this operation can cause relaxation of the sphincter muscles and fecal incontinence.

Painful bladder spasms that are rapid in onset and subside within a few minutes may be experienced during the first two to four days. They may be caused by movements of the catheter, controlled by antispasmodics, and eliminated by removal of the catheter.

When the patient has had a cystotomy tube in place, it is usually removed as soon as feasible and a dry, sterile dressing applied as needed. The urethral catheter is removed several days later. In other cases, the urethral catheter is removed after two to three days, depending on whether bleeding has ceased. Following the removal of either of these tubes, the time and amount of voiding are carefully noted and recorded. Urgency and dribbling may occur for several days after the removal, but the patient may be reassured that this is temporary. Perineal exercises are helpful in restoring bladder control. These include emptying the bladder and starting and stopping the urinary stream. The nurse should suggest to the patient who is ready for discharge that he limit his fluid intake during the evening in order to prevent nocturia—a problem that can cause him much anguish. She can be really helpful in preparing him for return to his family and former way of life by stressing the point that his present condition is transient and will gradually improve. The family should also be made aware of the facts and be encouraged to assist the patient by their understanding and love.

Palliative treatment is employed for patients whose physical condition is not amenable to surgery. This consists of the administration of estrogens. The prescribed dose is determined by the physician and the patient is maintained on this dosage. Although hormonal treatment is not curative, the relief of pain and obstruction caused by the cancer is often quite dramatic. Medical follow-up is important for the patient who is receiving hormonal therapy, since recent evidence indicates that emboli may occur. The patient should be told that his body fat will be redistributed and that breast enlargement will occur, so that these things will not disturb him unduly when they happen. Soon after medication is begun, the patient is able to return home and there, among his family and friends, can return to a reasonably full and active life.

CANCER OF THE TESTIS

Testicular tumors are very rare and arouse far more interest than their frequency justifies. Only about two thousand cases occur per year in this country, or about two in every 100,000 males in the population. Between 50 and 100 new cases of tumor of the testis are seen at Memorial Hospital each year. One interesting and unexplained fact about this tumor is that it has a definite predilection for whites over blacks.

The most common tumors of the testis are classified as germinal tumors, of which there are five groups. For the purposes of this discussion they will be divided into two main groups—seminoma and tumors other than seminoma. The latter include embryonal carcinoma, teratoma, teratocarcinoma, and choriocarcinoma. In addition to the pathologic classification relative to local morphology of the tumor, testicular tumors are staged according to their local extent. Stage A tumors are confined to the testis and epididymis. Stage B tumors are those which have metastasized only as far as the regional lymph nodes. Stage C tumors are those that have spread to areas outside of the regional lymph node area.

Diagnosis

The outstanding presenting manifestation of testicular cancer is a painless mass in the scrotum. Usually the patient notices it while he is showering or dressing. Occasionally, a patient presents with a symptom complex not unlike that of epididymitis and he may be treated for a period of weeks or even months for epididymitis before the true diagnosis becomes known. One systemic manifestation of testicular tumor is gynecomastia. This results from the fact that the tumor is capable of elaborating hormones that induce breast enlargement. Patients with metastatic disease may also exhibit this symptom, but enlargement does not necessarily mean that one is dealing with disseminated cancer. The most common sites of metastases are the lung, liver, and lymph nodes. Embryologically, the testes originate in association with the kidneys, which accounts for the fact that the lymph nodes that drain the testes are situated along the aorta and vena cava. And this fact, in turn, accounts for the treatment of the regional lymph node system either by radiation or surgery in this area, not in the groin. A testicular tumor does not spread to the groin under ordinary circumstances; it spreads to the retroperineal nodes that are associated with the kidney.

The clinical study of these patients includes urinary gonadotrophin assays, chest x-rays to rule out metastasis, and an intravenous pyelogram to check for ureteral deviation by retroperineal lymph node enlargement. A lymphangiogram is done and occasionally an inferior vena cavagram— also to check for lymph node enlargement.

Treatment

The treatment of testicular carcinoma is not well standardized. Admittedly, the best way to treat this disease is by removing the testis; there is no disagreement on this point. The major question that does arise is whether the regional lymph nodes should be treated by irradiation, or surgery, or both, and that question cannot be answered with the information now available. Various combinations of irradiation, surgery, and chemotherapy appear to have the capacity to control at least some of the symptoms in patients with distant metastases and, in such situations, the physician never gives up until he has exhausted all the possibilities.

The important point in the treatment of cancer of the testis is that this disease is curable although it is sometimes depressing to deal with because it occurs chiefly in young men. Some patients do die of it, but the overall cure rate is about 60 to 70 percent. Seminoma has a very good cure rate because, first of all, it is not an aggressive tumor, and secondly, it is amenable to successful treatment by irradiation. In the great majority of patients the survival rate is excellent. For patients with stage A seminoma, that is, a tumor that seems to be confined to the testis, the survival rate is at least 90 percent. Tumors other than seminoma and which appear clinically to be stage A tumors have a survival rate of at least 60 to 70 percent.

At Memorial Hospital, the recommended treatment for cancer of the testis, whether it be a stage A, B, or C tumor, is orchiectomy. This controls the primary tumor, establishes the diagnosis, and prevents further dissemination from the primary source. If the tumor is a seminoma, radiation is recommended unless there is wide dissemination at the time of diagnosis, and then treatment consists of varying combinations of irradiation and alkylating agents to which these tumors are very responsive. If the tumor is other than a seminoma, retroperitoneal lymph node dissection is advised. This is an abdominal operation, usually carried out transabdominally. Its major side-effect is that seminal emission is lost; thus, although these patients are not made impotent by the operation, they become infertile. Spermatazoa may be manufactured in the remaining testis, but the operation makes it impossible for the sperm to be ejaculated into the seminal fluid. When the tumor is resectable, the patient is treated with adjunctive chemotherapy. When it is not resectable, he is treated with a combination of irradiation and chemotherapy.

Comprehensive Nursing Care of the Patient with Testicular Cancer

The patient with cancer of the testis is usually young and in apparently good health. His only complaint is a mass or swelling in the scrotum, which may be accompanied by backache. He may have a history of trauma, and for this reason will ignore the swelling and expect it to go away spontaneously. Trauma is not usually the cause of the swelling, but it gives the young man an opportunity to confide in someone without embarrassment. The most logical person for him to turn to is his wife or parent, and together they seek medical advice, but the idea that the difficulty might be cancer probably never occurs to them. Then they find that this young person must be admitted to a hospital for an orchiectomy.

Routine laboratory and diagnostic tests, including a chest x-ray, which is particularly important in ruling out metastasis, are performed. A base line 24-hour urine specimen is collected for chorionic gonadotrophic assay, and will be repeated postoperatively if the results are positive. As the patient is prepared for surgery, it must be remembered that this relatively minor diagnostic operation represents an emotional heartbreak for all concerned. The resulting anxieties and reactions of the patient and his family must be handled with patience and compassion.

The surgery consists of making a small inguinal incision and removing the spermatic cord and testis. A biopsy is not done in these cases, since an incision into a malignant testicular tumor may cause local spillage and result in recurrence and metastasis to the inguinal nodes. If the exposed tissue is suspected of being malignant, the specimen, consisting of the testis, epididymis, and attached spermatic cord, is removed.

In the early postoperative period, the emphasis in nursing care is on measures to relieve pain and anxiety, since the definite tissue diagnosis is still pending. The tissue diagnosis will determine the treatment, which may be further surgery, irradiation, or chemotherapy using one or a combination of drugs. When the patient is told his diagnosis, just the fact that there are recognized methods of treating his disease, be they curative or palliative, is somewhat reassuring to him. The nurse must be aware of methods of treatment that might be used so that she will be able to clear up any misconceptions that the patient or his family may have.

Once the diagnosis of cancer is established, the surgical procedure utilized is a retroperitoneal lymph node dissection, since the route for metastasis of testicular cancer is usually lymphatic. The lymphatic network leading from the testis is complicated and, since metastasis may occur while the primary growth is still small, it is important for nurses to understand that while a nodal metastasis may occur in the supraclavicular area relatively early, it is not always proof of advanced disease.

Preoperatively, the nurse should familiarize the patient with what he may expect following his surgery. Many of these young patients are having their first hospital experience, and they are frightened and reluctant to move about much postoperatively. Teaching the patient preoperatively how to deep breathe and cough, and how to splint himself, and assuring him that although he will have pain after surgery this can be controlled with medication, will all help to ease his anxiety.

Postoperatively, accurate recording of vital signs is important because much of the node dissection was done in areas close to the large abdominal vessels. Any significant drop in blood pressure should be reported to the physician immediately. Dressings should be checked frequently; there will be some drainage through the drain site, but it should not be excessive. Accurate recording of intake and output is stressed. An indwelling catheter is usually in place for the first 24 hours. Because of the abdominal approach and the handling of the abdominal organs in this procedure, the patient also has a nasogastric tube so that gastric suction can be used to remove the gastric juice and decompress the stomach. Intravenous fluids will be given until the patient has bowel sounds and can tolerate fluids in adequate amounts.

The patient is often hesitant to move about, even though preoperative instruction was given. The nurse explains that activity will decrease the need for the nasogastric tube, and the patient may consider that possibility but still choose to remain in bed. Activity is necessary, because any handling of the intestines gives them an inertia that only exercise can overcome. As the patient moves about, the exercise makes him breathe more deeply and promotes the return of normal bowel sounds. Also, he becomes tired and will probably get a better night's sleep because of fatigue.

If the preoperative 24-hour urine for chorionic gonadotrophins was positive, a postoperative collection is obtained and, if it is still positive, there are probably distant metastases. Chemotherapy may then be used, either as a prophylactic or therapeutic measure. A combination of drugs is administered; the length of therapy is long; the side-effects are distasteful; but the long-term results are gratifying.

All of the nurse's skill and ingenuity will be taxed when, about ten days postoperatively, the patient is started on a drug that will make him feel worse than he did after his surgery. He will be nauseated, weak, listless, and his hair may fall out. All this results from his medical treatment, and he may have been told that it will have to be repeated at least every two months for two years. This is a difficult regimen for the patient to accept. The nurse must direct every effort toward providing the necessary supportive measures and skills needed to minimize the discomforting side-effects of the drug. She can assure the patient that his hair will grow back, sometimes curly, if it was previously straight. Weakness and listlessness can be accommodated; activity can be controlled or limited. If the patient is nauseated and the sight of food is revolting to him, supplementary feedings may be administered. Accurate intake and output records are kept in order to monitor the nutritional needs of the patient. Sometimes just the hydration and the chemical effects of the intravenous solution can make him feel better. Antiemetics are usually available on a PRN basis, besides being administered at a specified time prior to the administration of the chemotherapeutic drug. The nurse must also be aware of the toxic effects of the drugs used in chemotherapy; damage may occur to the various blood cells, bone marrow, and lymph nodes. Frequent laboratory studies, including a white blood cell count and a platelet count are made, and significant changes in cells are noted. Some of the drugs may produce oral or intestinal ulceration or irritation. In such instances, an antifungal suspension and a soothing mouthwash may be helpful. Diarrhea can also be controlled by medication. All in all, this is a difficult time for a young man who entered the hospital just three weeks previously for treatment of a small swelling.

Radiation therapy may also be used in conjunction with primary surgery, to destroy metastatic lesions. Patients receiving radiation often complain of a flu-like malaise, nausea, diarrhea, and anorexia. These symptoms are relieved by the use of antiemetics, tranquilizers, and constant reassurance. It is important for nurses to be aware of the fact that, due to the patient's youth, the castrating effects of the disease, and the generally poor prognosis, they may become more sympathetic than empathetic in their relationships with the patient. This does not help the patient at all. What he needs is mature understanding and judgment, tempered with kindness. After all, the nurse is helping to prepare him for a return to his community and normal activities, knowing that this very unpleasant treatment will probably be repeated often. If the initial episode is well handled, perhaps the patient will not dread the subsequent ones and can concentrate on the job of living.

SPECIAL CARE FOR THE PATIENT
WITH AN ILEAL CONDUIT

One who teaches self-care to patients who have an ileal conduit and who must wear an appliance throughout the rest of their lives, must consider many factors. First, patients' attitudes toward their self-image vary greatly. Many experience a change in personality and develop a negative attitude of complete or partial rejection of their situation. The patient who has been semi-comfortable and up and about after his operation will often show some form of rejection of the change in his body that the surgery created. One who has experienced lengthy periods of illness and suffered other symptoms associated with it, will usually have a more receptive attitude toward the change in his physical makeup. Being allowed to release his feelings through talking and questioning will help him to maintain the integrity of his personality. Having his queries answered in a straightforward way will help to relieve him of his present fears and any that he may entertain for the future. The stoma therapist has an important job in helping these patients make the necessary adjustments so that they can return to their preoperative activities in the community. (See Appendix A, p. 301.)

The second most important factor is that instruction in self-care must be geared to the patient's level of comprehension. Facts should be taught accurately, utilizing simple lay language, and the teacher should be constantly reassuring and avoid any statement that may cause the patient to reject the instruction. It is well to involve a member of the family early in the teaching program, because this person will provide important moral support to the patient after he goes home. Studies have indicated that the spouse is the one who most often furnishes the key to the patient's success or failure in adapting to his disability.

Instruction in self-care is presented in steps, and the reason for each step is explained fully. The patient who takes his own notes during instruction will find them helpful, and just doing this helps him to be less apprehensive. He may add his own notes to the instruction card (see Appendix B). However, each patient must be approached on an individual basis, because no two will react in exactly the same way to instruction.

The patient is first taught to prepare the appliance. Then he is shown how to apply two coats of tincture of benzoin to the flange (a round, thin head on the permanent appliance) of the clean appliance, followed by special cement or double-face adhesive (some patients are allergic to one or the other). A most important point for the patient to remember is that the valve must be closed when the appliance is put on or there will be spillage of urine which would not only be embarrassing to the patient but discouraging too. When the patient has taken his own notes, the second application of the bag usually goes quite smoothly.

The patient should be standing when applying the appliance but, if this is not possible, he should be sitting upright. He is told to protrude his abdomen (this stretches the skin and prevents wrinkling) so as to have a smooth base to which to attach the appliance. He holds the appliance and, looking down directly at the stoma, places the opening directly over the stoma, holds it there for a few seconds and then presses his fingers around the flange to secure it to the skin. Then he fastens the belt around his torso. Cleanliness is emphasized throughout the procedure. The patient is also taught how to clean the appliance (after removal) by using a little solvent on the flange, and then removing the solvent with soap and water or skin cleanser, and allowing the appliance to soak overnight in a detergent (Urikleen) or weak chlorine solution. The next morning it is rinsed and hung on a special rack to dry.

Immediately after his return from the operating room, the patient is given an accessory kit and appliance of the proper size and everything needed to apply and care for it. Permanent appliances have an attachment that can be used during the night, and the patient is encouraged to use it.

In all instruction regarding self-care, hygiene is stressed, particularly the necessity of frequent bathing and proper cleansing of the skin before attaching the appliance. The patient is also told that a sediment that feels like sand and which acts like sandpaper on the stoma, may collect in the bag. This is an alkaline salt and can be eliminated by a cranberry regimen— one or two glasses a day. Cranberry juice will also help to keep the appliance from developing a urine odor. Before he goes home, the patient is given detailed instructions about where and how to order equipment, and what he may use for substitutes should he run out of something. He is given at least a month's supply when he leaves the hospital. Patients from outside the United States are given a six-month's supply. The enterostomal therapist attends to this aspect of care.

One Patient's Reaction to Her Ileal Conduit

The content of this chapter was extracted from a tape recording of a symposium on urogenital cancer held at Memorial Hospital. Among the panel members were two patients who had ileal conduits constructed in the surgical treatment of their disease. The following statement of one of them points up the fact that, although this is a drastic and often image-shattering procedure, it is possible for one to survive it with dignity, grace, and humor.

Well, it has changed me. Like many of your patients, I was retired and looking forward to many things, and now I have taken up this unexpected—I won't call it a hobby exactly—different way of taking care of myself. And I can tell you there is one real consolation in this—more than a consolation. I am rather proud of myself that I can still learn new things. And also, I can laugh at myself, being so very awkward and having small disasters, and really, bedwetting at my age!

All of these things could make one angry, or could be turned into a new way of living and quite an adventure, I may say. Different perhaps from going on a safari, but interesting just the same.

I think the thing that struck me most was the miraculousness of having an ileal conduit constructed—knowing of course that it was a lifesaving thing—but I was really awed that I could have this thing done, and that it works.

Each of us will meet any crisis that comes up in his or her own way, but this is something learnable and that is what I think I am most proud of. Just to keep learning and growing and living is really very wonderful.

LONG-TERM MANAGEMENT OF THE
PATIENT WITH UROLOGIC CANCER

Plans for the patient's discharge are anticipated at the time he is admitted to the hospital. The main problem that faces the person about to undergo urologic surgery is fear—fear of death due to cancer, or rejection by his friends and family, of possibly being unable to hold down his job, or of inability to participate in his usual life activities. These threats to his self-image may give rise to either withdrawal or severe anxiety. Knowing that this is a unique experience for the patient, the team objective is to establish an atmosphere of trust and to develop an individualized care plan based on the patient's specific needs. The plan includes telling the patient, prior to surgery, what his operation will consist of, what he can expect in the postoperative period, and how it will be possible for him to live and carry on his former activities while wearing a permanent appliance—if that will be needed.

Before the patient goes home he is told to watch for excoriation of the skin which may result from improper application of the appliance, and for bleeding or edema of the stoma which may occur when the appliance rests on any part of the stoma. Also, he is told to report to his physician any untoward symptoms, such as unusual pain or diminished urinary output.

The patient's socioeconomic and cultural background will greatly affect his reactions and adjustments to his status postoperatively, and his family's reactions to him as well. A member of the clergy can often be helpful in assisting the patient to come to terms with his illness just by making it possible for him to discuss his fears with someone other than medical personnel. Thus, he may gain insight into his reactions to his illness before he goes home. The prime function of the nurse at this time is to help alleviate the patient's fears through guidance, logical discussion, and repetitive teaching which includes the family. If the patient will require assistance with self-care after he gets home, a referral to the Visiting Nurse Association is made. The referral should include information regarding medication that has been ordered for sleep or pain, the nature of the operation that was done, the type of appliance being used, the extent of activity the patient is capable of, and the patient's and family's reactions to his surgery.

On post-discharge clinic visits, the nurse will assess the patient's progress and reinforce the instruction in self-care that he was given while in the hospital. Constant reassurance is important to the patient's rehabilitation, and repetitive teaching cannot be over-stressed. When a family member accompanies the patient to the outpatient department, that person is included in the teaching. Unless the family, as well as the patient, accepts the alteration in the patient's body image and function, he may feel rejected and his progress will be slowed. He may have no appetite and will lose considerable weight. The nurse should encourage him to take small portions of some nourishment every two hours.

Emergency situations that may arise after the patient leaves the hospital include pain, hematuria, chills and fever, decreased urinary output, and distention. He should be instructed to call his doctor or the hospital for advice. If he calls the hospital, the nurse in charge of the genitourinary service will try to evaluate the extent of the emergency and advise the patient either to come to the hospital immediately, refer him to the physician, or schedule him for an early appointment in the outpatient department. The patient must be made aware of the importance of vigilant follow-up care and of the fact that the rehabilitation period continues until he is fully able to return to a life that is as normal as his situation will allow.

Follow-up outpatient department visits for Memorial Hospital patients are scheduled according to the patient's progress. Initially, it may be weekly, then every three to six months, and then annually.

In the long-term management of urogenital cancer, when there is recurrence of disease and increased debilitation, realistic goals must be set for the patient. Allowing him to ventilate his problems is helpful, and continued compassion and kindness go a long way in alleviating fears. His family often needs assistance to enable them to cope with the changing state of the patient's condition. As he becomes increasingly debilitated by his recurrent illness, the family becomes increasingly involved in providing the necessary care. Periodic conferences with the clinic (or outpatient department) staff are encouraged so that an evaluation can be made when problems such as the need for increased medication for pain arise. Financial assistance, and perhaps household assistance, may also be required to maintain the family unit. Sometimes transportation services need to be provided for patients who must get to the clinic for treatment. Whatever the state of the patient's health and whatever his needs, it is important for the nurse to help him to maintain as much independence as possible.

Frequently, patients with urogenital cancer will be referred to a social worker. Her relationship to these patients is unique in several ways. First, it involves not only the patient but his family as well. Second, it is a sustaining relationship that is maintained for as long as the patient and his family are in need of her assistance. Third, it demands that the social worker be able to grasp the patient's emotional status at any time, whether it be at a point of crisis or on a routine clinic visit. Also, it is a relationship that has to be viewed in the context of other relationships that have developed between the patient and various team members while he was hospitalized. The techniques that the social worker uses in her relationship with the patient must be geared to the special problems that arise in connection with his illness. Many of these patients are men who are on the verge of retirement, and often, especially early in the relationship, they have a strong need to ventilate angry feelings about having acquired such a disease at a time in their lives when they were looking forward to reasonable financial security and relaxation. All of them—young or old—are likely to have guilt feelings about having placed such a burden on their families. The younger patient is often the breadwinner for his family and, from a psychodynamic point of view, his masculine identity is linked to this role. Depending on how sturdily this role is linked to masculinity, the social worker may be able to help the patient find other ways of maintaining his identity as a male. If his masculine identity is linked to sexual potency, and the surgery or other treatment has made him impotent, he may be unable to feel potent in any other area. Again, depending on how much priority he places on this, the worker may help him to find ways to compensate for his sexual impotency. Often the worker will have the role of go-between until the patient and his family are able to communicate with each other about their feelings concerning the man's illness.

One of the most important messages that the social worker needs to convey to the family is that she will continue to be available to them after the patient's death, should that occur. Family members often feel very angry toward medical personnel after the death of a relative and they need to talk to someone outside about these angry feelings. They may also tend to blame themselves for not having been able to save their loved one and, consequently, feelings of guilt add to their grief. The social worker's availability to the family continues while they begin to come to grips with both the painful feelings and the practical problems precipitated by the patient's illness.

QUESTIONS AND ANSWERS

Q. How much does the physician tell the patient who has urogenital cancer?

A. In most cases treated at Memorial Hospital, the patient is told that he has a malignant tumor and exactly what the physician plans to do about it. Because of the anatomic area involved, this is a medicolegal necessity quite apart from medical ethics. Informed consent is now mandatory. The patient must know what is going to be done and why, and what the risks and ill effects are. For example, a patient who is going to have a cystectomy for cancer of the bladder is told that he will lose his normal urinary function and his sexual function. If he is going to have a radical prostatectomy, he is told that he will lose his sexual function, and possibly his urinary control and if he is going to have a node dissection for testicular tumor, he must be told that he will probably be infertile but his sexual mechanics will be normal otherwise. The physician is perfectly frank with the patient in terms of what his diagnosis is, what will be done about it, and what the complications or unfortunate effects of the various procedures are.

Q. Is there any correlation between undescended testes and the development of testicular tumor?

A. The incidence of testicular tumor is 10 to 40 times higher in men with an undescended testis than in men with normally descended testes. The incidence of tumor of the testis is about 1 per 100,000 men, but if you consider only men in the age group in which this tumor is likely to occur, the incidence is probably about 1 in 20 to 30,000. Then if you multiply this rate by 10, it becomes apparent that a man with an undescended testis has about one chance in 2,000 or 3,000 of developing cancer of the testis. So that undoubtedly there is a relationship. Furthermore, if a patient has a tumor in one testis, there is almost a 25 percent chance that he already has, or will get, a tumor in the other testis, a risk that is high enough to justify prophylactic castration. It should be stated here that the consensus among physicians is that a testis in an abnormal position is not more prone to develop tumors simply because of its abnormal position, because the incidence of testicular cancer is not changed when the testis is brought into normal position.

Q. Is smoking a factor in the etiology of cancer of the bladder?

A. A number of epidemiological studies have been done here and abroad that indicate that bladder cancers are approximately twice as common in smokers as in non-smokers. In other words, the risk of bladder tumors is presumably doubled in smokers. However, epidemiological studies in the Scandinavian countries and in the United Kingdom have not borne out these statistics. In any case, the correlation between smoking and the development of bladder cancer is nowhere nearly as spectacular as that between smoking and lung cancer.

Q. Is chronic cystitis a predisposing factor in cancer of the bladder?

A. There is probably some increase in the risk of cancer in people with chronic bladder inflammation of any sort, just as there is an increased risk of cancer in smokers over non-smokers. However, many people who have chronic cystitis over many years do not develop bladder tumors.

Q. Do patients with renal carcinoma require hemodialysis pre- or postoperatively?

A. Generally, no. The tumor is removed by removing one kidney, and the other kidney is sufficient to support life. Should a recurrence or a new tumor arise in the remaining kidney, a partial nephrectomy would be carried out, but this is not usually done unless the remaining part of the kidney is adequate to sustain life. However, if such an operation is done, it is possible that hemodialysis will be needed to tide the patient over the postoperative period.

Q. What endocrine treatments are helpful in patients with metastatic prostatic cancer?

A. Estrogen therapy or castration, or a combination of these, have approximately the same effect in ameliorating the course of metastatic prostatic cancer.

For many years, Estinyl was used in doses of one-half milligram per day; this would be the equivalent of about 10 to 30 mg of diethylstilbestrol. Recent evidence suggests that such large doses are not necessary to obtain a good remission, and that the adverse effect they may have on blood coagulability could lead to an increased risk of thromboembolism. At Memorial Hospital, the current recommendation is Estinyl, .05 mg a day, or stilbestrol 1 mg per day. There is no evidence at present to suggest the superiority of one estrogen over the others, nor is there any acceptable evidence of the superiority of large doses over small doses.

For patients who have relapsed following conventional endocrine therapy, symptomatic remissions can sometimes be achieved by hypophysectomy, by corticosteroids and sometimes by progestational steroids; usually all of these receive some trial in the patient who has relapsed following conventional therapy.

Q. What is the recommended treatment for a patient with a kidney tumor and metastasis to the femur?

A. This situation presents a difficult problem for the physician. There are a few cases on record in which a kidney tumor and a solitary metastasis have been removed. Unless the patient wants to take the risk of going the whole way with treatment on the possibility that he might be cured, a nephrectomy would be done and the metastatic lesion would be treated with radiation or cryosurgery. If he wants the ultimate in treatment, he would have a leg amputation. In some cases, an arm has been removed because of pain in a metastatic lesion in the upper end of the humerus. But in general, the prognosis for a patient with even a single metastasis is poor.

Q. Do any problems with wound healing arise when the patient is given radiation before a cystectomy?

A. No major problems develop unless the surgeon does extensive debriding. The closure is done with steel wires and, occasionally, with silver retention sutures.

Q. What is the main problem that arises for patients on ileal conduits?

A. Difficulty with the appliance is the main problem. Often the appliance leaks and the patients have to be re-taught the procedure of applying it properly.

Q. Should indwelling bladder catheters ever be clamped and if so, under what circumstances?

A. There is no reason for clamping a catheter except, perhaps, when the patient is being moved from the operating room to the recovery room; also, if the bag is not applied immediately, a plastic plug may be used temporarily. Occasionally, a patient does not want a bag and can handle an indwelling catheter by using a plastic plug which he removes when necessary and allows the urine to drain out. A nephrostomy or ureterostomy tube should *never* be clamped.

Q. What does a clinic patient do when a problem arises other than at clinic time?

A. Usually, the patient will call the hospital and is connected with the evening supervisor who will, in turn, get a doctor on the genitourinary service to take care of him if it is an emergency situation.

APPENDIX A

MEMORIAL SLOAN-KETTERING CANCER CENTER
DEPARTMENT OF NURSING
INSERVICE EDUCATION

Accessory Kit Supplies

Green plastic tote box
Tincture of benzoin
Antibacterial skin cleanser
Solvent
Skin bond cement
Dusting powder
Paper tape
Karaya powder
Alcohol swabs
Gauze sponges 4 x 4
Urikleen or similar deodorizer
Plastic drying rack for appliance
Bongart bags (emergency use)
Stoma measuring guide

Care of Appliance

1. Remove cement from face plate with a little solvent.
2. Wash appliance with mild soap and water. Use Urikleen or similar deodorizer as final rinse or overnight soak.
3. Put cleaned appliance on plastic hanger and dry away from heat.
4. Wash belt when soiled with mild soap and water. Rinse well and dry away from heat.

KEEP THIS REFERENCE CARD IN GREEN ACCESSORY KIT

Application of Appliance (Grick's, Perma, Marlen or similar)

I.   *Prepare Appliance*
  A. Apply one or two coats of tincture of benzoin to flange of clean appliance.
  B. Apply cement or double faced adhesive disc to flange of bag.
  C. Close outlet valve and set the prepared bag aside.

II.   *Prepare Skin*
  A. Have patient in standing position when possible. Empty bag.
  B. Remove old appliance carefully using a small amount of solvent.
  C. Remove old cement or adhesive from skin with a minimal amount of solvent.
  D. Remove solvent with antibacterial skin cleanser and water. Dry skin.
  E. Hold rolled gauze wick over stoma while preparing the skin.
  F. Apply two coats of tincture of benzoin or similar skin preparation to skin around stoma. Fan dry the skin.
  G. Use small Karaya seal or Karaya powder to area surrounding stoma.

III.   *Apply Appliance*
  A. Have patient protrude his abdomen and center the new appliance from the bottom upwards to assure proper fit.
  B. Apply pressure evenly to assure a good bond. Snap waist belt to hooks on face plate of the appliance.
  C. Dust edges around face plate with talcum if skin cement was used as the bonding agent.

KEEP IN GREEN TOTE BOX
ILEOSTOMY OR ILEAL CONDUIT INSTRUCTION CARD

APPENDIX B

MEMORIAL SLOAN-KETTERING CANCER CENTER
DEPARTMENT OF NURSING
INSERVICE EDUCATION

Return to Enterostomal Therapist   KEEP IN NURSING CARE
(upon discharge)   KARDEX

Name_____   Unit_____

Ileal Conduit or Ileostomy Check List

Stoma Care: *Equipment:*

                               Date/Nurse   Nurse/Date

Observed by patient   Care of equipment
Observed by family   Night drainage
Performed by patient   Procur. of supplies
Performed by family   Green access. kit
Appliance: *Miscellaneous:*
Temporary name   Ostomy hygiene
Permanent name   Follow up care
Patient applied   V.N.S. referral
Family applied   Dietary management
Seen by volunteer
Patient applied
Appliance

Points to Be Discussed with Family Member, Volunteer, Patient and Nurse
at Patient's Bedside
1. Travel and travel kit.
2. Management of common skin problems.
3. Activities permitted and prohibited.
4. Wardrobe and underwear.
5. Resumption of social activities (sexual if applicable).
6. Odor control.
7. Maintenance of good hydration to prevent crystals and stones.
8. Availability of hospital personnel to help with problems arising after hospital discharge (emergencies).
9. Thoughts and feelings about the changed body image.
10. Return to work and what to tell family and friends.
11. Discuss the operative procedure generally.
12. Need for privacy during appliance change.
13. Need for discussion of ostomy with family and friends.

SUGGESTED READINGS

Books

Bouchard, Rosemary. *Nursing Care of the Cancer Patient.* St. Louis: Mosby, 1967.

Conn, Howard F. (Ed.). *Current Therapy.* Philadelphia: Saunders, 1964.

Glenn, James F. (Ed.). *Diagnostic Urology.* New York: Hoeber Medical Division, Harper and Row, 1964.

Glenn, James F. and William H. Boyce. *Urologic Surgery.* New York: Hoeber Medical Division, Harper and Row, 1969.

Keuhnelian, John G. and Virginia E. Sanders. *Urologic Nursing.* London: Macmillan, 1970.

Marshall, Victor F. *A Monograph for the Physician: The Diagnosis of Genito-Urinary Neoplasms.* American Cancer Society, 1963.

Marshall, Victor F. *Textbook of Urology,* 2nd ed. New York: Hoeber Medical Division, Harper and Row, 1964.

Moroney, James. *Surgery for Nurses.* London: Churchill Livingstone, 1971.

Raspe, G. and W. Brosig (Eds.). *International Symposium on Treatment of Carcinoma of the Prostate.* Oxford: Pergamon Press-Vieweg, 1971.

Roen, P. B. *Atlas of Urologic Surgery.* New York: Appleton-Century-Crofts, 1967.

Sawyer, J. R. *Nursing Care of the Patients with Urological Disease.* St. Louis: Mosby, 1970.

Smith, Donald R. *General Urology,* 5th ed. Los Altos, Calif.: Lange Medical Publications, 1966.

Starzl, Thomas E. *Experience in Renal Transplantation.* Philadelphia: Saunders, 1964.

Whitehead, Sylvia. *Nursing Care of the Adult Urology Patient.* New York: Appleton-Century-Crofts, 1970.

Periodicals

Ansell, Julian S. "Catheter Care," *Journal of Urology, 89:*940-44, June, 1963.

Blandy, John. "Urinary Bladder Substitution and the Nursing Care Involved," *Nursing Mirror, 122:*5-10, July, 1966.

Bloedorn, F. G. et al. "Radiotherapy in the Treatment of Cancer of the Bladder," *Southern Medical Journal, 60:*539-544, May, 1967.

Bois, Marna S. et al. "Nursing Care of Patients Having Kidney Transplants," *American Journal of Nursing, 68:*1238-47, June, 1968.

Bonnell G. E. "Urologic Investigative Procedures," *Canadian Nurse, 59:*825-28, September, 1963.

Christopher, Nancy. "Postoperative Care Following Nephrectomy," *Canadian Nurse, 59*:838-39, September, 1963.

Cooper, H. G. "Treatment of Genito-Urinary Tuberculosis," *Journal of Urology, 86*:719-27, December, 1961.

Cox, C. E. and D. R. Smith. "Neoplasms of the Kidney and Adrenal Gland," *California Medicine, 100*:351-357, May, 1964.

Craig, Ilsa. "Collecting Specimens of Urine: The Nurse Holds the Key to Diagnosis of Infections," *Nursing Times, 62*:531-32, April 22, 1966.

Creevy, C. D. "Reactions Peculiar to Trans-Urethral Resection of the Prostate," *Surgical Clinics of North America, 47*:1471-1472, December, 1967.

Culp, O. S. "Radical Perineal Prostatectomy: Its Past, Present, and Possible Future," *Journal of Urology, 98*:618-626, November, 1967.

Davis, Joseph E. "Drugs for Urologic Disorders," *American Journal of Nursing, 65*:107-12, August, 1965.

Dick, Vernon S. "Carcinoma of the Prostate Gland with Metastases," *Surgical Clinics of North America, 42*:771-97, June, 1962.

Downing, Shirley R. "Nursing Support in Early Renal Failure," *American Journal of Nursing, 69*:1212-16, June, 1969.

Ellis, William J. and John T. Grayback. "Sexual Function in Aging Males After Orchiectomy and Estrogen Therapy," *Journal of Urology, 89*:895-99, June, 1963.

Enty, Harold F. "Fibrinolysis: A Complication of Transurethral Resection of the Prostate Gland," *Journal of Urology, 91*:671-75, June, 1964.

Felix, Kathleen S. "Total Patient Care: The Team Approach in Transplantation," *Nursing Clinics of North America, 4*:451-60, September, 1969.

Flint, L. D. et al. "Radical Prostatectomy for Carcinoma of the Prostate," *Surgical Clinics of North America, 47*:695-705, June, 1967.

Geist, Dorothy I. "Round the Clock Specimens," *American Journal of Nursing, 60*:1300-1302, September, 1960.

Glantz, G. M. "Cystectomy and Urinary Diversion," *Journal of Urology, 96*:714-717, November, 1966.

Grabstald, Harry. "Cancer of the Prostate," *CA—A Cancer Journal for Clinicians, 15*:1-22, 1965.

Juzwiak, Marijo. "Nursing the Kidney Transplant Patient," *RN, 31*:34-41, May, 1968.

Kassilman, Mary J. "Nursing Care of the Patient with Benign Prostatic Hypertrophy," *American Journal of Nursing, 66*:1026-30, May, 1966.

Kaufman, J. J. "The Diagnosis of Testicular Tumors," *CA—A Cancer Journal for Clinicians, 17*:2-6, January-February, 1967.

Kaufman, J. J. "The Treatment of Testicular Tumors," *CA—A Cancer Journal for Clinicians, 17*:2-6, March-April, 1967.

Kelly, Ann and Goffredo Gensini. "Renal Arteriography," *American Journal of Nursing, 64*:97-99, February, 1964.

Kunin, Calvin M. and Regina C. McCormack. "Prevention of Catheter Induced Urinary Tract Infections by Sterile Closed Drainage," *New England Journal of Medicine, 274*:1155-61, May, 1966.

Laskowski, T. Z. et al. "Combined Therapy: Radiation and Surgery in the Treatment of Bladder Cancer," *Journal of Urology, 99*:733-739, June, 1968.

Leopold, Alice. "Psychological Problems in Hemodialysis," *RN, 31*:42-45, May, 1968.

MacKinnon, Harold A. "Urinary Drainage: The Problems of Asepsis," *American Journal of Nursing, 65*:112, August, 1965.

Miller, Opal. "Nursing Care After Pelvic Exenteration," *American Journal of Nursing, 62*:106-107, May, 1962.

Mohammed, Mary R. B. "Urinalysis," *American Journal of Nursing, 64*:87-89, June, 1964.

Mossholder, Irene B. "When the Patient Has a Radical Retropubic Prostatectomy," *American Journal of Nursing, 62*:101-104, July, 1962.

Murphy, F. J. and S. Zehman. "Ascorbic Acid as a Urinary Acidifying Agent," *Journal of Urology, 94*:297-303, September, 1965.

Patricia, Sister M., and Loyola C. Floyd. "Nursing Care in Prostatectomy," *Canadian Nurse, 59*:833-35, September, 1963.

Samellas, W. "Urinary Control Following Radical Perineal Prostatectomy," *Journal of Urology, 95*:580-583, April, 1966.

Scott, R. "Needle Biopsy in Carcinoma of the Prostate," *Journal of the American Medical Association, 201*:958-960, September 18, 1967.

Tavel, F. R. et al. "Retroperitoneal Lymph Node Dissection," *Journal of Urology, 89*:241-245, February, 1963.

Thomson, Gretchen. "After Renal Surgery," *American Journal of Nursing, 61*:106-107, September, 1961.

Ungvarski, Peter. "Mechanical Stimulation of Coughing," *American Journal of Nursing, 71*:2358-61, December, 1971.

Whitmore, Willet F. "The Treatment of Bladder Tumors," *Surgical Clinics of North America, 49*:349-370, April, 1969.

Wilson, T. H. et al. "Aggressive Approach to Metastatic Testicular Teratocarcinoma," *Journal of Urology, 96*:239-242, August, 1966.

Radiation Therapy—
A Treatment Modality
for Cancer

Regional Medical Program — Oncology Nursing Seminar

on

NURSING MANAGEMENT OF PATIENTS
RECEIVING RADIATION THERAPY

Seminar Leader

Giulio J. D'Angio, M.D.

Seminar Participants

Giulio J. D'Angio, M.D., Chairman, Department of Radiation Therapy

Basil S. Hilaris, M.D., Assistant Attending Radiation Therapist, Department of Radiation Therapy

Roberta Klein, M.S.W., Assistant Director Social Service Department

Jean P. MacNeill, Chief Technologist, Department of Radiation Therapy

Louis Maddalone, Mold Room Technologist, Department of Radiation Therapy

Katherine Nelson, R.N., Ed.D., Associate Professor of Nursing Education, Teachers College, Columbia University

Carol Reed, R.N., B.S., Staff Development Coordinator, Department of Nursing

Prenella Roberts, R.N., Head Nurse, Department of Radiation Therapy

Jean M. St. Germain, M.S., Attending Physicist, Department of Medical Physics

Until fairly recently, the administration of radiation therapy was considered a simple procedure that could be carried out by a physician without help from anyone else. Today, the operation of any department of radiation therapy involves smooth interaction with many other departments and their representatives including physicians, professional nurses, pathologists, internists, radiation technologists, biologists, engineers, and social workers. All of these departments and people must contribute their special knowledge and skills to produce a radiation therapy department that functions smoothly and effectively.

The radiation therapist (an M.D. who specializes in radiation therapy) must be knowledgeable in the field of physics and have an understanding of radioactivity. People are sometimes awed by what radiation means, what it entails for the patient, and what it can mean in terms of exposure hazards for personnel who work with patients receiving radiation. Actually, it is a form of therapy that is very efficient in managing patients with cancer—one of the gentlest ways of treating this disease, in fact. There are problems connected with its use, of course. Some of them are concerned with the actual techniques employed and the medical aspects of the care that is delivered. Others are concerned with such peripheral matters as the problem of getting the patient to and from the hospital for treatment.

The effects of radiation are initiated by the interaction of x-rays or gamma rays with the orbital electrons of the tissue atoms. The result of this interaction damages the DNA and may cause cellular death at the time the cell is about to divide. As the mitotic process progresses, the chromosomes tend to clump and form a bridge between the two potential daughter cells. When radiation is applied, complete division at this bridge is aborted. This effect on cells is clinically observable in a reduction in the size of a tumor after it has been irradiated.

Cells that are most active mitotically are also the most radiosensitive. These are the cells that are involved in malignant lymphomas, leukemia, undifferentiated squamous cell carcinoma, and such germinal tumors as seminomas and germinomas. Moderately radiosensitive tumors include the well-differentiated squamous cell carcinomas of the skin and mucous membrane, adenocarcinoma, and some sarcomas. Relatively radioresistant tumors include osteogenic sarcomas, malignant melanomas, and some gliomas. Radiosensitivity cannot be taken as an indication of curability of a cancer, however, because often the most radiosensitive lesions show marked anaplasia, aggressive growth, and wide dissemination. Actually, the chance for cure by radiation therapy depends mainly on the location and accessibility of the tumor, its size and biologic behavior, and probably immunological factors as well.

Whether radiation is used with intent to cure or to palliate, alone or in combination with other treatment modalities, it has a major role in the management of cancer. In fact, some time in the course of treatment, 50 percent of cancer patients can benefit from radiation therapy. About half of these are treated for cure and about half for palliation. Cure is often obtained, but when this is impossible, the patient's longevity is made infinitely more comfortable by this simple, painless, easy to administer therapy that causes relatively little upset. In many cases, radiotherapy is combined with other modalities with very good results.

MODALITIES AVAILABLE

At the very outset, it is necessary for the physician to decide which modality or combination of modalities will be most likely to benefit the patient, and whether the objective is to cure or to palliate. Cancer of the cervix is the classic example of lesions that are treated by radiation with the intention of obtaining a cure. On the other hand, radiotherapy for cancer of the esophagus is usually given for palliative purposes since, in most cases, the disease is so far advanced by the time the diagnosis is made that cure is impossible. The objective in either case is to deliver a cancericidal dose of radiation to the tumor with the least damage to the surrounding tissues. In outlining a treatment plan, the radiation therapist considers many factors: the general status of the patient; the type, location, and volume of the tumor; and the expected reaction of the tumor to radiation. These, and other physical and biological factors govern the selection of the type and dose of radiation that is prescribed.

Therapeutic radiation is provided by a wide variety of equipment, the various units being capable of generating a broad spectrum of wave lengths with varying penetration characteristics. Isodose charts show the penetration of the beam for a given energy and help verify the suitability of the type of radiation chosen for the particular tumor being treated.

A low-voltage (100 kilovolt) unit is suitable for treating superficial thin lesions such as basal cell carcinoma. It produces soft x-rays of low penetration which deposit most of their energy in the first few centimeters of tissue. The energy from such a unit is quickly absorbed and does not penetrate much beyond the superficial tissues. The megavolt machines in the 250-300 kilovolt range produce x-rays that penetrate somewhat deeper and are useful for treating superficial thick lesions such as tumors of the parotid gland. As the machines step up to a million volts, two million, or even six million, the depth of the penetration of the x-rays becomes correspondingly greater. The betatron produces 35- or even 45-million-volt electron x-rays.

The low-voltage (100 kilovolt) unit delivers approximately 8 percent of its maximum dose at a depth of ten centimeters. At this same level, the 250-volt machine delivers approximately 35 percent, the 2-million volt machine delivers 50 percent, the 6-million volt machine delivers 70 percent, and the 35-million volt betatron delivers 85 to 90 percent of their maximum doses. Thus, the penetration achieved with the betatron permits treatment at depths beyond the reach of the lower energy beams and is useful for treating areas of the body that are quite thick, and for treating very large people. At the higher energies, the edges of the beam are sharp; the rays are not scattered either laterally or backward by the irradiated tissues as is the case with low-energy radiation in which there is significant scatter outside of the field. This confines the radiation more precisely to the treated area. Also, the maximum dose is not reached at the skin surfaces but at varying depths beneath it, so that skin reactions are not a limiting factor.

High-energy ionizing radiation can be obtained from such radioactive isotopes as cobalt-60 which is similar in penetration to the x-rays produced by the 3-million-volt generators. The gamma radiation from isotopes is indistinguishable from the electrically produced x-rays of the same energy value. Over 80 percent of the high-energy units in use today are cobalt-60 units.

The quantity of emitted energy is expressed in roentgens which represent a specific amount of energy. However, the amount of the dose that is absorbed varies with the composition of the tissues and the type of radiation being utilized. With the low-energy units there is considerable difference in the absorption rate of soft tissues and bone—the denser skeletal tissues absorb more of the dose. At higher energies, the absorption differential does not exist, and the amount of energy absorbed by bone and soft tissues is approximately the same. This allows treatment with cancericidal doses in the vicinity of bone without producing bone damage. Also, the finite range of the high-energy beam permits one to give a dose to a tumor that is over a bone and stop just short of the bone. Hence it is very useful in treating tumors in growing children where it is particularly desirable to achieve maximum effect on the tumor while minimizing the effect on the surrounding normal tissues. There is no qualitative difference between the beam from a betatron and that from an x-ray machine. The difference lies in their differing degrees of penetration.

Radiotherapy also employs several types of radioactive materials. The first distinction among these types involves the difference between radioactive nuclides that are concentrated because of physiologic processes, unsealed sources that are introduced in hollow cavities, and the sealed sources, such as radium, that are inserted into tissues. The second distinction is made according to whether the implant is temporary or permanent. A permanent implant (including the use of radioactive seeds or wire material) is what its name implies, and is utilized in the treatment of surgically nonresectable tumors and certain types of superficial lesions that lend themselves to this kind of treatment. A temporary implant is put into place for a specified period of time and then withdrawn, and the patient no longer contains any radioactive material.

Radiation itself may be divided into types, and the two types most frequently used in medical therapeutics are beta and gamma radiation. Beta radiation generally has a very short range; that is, rays travel only a short distance before their energy is dissipated. This is very useful information for the nurse. For example, when a patient is being treated with phosphorous-32, a pure beta source, his body becomes the nurse's shield. Consequently, when a pure beta emitter is used, it is generally considered that there is virtually no external radiation hazard. On the other hand, when gamma radiation, particularly the so-called hard gamma radiation, is being employed, the nurse must rely on the simple inverse square relationship to determine the distance at which she must work to avoid radiation exposure. Nuclides that emit gamma rays are of two types—the hard and the soft gamma emitters. Hard gamma emitters can be compared to high-voltage x-ray machines that produce a penetrating type of radiation. In this instance, the nurse must rely on distance for protection. The soft gamma emitter may be likened to the low-voltage x-ray machine which produces rays with a limited amount of penetration, and the nurse can make use of the patient's body as a shield to attenuate some of the radiation before it reaches her. When a hard gamma emitter is used, no attenuation, or at least very little, is provided by the patient's body.

Half-life is a quality of isotopes that the nurse should know about. Half-life is defined as the rate of decay of isotopes according to the time it takes for them to lose half of their strength. Half-lives vary from fractions of seconds to billions of years. One of the most commonly used isotopes is radium-226 which has a half-life of 1620 years. On the other hand, iodine-125 has a half-life of 60 days, and thus can be used for a permanent implant.

Half value layer (HVL) is a term used to express the amount of material that must be interposed between the nurse and the source of radiation in order to reduce the exposure by one-half. For iodine-125, a soft gamma emitter, the half layer value is 1/1000 of an inch of lead or less. For radium-226, a hard gamma emitter, the half value layer is about half an inch of lead. Thus it can be seen that it is very important for the nurse to know about the properties of the various radium nuclides and to understand what is involved in terms of her own protection.

Remote After-Loading

An improvement in the use of radioactive implants is a technique that is called *remote after-loading*. The patient comes to the radiotherapy department, and an applicator is inserted and connected with plastic tubes to a lead safe installed in the wall of the treatment room. Up to this point there is no radioactive source in the patient. From outside the room, the technologist and the therapist can direct radioactive sources mechanically from the lead safe into the applicator. The advantage of this technique is that the patient does not have to be hospitalized. These are high-intensity sources with treatment times generally less than one hour, as opposed to the 24- or 48-hour treatment time that is needed when radium-226 is used. Additionally, there is no exposure to the radiation therapist, the radiation therapy technologist, or nursing personnel. Consequently, it is to be hoped that the technique of remote after-loading will become widely used.

THE CARDINAL RULES OF
RADIATION PROTECTION

The nurse who cares for patients who are receiving an internal dose of radiation through implantation of a radioisotope needs to observe, at all times, the rules for radiation protection. That is, she needs to know, how to utilize the principles of time, distance, and shielding. The principle of time means simply that the less time the nurse spends with the patient, the less time she is exposed and the less radiation she receives. This does not mean that these patients must be neglected. Good organization is the key to giving the amount of care that is necessary. The nurse needs to plan ahead, to work rapidly, and to do as much as she can away from the bedside. But she should be sure to explain to the patient why these precautions are necessary. She should not linger unnecessarily at the bedside; at the same time, it is important not to shun the patient or to show reluctance to enter the room. Nursing assignments should be rotated, so that no one nurse is consistently exposed over several days. Most well-instructed patients are very considerate of the nursing staff and other attendants, and they often advise personnel about the hazard before they enter the room or if they remain too long at the bedside.

The principle of distance means that the dose rate decreases as the distance from the source of radiation, or the patient, increases. Consequently, the nurse should not linger close to the patient when it is not necessary. When giving nursing care, she should try to stand as far from the source of radiation as possible, depending on the area of the implant. For example, if the patient has a vaginal applicator in place, the nurse should do as much as she can while standing at the head of the bed. When caring for a patient with seeds implanted in the head and neck, it may be possible for her to do much of her work while standing on the opposite side or at the foot of the bed. The principle of shielding implies specifically that the presence, thickness, and kinds of barriers that are placed between the worker and the source of radiation will affect how much radiation the nurse receives. When the dose rate is considered very high, lead shields can be provided for the bedrails or the nurse can wear a lead apron when caring for patients being treated with radionuclides of low energy equivalence.

Patients who are being treated by radioactive implants need an extraordinary amount of reassurance. All personnel should make a special effort to speak to these patients as they pass the door, or wave to them, so they won't think they are being shunned. By spending just a little time with them, the nurse can convey the idea that there is someone to whom they can turn when they feel completely overwhelmed by what is happening to them. Being allowed to have visitors will help to improve a patient's morale, but family members must be told why they will be instructed to remain at a prescribed distance from the patient, why children and pregnant women should not enter the room, and why visits must be limited according to the radiation levels in the room.

In several situations, because of the isotope being used, specific nursing implications exist. For instance, after a patient has had colloidal phosphorous-32 instilled and is returned to the nursing unit, it is essential that he be turned every 10 to 15 minutes for the first two hours to ensure good distribution of the fluid. The patient with a radium or cobalt implant needs special understanding and reassurance from the nursing staff. She is usually on bed rest for 48 to 72 hours, has a Foley catheter in place that needs to be watched to see that it does not become plugged, is on a low residue diet, and is given medication to induce constipation. "Pericare" is not given to these patients although perineal pads may be changed as necessary. Douches are usually ordered after vaginal applicators are removed.

After a temporary implant has been inserted, a tag is affixed to the patient's chart indicating what the exposure rate is at the surface of the patient's body and what it is at one meter from his body, as well as the rate at which the exposure drops. The patient remains in the hospital and in a single room until the nuclide is removed. The tag that is inserted in the patient's chart following implantation of a permanent source differs from the one for a temporary implant in that it not only identifies the nuclide and its exposure rate, but states how long the patient must remain in the hospital and how long he must remain in a single room. These dates are based on the readings that are taken at one meter, since beds in hospital wards are approximately one meter apart and the patient in the next bed should be protected from excessive exposure to radiation. So it is the radiation safety officer or his representative who calculates the date beyond which the radionuclides will have decayed to the point that special precautions are no longer necessary on the part of personnel working with the patient.

At Memorial Hospital, the physics department has the overall responsibility for radiation protection, and the health physics officer keeps an eye on all involved personnel to make sure that no one receives unnecessary exposure.

Film badges are generally assigned to all personnel working in the radiation therapy unit. Some people assume that this badge protects them from radiation, and of course it doesn't. A film badge is simply a piece of masked film worn like a badge by nuclear workers. It is darkened by nuclear radiation, and thus radiation exposure can be checked by inspecting the film. All it is meant to do is to quantitate the radiation the person wearing it receives.

Planning for the Patient's Discharge

Some patients go home while still containing a therapeutic amount of a radionuclide. Such a patient should be interviewed by a member of the radiation department staff who will tailor instructions to meet the particular needs of the patient. If he is a young man with children at home the information he needs will be different from that needed by an older person who may live alone, or who at least would not have young children at home that would be exposed to any radiation hazard. On the other hand, if the older patient has grandchildren who visit him regularly, he should be told about the importance of distance in avoiding exposure. At Memorial Hospital, these patients are given a printed form containing information they may need in order to cope with any problem that may arise after they get home (see Appendix A, p. 331), and also the telephone number of the radiation officer they can call if a particular question comes up. A common misconception is that the patient who contains radioactive material contaminates everything he touches. Family members sometimes ask whether their relatives can sit at the dining table with the family, use the same utensils or sleep in the same bed with another person. They wonder too about shaking hands with him or kissing. Therefore, the printed form is helpful to the family as well as the patient. Sometimes a patient who has an implant of iodine-125 is given a shielded bandage that consists of a piece of lead foil inserted into the bandage which will completely shield out all gamma radiation that might otherwise reach a person standing next to him. When the patient knows that he does not present an external hazard to anyone he comes in contact with, he is more likely to circulate among others and have some social life instead of feeling that he must keep himself isolated.

Another misconception is the idea that a patient who has an implant of radium-226 will contaminate pads or dressings and that the excreta is also contaminated. This is not true. No secretions or discharges from the person being treated with a sealed source are contaminated. The external hazards that exist with these patients are those that must be minimized by applying the simple concepts of time and distance. Another problem that sometimes occurs is that a radiation source may become dislodged. Therefore, a protective lead container should be kept in the patient's room so that if a source does become dislodged, it can be picked up with a forceps, put into the container, and the appropriate radiation safety officer or radiation therapist called for instructions as to how to treat both the source and the patient.

Phosphorus-32 is an isotope that, fortunately, produces only beta radiation. It is used commonly to control effusions. The radionuclide in colloidal suspension is introduced directly into the hollow cavity affected. So long as there is no seepage or drainage, the patient does not present a radiation hazard to anyone working with him because of the limited range of the beta radiation. However, if he has a previous wound, say from a chest tube, and this is still draining, the fluid will be contaminated. There may also be seepage from the wound site. Therefore, Evans blue dye is added to the P^{32} and, since this is easily visualized on dressings and linen, the nurse is instructed to watch for blue staining and to call the radiation therapist or radiation safety officer on duty for advice as to what to do in a particular case. The nurse should wear gloves whenever handling any material that is contaminated or suspected of being contaminated to protect herself. (Radionuclides in solution can be given parenterally or by mouth.)

Fifty percent of iodine-131 will be excreted within 24 hours, most of it in the urine and the rest in saliva and sweat. If urine is to be collected from such a patient, a shielded container should be used and the patient instructed to collect the specimen himself. He is also given paper utensils to use for a specific period of time and these, along with the linen and bed sheets, are collected in such a way that they can be checked for contamination.

THE MULTIDISCIPLINARY MANAGEMENT OF THE PATIENT RECEIVING RADIATION THERAPY

Role of the Radiation Technologist

The fact that one out of every two patients with cancer needs radiation therapy points up the need for more trained personnel, particularly radiation technologists. The role of the technologist is primarily to relieve the radiation therapist of many of the responsibilities that he formerly carried alone. The technologist is now the one who sets up the patient for treatment and is responsible for making certain that the radiation is directed to the locus of the tumor and nowhere else. Until the last few years, it was necessary for these functions to be carried out under the supervision of the radiation therapist. Before 1968, training in radiation technology was largely empirical. In that year, however, the American Medical Association specified the requirements for schools of radiation technology. Now there are several such schools in the United States, the one at Memorial Hospital having been started in October, 1970.

Regardless of the fact that nurses and other personnel try to allay the patient's fears about radiation therapy, many of them come to the department quite frightened. The treatment room has many pieces of large and complicated equipment, some of which hang directly over the patient as he lies on the treatment table. The technologist positions him and talks to him about the machine and the treatment—how long it will last, and what he can expect. He is assured that there will be no pain, that he will be under constant observation via audio and visual communication aids. Sometimes the patient must wait a relatively long time after he arrives in the treatment room while the dose is being computed and equipment is being adjusted to fit the exact specifications drawn up by the therapist. During this time, the technologist gives the patient continuous support. After he is positioned he is made as comfortable as possible with sandbags, pillows, or whatever else is needed to keep him from moving about. Soft music is piped into the room (at Memorial Hospital) to make the time seem less long. Children are likely to be a little upset the first time they come to the treatment room although, on the whole, they are very cooperative. When they are shown the television camera they seem to enjoy the thought of being on TV. They smile at the camera and really enjoy the two minutes or so that they are being treated. After the first treatment, most patients are much more relaxed about it.

While the treatment is being given, the technologist watches the machine to see that it functions properly. If anything seems the least bit out of order, the engineers are called to check and make any needed adjustments. (The machines are very expensive—a cobalt machine costs over $100,000, and a new x-ray tube can cost thousands of dollars.) The technologist must also be on the alert for any special instructions that have been given by the doctor. For example, if blood work has been ordered, the technologist must make sure that the work has been done and that the doctor has checked the results and approved going ahead with the treatment. If a patient is to be changed from a cobalt therapy machine that is practically noiseless to a generated source where electrical hum at least is to be heard, he should be warned in advance of the difference so as not to become unduly alarmed by the change in noise level. If he is to be treated for the first time with a machine that rotates, he should be told about this as well as the reasons for it; it is enough for most patients to know that the rotating machine delivers the maximum dose of radiation to the tumor and still spares the surrounding tissues. Whenever possible, the same technologist is assigned to a patient for as long as he comes to the department for treatment, and thus an atmosphere of understanding and good rapport is established. The patient often confides in the technologist when he thinks his complaints or requests are too trivial to bother the doctor about. Sometimes, these are complaints that need to be reported to the doctor or the nursing department so they can be handled by the proper personnel. In summary, the technologist should be tactful but not indifferent, cheerful but not facetious, sympathetic but not obtrusive.

Role of the Mold Technologist

Among the specialists on the team that cares for the patient receiving radiotherapy is the radiation mold technologist. A mold is a customized, protective shell that is usually made of laminated plaster of paris and is fitted onto the patient when he is receiving radiation. The purpose of the mold is to ensure that the correct area is irradiated while the surrounding tissues are protected from the effects of the rays. Sometimes these molds are made of an acrylic resin or a clear plastic which is transparent. The mold is a very important factor in radiation therapy, especially in treating small volumes such as pituitary adenomas where a very small gland is affected and the area to be irradiated is very small also. It allows for greater precision in the application of radiation.

The patient is positioned and the area to be irradiated is outlined by the radiation therapist. Then the mold is made right on the patient's body with whatever material is chosen, and small portals are cut in the mold to allow the beam to be directed to the precise area to be treated. The mold may be used on successive days without alteration and the technologist is assured that the beam will always be directed to exactly the same area. For children, a little space suit may be constructed which will restrain them in exactly the same position every day and the treatment can be repeated with the knowledge that the beam will always be directed to the desired area and nowhere else.

Not all patients require molds; they are needed mostly for patients receiving radiation to the extremities or to the head and neck. Each mold is customized, so they are not transferable from one patient to another. It takes about two hours to make a mold after the patient arrives in the treatment room. The cost depends on the material used. Plaster of paris molds cost between $4 and $5, while the transparent plastic ones can cost as much as $30 to $40. In any case, the cost is small compared to the precision gained by their use.

The molds are also usable for patients receiving radionuclear therapy. For example, if an area of the tongue is being irradiated by an implant of suitable type, a mold made of acrylic with a lead insert can be placed between the tongue and the hard palate to protect the surrounding tissues. The nurse can remove the mold when necessary for giving certain kinds of care and then replace it immediately.

Role of the Nurse

The nurse who works in the radiation therapy department is responsible for maintaining a very high level of patient care. She helps prepare the patient for therapy and gives constant support. She is the liaison between the radiotherapist and the technologist. She is the professional person who is closest and most frequently in contact with the patient, and should spend as much time as is needed to reassure him and to explain thoroughly what is going to happen to him, the reason for the red markings on his skin, what he can expect to experience on arrival in the radiation department, and why good skin care is so important after radiation treatment. The patient may have many misconceptions about radiotherapy as a result of what he has read or been told by well-meaning friends or other patients. By being receptive and showing friendly concern and understanding, the nurse can create an atmosphere that is conducive to free expression of any fears or misunderstandings the patient may have. If she discovers needs that she herself cannot satisfy, she can convey this information to the physician, or channel them to the specialists in other departments such as the social service department.

During the initial examination, many patients are terrified, not only because they do not know what is going to happen to them, but also because they have the feeling that this is "the end of the road." For some reason, many people view radiation therapy as a "last-ditch" procedure that implies imminent death. Whenever the nurse discovers this attitude in a patient or his family she tries to correct it. The patient is given a small booklet that contains basic information about radiation therapy. For example, it tells about the reduction in white cells or platelets that may occur, and the reasons why therapy is not undertaken until blood studies are completed. It also contains simple instructions about such things as how to care for the skin after treatment and why soap and water should not be used on the treated area.

Reactions that may develop during radiation are not stressed, because this may lead to worry that actually can help produce such reactions as nausea and vomiting. Because he is usually both frightened and weak, every effort should be made to keep the patient calm and he should get as much rest as possible. If he is an outpatient and lives a considerable distance from the treatment center, it is advisable for him to try to locate somewhere nearby so he will not have to make long trips to and from the center. As the treatment progresses, the patient will have a certain amount of malaise and will lose his appetite. He is strongly encouraged to take plenty of fluids and is given a high protein, low carbohydrate diet to which protein supplements are often added. Accurate intake and output records must be kept, since the patient may become dehydrated and mildly or severely anorectic during the therapy. Adequate fluid intake is also of value in helping to prevent the onset of uremia.

Many patients react to radiation by becoming nauseated and by vomiting. The reasons for this are not clear. With the advent of the tranquilizers and antiemetics, these problems have been greatly lessened. Many patients are routinely placed on such drugs before treatment, and kept on them for a time afterwards. Every effort should be made to develop a schedule that will lessen any discomfort for the patient who is receiving this kind of therapy. For example, if he will be receiving therapy in the late morning, arrangements should be made for him to have a high calorie, high protein breakfast of things he likes to eat, since he will probably not feel like eating for the rest of the day after the treatment. He should be bathed before the treatment and his bed made while he is in the therapy department so that he will be able to rest immediately after he returns to his room. Antiemetic medication should be given long enough ahead so that it becomes effective before treatment; it will not do him much good if he gets it while en route to the treatment room.

The nurse needs to be aware of several specific reactions that the patient might have following radiation therapy, including first of all, the signs and symptoms of leukopenia. Large amounts of radiation depress bone marrow and this often results in an associated anemia. The significance of the white blood count and hemoglobin determinations needs to be stressed, and the nurse must see that these tests are carried out. Such local effects as erythema and loss of hair should be watched for. Mucosal reactions may sometimes involve the mucous membrane of the mouth or of the gastrointestinal tract. The patient who is receiving radiation to the head and neck often develops a mucositis; the mucous membrane of the mouth and pharynx becomes very red and there is increased secretion of mucus. On about the tenth or fifteenth day following treatment, a thick white membrane forms and the patient develops a cough, sore throat, dysphagia, and intense dryness of the mouth. Many nursing measures can be taken to alleviate these conditions, the emphasis being on good oral hygiene and proper nutrition and hydration. A mild saline or a salt and soda bicarbonate solution may be used as a mouth wash and gargle several times a day. Oral irrigations may also be helpful. Various agents that have a surface anesthetic effect may be ordered to relieve throat pain; for example, xylocaine or benzocaine lozenges. Soft foods with low salt content are easier to swallow, and patients often enjoy cold frozen foods. Carbonated beverages will help relieve dryness of the mouth. Good oral hygiene is essential at this time; in fact it should be maintained throughout the course of therapy.

Treatment to the larynx may produce an edematous condition that can result in severe narrowing of the air passages. Hence, any complaints of dyspnea should be reported immediately. Treatment of the esophagus may produce an esophagitis and the patient may say that he simply cannot swallow, or that the food "sticks." A soft diet with a high protein, high calorie supplement may be required. Antacids, either plain or combined with a topical anesthetic, may be ordered.

The patient who is receiving therapy to the pelvis and abdomen must be observed for symptoms of proctitis or cystitis—pain or a sensation of burning on voiding, or the appearance of blood in the urine. In such cases, medication that has an analgesic effect on the urogenital organs will probably be ordered. If diarrhea develops, a soft, low residue diet and appropriate medication are ordered.

Skin reactions are always anticipated, and this is why soap and water should be used with great caution. If the area gets wet, warn the patient not to wash or scrub it; otherwise it could become quite irritated. Rubbing alcohol, talcum powder, skin creams, ointments, heating pads, or hot water bottles should not be applied to treated areas unless ordered by the radiotherapist. Restricting garments such as brassieres, girdles, and collars or garments that are starched tend to irritate the skin. Nylon garments should not be worn because they are not porous; they tend to keep the skin wet and this causes breakdown. Male patients receiving treatment to the head and neck should shave with an electric razor not oftener than once a week. The treated area should not be exposed to sunlight during the treatment period, or for a year or more afterward. This is because the effects of radiation on the skin are similar to the effects of the sun's rays. To the naked eye the irradiated skin may appear red or blistered just as it does in sunburn but, actually, the loss of skin and tissue may be quite sizeable if the area is exposed to the added insult of rays from the sun. The patient who expects to be exposed to the sun is advised to use a protective cream such as Uval. Adhesive tape should never be used, because the skin is very sensitive and will come off with the tape. Microderm, Telfa pads, or a nonirritating type of paper tape may be used to secure dressings in place.

For patients who have a mild skin reaction, that is, simply a pinking or blushing of the skin a week or two after treatment has been instituted, corn starch is applied two or three times a day. Talcum powder should not be used because it contains an abrasive. The patient who has a moderate skin reaction to radiotherapy develops a bright red erythema, and also experiences a suppression of the sweat glands, temporary or permanent epilation, and dry desquamation. For this last condition, careful supervision by the physician is necessary; he will order ointments or corn starch as the situation demands. A severe skin reaction results in purple erythema, suppression of sweat glands, permanent epilation, and moist desquamation. In pelvic cases, reactions in deeper structures may also appear, such as inflammation of the pelvic mucous membrane and cystitis with painful micturition. In treating these patients, a positive pressure machine may be used two or three times a week to spray the area with a half strength solution of hydrogen peroxide, or half strength Dakin's solution followed by saline solution. An ointment may be ordered. It may contain steroids, antibiotics, and other agents as required by the particular patient. In severe reactions, necrosis often occurs and, again, the best way of cleansing the area is to use a positive pressure spray with water or half strength Dakin's solution followed by saline solution. To break down necrotic tissue, a half strength acetic acid spray is sometimes used, or one of the gels. Ointments and dressings are applied as ordered, but never adhesive tape or paper tape. Sometimes, the patient is wrapped in a sweater made of Surgifix which keeps tape off the skin. Most importantly, the skin should never be cleansed by rubbing or any kind of friction, and large dressings should be used to keep it dry and clean. Skin folds should always be separated, otherwise severe maceration will occur. For both inpatients and outpatients, the dressings are done in the radiation therapy department, because the radiation therapist wants to see the patient every day.

In summary, the nurse must have a thorough knowledge of what radiation therapy means; the forms in which it may be administered; the reasons for its use; the potential hazards for the patient, for herself, and for others; and she must know how to properly interpret this information to the patient and his family. She needs to be familiar with the procedures relating to the use of isotopes that are used in the hospital where she works, and know whom to contact in the event of contamination of the room, linen, clothing, and so forth. She must be familiar with the techniques used to control contamination and the internal hazards presented by radioisotopes; the procedure to follow when contamination is suspected; how to handle, store, and dispose of excreta; and how to dispose of such contaminated articles as bed

linen, clothing, and towels, both before and after they have been checked by
the radiological safety officer. What she knows and how well she can interpret what she knows is very important in allaying the fears of the
patient who is undergoing treatment, and in protecting the patient as well
as others in the immediate environment.

Role of the Social Worker

Although many patients who undergo radiation therapy for cancer appear
to have a great deal of inner strength in addition to the support they receive
from the excellent nursing care they get, and from their families, some of
them do have problems that require the services of specialists outside of the
medical and nursing staff. Cancer is a life-threatening disease that arouses
many emotions within patients and their families, and often the services of
a social worker are needed to help them cope with the presenting problems
and the disturbance of normal relationships.

When the patient first learns that he is to have radiation his reaction is
one of depression, because this confirms that he really does have cancer, or
that the cancer has spread. Many of these patients are being managed on
an outpatient basis and when they learn that they must travel to a treatment
center every day, or at least several times a week, serious tensions develop.
For instance, if the patient who lives in Poughkeepsie must get to a treatment center in New York City, he has a round trip of 160 miles. If he can
sit up, perhaps he can get someone to drive him back and forth, but this
is very tiring for a person who is probably already quite weak. If he cannot
sit up and must travel by ambulance, the cost will be between $130 and $150
for the round trip. The chances are that he cannot be admitted to the
hospital because of the shortage of beds and the fact that acutely ill patients
are given priority. The answer to the suggestion that the patient be treated
elsewhere is that often there are no "elsewhere" comparable facilities nearby
for treatment he needs. Thus, the problem of transportation makes it difficult to follow patients who have been treated in city hospitals and discharged
to their homes, or to undertake their treatment as outpatients. Memorial
Hospital contracts for a limousine service that brings over 150 radiation and
chemotherapy patients in from the five boroughs of the city every week.
They must be "sit up" patients and no relative can travel in the car with
them. For patients who cannot sit up, other means of travel must be found.
Medicare does not allow funds for this; major medical policies sometimes
do. The American Red Cross may offer some help but cannot furnish
transportation more often than once a week.

The second problem that often arises is the cost of treating a patient with cancer. Most families are not protected by insurance except those who have major medical insurance. The husband may have to give up his work to stay home and care for his wife. If it is the husband who is ill, of course his earnings stop. Medicare does not help these people. However, if over one-fourth of the family income must be spent on the patient's care, he will immediately come under Medicaid coverage. This helps with the medical bills but does not help support the rest of the family. (Fortunately, cancer has been included under Medicaid as a catastrophic disease.) Sometimes a homemaker can be secured, but the family may not be able to meet this cost. Cancer Care and the American Cancer Society are two agencies that may be of some assistance to patients who live in the New York area. For example, Cancer Care will often pay part of the cost of transportation if the patient lives within a 50-mile radius of the city, part of the nursing care and part of the drug costs, as well as homemaker costs for middle-income patients who have advanced disease. The American Cancer Society often helps by supplying homemaker services, but it often takes weeks to find such a person. This agency also is able to provide some nursing care, dressings and prostheses for patients within a 50-mile radius. As to living costs for the patient and his family, the only resource is social security for the older patients and welfare for others.

One expense that sometimes occurs with a patient receiving radiation is the cost of a wig, since many patients suffer permanent epilation following radiation. The wigs now being made of dynel and other synthetic materials are less costly than human hair, and some organization can usually be found that will purchase wigs for patients. Children, especially, feel embarrassed to be seen after their hair has fallen out and it is very important for them to be fitted with wigs.

The social worker, helping patients and families to overcome the many problems precipitated by illness and treatment, may assist the patient in detecting and accepting the need of a specific resource. An appropriate source will be sought, as part of a total plan to help the patient come to grips with both emotional and practical problems.

QUESTIONS AND ANSWERS

Q. How much preoperative radiation is now being given and for what conditions?

A. Preoperative radiation is under investigation in many cancer treatment centers in many parts of the world. The reasons for using it are that it may make the excision of the tumor easier and more efficient, and that any tumor cells that might be dislodged during surgery will tend not to be viable after the radiation. This technique has not been universally successful but it is believed that it may make it possible to remove tumors that would otherwise be inoperable by bringing under control the "tentacles" so that the central mass can be removed. Patients with head and neck cancer seem to have benefited most by this treatment.

Q. Are laser beams being used in radiation therapy?

A. The use of the laser beam is under investigation in several institutions. Its effect is mostly the result of heat that is produced by the beam. It is suitable for rather special situations; for example, in treating melanomas of the eye.

Q. When is hyperbaric oxygen used in conjunction with radiotherapy?

A. Hyperbaric oxygen means breathing oxygen under increased pressure. It is under study to determine whether a greater effect than usual can be achieved with a given dose of radiation.

For the maximum effect of radiation to be obtained in the tissues there must be a reasonably high concentration of oxygen at the locus where the radiation and the cell interact. In areas where oxygen concentration is low, necrotic areas for instance, the oxygen concentration is low and the effects of radiation are correspondingly low. There are also gray areas that are not completely lacking in oxygen but which still do not have a good blood supply. When more oxygen is forced into the blood serum because of the increased pressure, more oxygen can be delivered to the cells than through the hemoglobin alone, and thus the oxygen tension at the site of interaction between the x-rays and the cells is increased.

Some clinical trials have been more promising than others. Encouraging results have been obtained in some cases of head and neck tumor.

Q. Is it possible to predict in advance whether late radiation reactions such as necrosis will occur?

A. Yes, late radiation reactions can be predicted because they are dose related. There is a dose limit beyond which the tissues will suffer irreparable damage, and one can predict with confidence that a certain number of patients will suffer bone necrosis, or damage to the brain, spinal cord, or some other organ. The physician must decide whether to take the calculated risk, and whether the risk is within the compass of possible cure. In the case of an arm or leg, he may have to decide whether to amputate at once or take the chance of the patient losing the limb from the aftereffects of radiation. The risks have been lessened recently by our greater understanding of the limits of the human body and of specific structures to radiation. In addition, the use of super-voltage machines instead of the low-voltage ones has made it possible to treat tumors near bones with less damage to the bone itself.

Q. How long do radiation treatments usually last?

A. The average treatment lasts from two to four minutes; sometimes five minutes. The time depends on several factors such as the beam that is used. Most of the time that the patient spends in the treatment room is taken up with getting him precisely in position. The actual time spent under the machine is very short.

Q. How often are treatments given, and who decides this?

A. The radiation therapist decides on frequency of treatments. Most often, treatments are given five days a week.
If the patient lives at a distance he may receive treatments on Monday, Wednesday and Friday to avoid making a long trip every day.

Q. Is there any pain or other sensation connected with treatments? Or immediately after the machine is turned off?

A. No.
Some patients say they have a peculiar burning sensation on the skin but this is thought to be a psychological reaction.

Q. When a patient has been treated with say, 4000 rads, what happens in terms of time thereafter? Is the patient radioactive in any way?

A. Once the machine is turned off or the implanted radium is removed, there is no further radiation within the patient. The patient, having been "hot" is now "cold." The radiated tissues will never be the same in the sense that there is a residual effect on the cells, and the higher the dose the greater the residual effect. The tissues approach normal in a matter of months but subtle changes can be detected either grossly or microscopically thereafter.

Q. Is there any correlation between age and the effects of radiation?

A. Age does not appear to be a factor in response to irradiation. Young people generally have better circulation, particularly to the limbs and distal parts of the body than older people, many of whom have arteriosclerosis, so it would be expected that the cells of younger people would respond better. The state of the tissues may also differ between the young and the old; that is, the older persons's tissues have less reserve and so are more likely to suffer damage after the passage of time following radiation. Growth and development of children is severely affected by radiation, however. In general, the younger the child and the higher the dose, the more pronounced the effect.

Q. Is radiation being used in the treatment of plantar warts?

A. Not as much as formerly. Even though low-voltage machines are used and the beam does not penetrate beyond the superficial layers of skin, some people react unfavorably and large ulcers may develop that require plastic surgery and reconstruction.

Q. Is radiation therapy ever used for benign tumors?

A. Not usually.
There are some lesions, however, that are histologically benign but which are nonetheless malignant in that they kill the patient. For example, hemangioma—the familiar strawberry birthmark on the skin of a newborn or young child—is usually trivial except for its unsightly appearance. But when the same kind of lesion appears on the larynx, it can close off the larynx and the child will die. Conditions of this kind can be controlled by radiation, but skilled judgment, expertise, and experience are required of the physician who makes the decision to use this modality.

Q. Is it possible for a patient with Hodgkin's disease to develop cancer of the skin in an area previously irradiated?

A. Yes, but it is by no means common.
Radiation is the treatment par excellence for early Hodgkin's disease and it would not be considered wise to withold radiation on the off chance that the patient would develop skin cancer ten years hence; but some of these patients do live long enough to develop the secondary problems of treatments that were given many years earlier.

Q. What problems arise when giving radiation therapy to children?

A. Not many arise.

On the whole, children behave very well in the treatment room when they have been properly prepared beforehand. Perhaps one in 30 will need to be restrained. They seldom move about or out of the treatment field, and the technologist seldom needs to go into the room to make sure they are still properly positioned. Sometimes a very small child is restrained by one gentle strip of Ace bandage to immobilize the joints, but this is unusual.

Q. Are parents of children who receive radiotherapy given any special instructions?

A. They are given printed information when the child first arrives in the radiotherapy department. Usually the parents are so apprehensive and nervous that it is better not to dwell too much on what will happen, and just take care of the problems as they arise.

Q. How early can Wilms' tumor be detected and what is the effect of radiation on this tumor?

A. Wilms' tumor can be seen in the newborn or even in a fetus. Peak incidence is at about two to three years of age. Children of this age are very susceptible to radiation, they still have most of their growing years ahead. The use of supervoltage machines has minimized the deleterious effects of radiation on the bones because there is less absorption of the rays by bone. Most babies that are seen with this condition have relatively restricted tumors, so the practice often is not to irradiate them. But radiation therapy is sometimes necessary and lifesaving.

The survival rate in Wilms' tumor has changed from 20 percent to 80 percent in the last generation due to expert care, excellent pediatric surgery, improved nursing care, and more proficient anesthesiologists, radiation therapists, and chemotherapists. Only about 500 cases are seen in the United States in a year's time, so many institutions are not equipped to handle such cases. The child with this condition should be sent immediately to the nearest oncologic pediatric center because the chances for survival are cut in half if the child is treated first by personnel who have had little experience in treating this condition. The survival rate seems to be higher when children with more advanced tumors are treated with radiation in addition to surgery and chemotherapy. The radiation may limit metastatic spread of the tumor by destroying any cells that might have been left behind at surgery or that might have been disseminated during surgery.

Q. Can cancer of the breast be cured by irradiation alone?

A. Yes, but probably not as often as indicated in some of the recent literature. It is not yet to be considered a suitable substitute for radical
mastectomy.

Q. How many courses of radiation can a patient with cancer of the breast,
for example, safely be given without being harmed more than helped?

A. Whether a person is harmed or helped by repeated courses of radiation
depends on the kind of radiation given, the dose, how it is administered,
and how large the field is. Each patient must be assessed individually
and the physician must decide whether to take a calculated risk of
harming the patient by ordering radiation when there is no chance for
survival without it.

Q. Why is malignant melanoma radioresistant and what is the treatment for
it?

A. When one says that malignant melanoma is radioresistant it means that
it is resistant in relation to the tissues around it. That is to say that if
the dose is heavy enough to have an effect on the lesion, it will also
destroy skin, bone, and muscle.
The preferred treatment at present is surgical excision and appropriate
node dissection of local parts which results in an average survival rate
of about 40 percent, even when local lymph nodes are involved.
Chemotherapy has so far proved disappointing in the treatment of this
disease.

Q. What special instructions are given to pregnant nurses who work in
radiation therapy units?

A. It is a general rule that a nurse who is pregnant is not assigned to such a
unit or to the care of any patient who has received a therapeutic dose
of a radioactive substance.

APPENDIX A

RADIATION THERAPY AT
MEMORIAL SLOAN-KETTERING CANCER CENTER

You no doubt wish to learn more about the treatments planned for you. The treatments themselves take but a few minutes. They are usually scheduled on a 4-times-per-week basis, but because each treatment program is planned individually for every patient, other time schedules are sometimes followed. The doctor, technologists and nurses looking after you will give you specific details and will also let you know the total number of treatments planned as soon as this information can be calculated. Additional treatments may be added or rest intervals may be prescribed by your doctor. Please do not be alarmed by deviations from the original plans.

Radiation therapy treatments present no hazard to anyone with whom you come in contact. Irradiation causes no pain or discomfort of any kind during your treatments. In fact, it is doubtful that you will have any unusual sensations, although an occasional patient will describe a "warm feeling." The appearance of the skin in the treated area may change after several days of treatment. There may be reddening very similar to that which follows exposure to the sun. Under certain circumstances the skin may actually look and feel sunburned. Should this happen you should avoid irritating your skin. For example, it is better to wear loosely fitted clothing and gently sponge the skin while bathing. Please do not scrub your skin with a washcloth or brush; this refers only to the skin being treated. The treated skin, since it becomes more sensitive, requires more care in order to prevent irritation. Do not apply heat to the treated skin. Do not apply any chemicals to the skin other than those prescribed by your doctor. Corn starch powder may be used liberally if the skin is not broken or cracked (as would occur in case of sunburn). However, if at any time your skin appears to blister or crack, please come to the examining room and ask for your doctor, who will advise you regarding skin care. Remember that excess sun exposure, hot water bottles, heating pads and unprescribed skin medication are to be avoided. The radiation therapy staff looking after you will answer any questions you may have.

Some patients receiving therapy to the abdomen may experience diarrhea or have an upset stomach as treatments go on. If you should have any troubles of this kind, do not hesitate to ask the staff for medications and dietary recommendations.

If you are being treated in areas near the upper chest, neck and mouth, you may expect soreness of the throat or a lump-like feeling on swallowing as treatment progresses. Also your saliva may become thick and foods and liquids may lose their taste. Please make every effort to maintain your diet during this time even though it may be difficult to eat and drink. These symptoms will begin to subside shortly after completion of your treatments. Adequate fluids and a high calorie, high protein diet is recommended. The staff will answer your dietary questions for you.

You may find that you tire more easily during the course of treatment, therefore you will have to get adequate rest and regulate your activities accordingly.

Each patient on radiation therapy will see their doctor once a week in "Status Check" Clinic. It is usually in the morning, and it will give your physician time to see the progress of your treatments. You will also have time to ask questions of the staff.

Please feel free to ask the members of the staff any questions you may have. After your treatments are completed, you may be asked to return for follow-up visits from time to time.

Care of Skin During and After X-Ray Treatment

Usually the skin becomes reddened (similar to sunburn) two or three weeks after the start of radiation therapy.

Please observe the following:

Instructions:

1. No water or soap on the treatment area until doctor's permission.
2. No massage, rubbing or friction of any kind on the skin.
3. No hot water bags or heating pads.
4. No ointment or other medication in the treated area unless prescribed by your attending physician in the radiation therapy department.
5. Do not expose treatment area to the sun.
6. Apply corn starch powder on the skin three times a day.
7. If the skin reaction becomes moist in character, notify your attending physician in the Department of Radiation Therapy. Corn starch powder is discontinued at this stage.

Radiation Therapy Staff
MEMORIAL HOSPITAL
New York, New York

SUGGESTED READINGS

Books

Bacq, Z. M. *Fundamentals of Radiology*. New York: Pergamon, 1961.

Barnes, P. and D. Rees. *Textbook of Radiotherapy*. Philadelphia: Lippincott, 1972.

Behrens, Charles F. et al. *Atomic Medicine*. Baltimore: Williams & Wilkins, 1969.

Bierwaltes, W. H. et al. *Clinical Use of Radioisotopes*. Philadelphia: Saunders, 1957.

Benna, R. and R. Rawson. "Treatment of Thyroid Cancer with Radioactive Iodine," in *Nuclear Medicine*, New York: McGraw-Hill, 1965.

Bouchard, Rosemary. *Nursing Care of the Cancer Patient*. St. Louis: Mosby, 1967.

Burton, M., Ed. *Comparative Effects of Radiation*. New York: Wiley, 1960.

Buschke, F. and R. Parker. *Radiation Therapy in Cancer Management*. New York: Grune & Stratton, 1972.

Cancer Management. A special Graduate Course on Cancer Sponsored by the American Cancer Society, Inc. Philadelphia: Lippincott, 1968.

Early, Paul J. et al. *Nuclear Medicine and Technology*. St. Louis: Mosby, 1969.

Ebert, R. V. "Radiation Pneumonitis," in Cecil-Loeb, *Textbook of Medicine*. Philadelphia: Saunders, 1969.

Etter, Louis E. *The Science of Ionizing Radiation*. Springfield: Charles C Thomas, 1965.

Hilaris, Basil S. *A Manual for Brachytherapy*. New York: Memorial Hospital Department of Radiation Therapy, 2nd ed., 1970.

Kurstine, I. *Effects of Ionizing Radiation on the Digestive System*. New York: Elsevier, 1963.

Nealon, Thomas F., Jr., Ed. *Management of the Patient With Cancer*. Philadelphia: Saunders, 1965.

Overman, R. T. *Basic Concepts of Nuclear Chemistry*. New York: Reinhold, 1963.

Quimby, E. *Radioactive Isotopes in Medicine and Biology*. Philadelphia: Lea and Febiger, 1962.

Quimby, E. *Safe Handling of Radioactive Isotopes*. New York: Macmillan, 1960.

Schultz, V. and A. W. Klement, Eds. *National Symposium on Radioecology*. New York: Reinhold, 1963.

Schwartz, E. E., Ed. *The Biological Basis of Radiation Therapy*. Philadelphia: Lippincott, 1966.

Smith, Dorothy and Claudia Gips. *Nursing Care of the Adult Patient.* Philadelphia: Lippincott, 1969.

Sutton, Audrey. *Bedside Nursing Procedures.* Philadelphia: Lippincott, 1965.

Tievsky, G. "Radiation Enters the Cell," in *Ionizing Radiation.* Springfield: Charles C Thomas, 1962.

Periodicals

Ariel, I. et al. "Intracavitary Administration of Radioactive Isotopes in the Control of Effusions Due to Cancer," *Cancer, 19*:1096-1102, August, 1966.

Augenstein, D. "Hyperbaric Oxygen Radiation Therapy," *Nursing Forum, 7*:324-335, No. 3, 1968.

Bloedorn, F. "Principles—Indications and Prospects for Preoperative Irradiation," *Cancer, 17*:70-73, April, 1967.

Boeker, E. "Radiation Safety," *American Journal of Nursing, 65*:111-113, April, 1965.

Boeker, E. "The Nurse in Radiation Hazards," *Nursing Clinics of North America, 2*:23-34, March, 1967.

Chamberlain, R. "Radioactive Therapy Trends from Art to Science," *Radiologic Clinics of North America, 1*:265-270, April, 1963.

Chu, Florence. "Radiation Treatment of Breast Cancer," *Clinical Obstetrics and Gynecology, 9*:221-234, March, 1966.

Corey, P. and R. Benna. "Progress in Radioactive Isotope Scanning," *Medical Clinics of North America, 50*:689-700, May, 1966.

Dunn, R. "Diagnostic Radioisotopes," *Hospital Medicine, 1*:30, February, 1965.

Forbes, M. Allen, Jr. et al. "Benzophenone as a Sunscreen," *Southern Medical Journal, 59*:321-324, March, 1966.

Forer, M. "Radiation and Health," *Nursing Science, 1*:350, December, 1963.

Greenberg, E. et al. "Bone Scanning for Metastatic Cancer With Radioisotopes," *Medical Clinics of North America, 50*:701, May, 1966.

Henschke, Ulrich K., Basil S. Hilaris, and G. D. Mahan. "Afterloading in Interstitial and Intracavitary Radiation Therapy," *The American Journal of Roentgenology, Radium Therapy and Nuclear Medicine,* Vol. XC, August, 1963.

Hilkemeyer, R. "Nursing Care in Radium Therapy," *Nursing Clinics of North America, 2*:83-95, March, 1967.

Hodges, L., and Hold. "Radiology for Medical Students," *Chicago Yearbook Medical Publishers, Inc.,* 4th ed., 1963.

Isler, Charlotte. "The Nurse and the Patient," *RN, 34*:48-51, March, 1971.

Kautz, H. D., R. H. Storey, and A. J. Zimmerman. "Radioactive Drugs," *American Journal of Nursing, 64*:124, January, 1964.

Kendall, E. B. "Care of Patients Treated with Sealed Sources of Radioisotopes," *Nursing Clinics of North America,* 2:97-105, March, 1967.

Kuhl, D. "Radioiodine Scanning in Diseases of the Thyroid Gland," *Radiologic Clinics of North America,* 1:101-114, April, 1963.

Lieben, J. "The Effects of Radiation," *Nursing Outlook,* 10:336, 1962.

Millburn, I. et al. "Treatment of Spinal Cord Compression from Metastatic Carcinoma," *Cancer,* 21:447, March, 1968.

Miller, A. "The Nurse on the Radiological Team," *American Journal of Nursing,* 64:128, July, 1964.

Prosnik, L. R. "Treatment for Malignant Disease" (Part I), and "The Nurse and the Patient" (Part II), *RN,* 34:42-51, March, 1971.

Puck, T. T. "Radiation and the Human Cell," *Scientific American,* 202:142-153, April, 1960.

Ring, A. "Cobalt-60 Teletherapy," *Hospital Progress,* 47:111, August, 1966.

Selby, B. "Proper Preparation of a Patient for X-Rays," *Hospital Medicine,* 1:17, October, 1964.

Sutton, M. "Treatment of Cancer by X-Rays," *Health,* 7:42-43, Winter 70/71.

"Symposium on Radiation Uses and Hazards," *Nursing Clinics of North America,* 2:1, March, 1967.

Tudway, A. "Place of Radiotherapy in Treatment of Malignant Disease," *Nursing Mirror, 121,* January 14, 1966.

Wildermuth, O. "The Case of Hyperbaric Oxygen Radiotherapy," *Journal of the American Medical Association, 191:*986-990, 1965.

Windeyer, B. "Modern Trends in the Treatment of Malignant Disease," *Nursing Mirror, 135:*11-15, July, 1972.

Zaino, H. "Eliminating the Hazards from Radiation," *American Journal of Nursing, 62:*60, April, 1962.

The Professional Nurse
and Chemotherapy

Regional Medical Program — Oncology Nursing Seminar

on

THE PROFESSIONAL NURSE AND CHEMOTHERAPY

Seminar Leader
Irwin H. Krakoff, M.D.

Seminar Participants
Susan Blecker, M.S.W., Social Worker
William Elstein, M.D., Resident Neuropsychiatric Service
Irwin H. Krakoff, M.D., Chief, Medical Oncology Service
Burton J. Lee, Jr., M.D., Assistant Coordinator, Department of
    Medicine, Memorial Hospital Regional Medical Program
Barbara Livingston, R.N., Nursing Supervisor
Eileen Somerville, R.N., Head Nurse

Chemotherapy is currently one of three major disciplines employed in the treatment of cancer. For many types of cancer, surgery and radiotherapy have long been the preferred methods of treatment. However, it has also long been obvious that many cancers are not amenable to treatment with either of these two modalities. This may be due to the fact that certain types of cancer—the leukemias and lymphomas, for example—are widespread by the nature of the disease or involve an entire system of the body. Or, a primary tumor, before original treatment, may have spread beyond the bounds of optimal treatment with surgery or radiation. In addition, many patients are subjected to surgery or radiation in the hope of a cure, but their disease may recur and then treatment by these means may no longer be possible. Thus, a large group of patients with cancer has furnished the incentive for developing a systemic means of treating this disease. Until very recently, "systemic" has meant chemotherapy or treatment with drugs. Currently, at Memorial Hospital, concerted efforts are being made to find ways to invoke or augment immune defenses as part of the systemic approach to the treatment of cancer. Although promising, these efforts are still in the experimental stage.

Chemotherapy, too, is still largely an experimental discipline, but studies that have been done over the last one hundred years have resulted in the development of chemicals that have proved helpful in the management of certain kinds of cancer. Somewhat over a century ago, about 1860, potassium arsenite (Fowler's solution) was found to have some effect on various neoplasms and was used systemically as a method of treatment— not very successfully as we now know. Between about 1860 and the 1940's there was relatively little investigation or development in the field of chemotherapy, and no important developments in the treatment of cancer.

During World War II, a group of biologists, physicians, and chemists working with the chemical warfare service of the United States Army (largely at the Edgewood Arsenal in Maryland) were charged with studying various poison gases, specifically as to the feasibility of their use in both offensive and defensive warfare. This investigative group was most concerned with mustard gas, of which nitrogen mustard is a derivative. Nitrogen mustard was studied in great detail and found to inhibit the growth of proliferating cells and, as a result of this discovery, was introduced as a candidate for treatment of cancer. Even while the war continued, nitrogen mustard was being tried out clinically. Information about the studies and trials of mustard gas did not become public, however, until the end of the war when it was declassified and several papers were published indicating that this chemical could be useful in the treatment of certain kinds of cancer. It became the prototype for a large group of compounds now being used for that purpose—triethylene melamine (TEM), triethylenethiophosphoramide (Thio-Tepa), and chlorambucil (Leukeran), for example.

In 1948 it became apparent that some of the folic acid derivatives could also be effective against certain types of cancer. Aminopterin came first, then amethopterin (now called methotrexate).

Practically all of the substances used in chemotherapy have been developed in the years since 1945. In fact, more such substances have been developed in the last ten years than in all previous history. This kind of drug development, and the results achieved from the use of these drugs, is most encouraging.

Literally hundreds of substances have gone through simple screening tests in the search for agents with antitumor activity. Some of the substances come from pharmaceutical houses or a chemical supply company's shelf. They may be soil filtrates or bacterial by-products. They may be studied in transplanted rat tumors, in mice or rats with leukemia, in developing chick embryos, in bacteria growing in a test tube, or in cells growing in culture. When the ability of an agent to inhibit some kinds of tumors in some kinds of animals is demonstrated, it is carefully studied in larger animals to determine the kinds of toxicity one can expect from its use in humans and, roughly, the dosages that might be tolerated. The next move is to go to the bedside where the researcher works first with cancer patients whose disease is far advanced. If the drug proves to have some usefulness in such situations, the researcher goes on to make a broader assessment of the compound's effectiveness.

Conventionally, the phases of these studies have been identified as Phase I, II, and III. In a Phase I study, the objective is to establish the tolerated dosage in terms of toxic and therapeutic effects. A Phase II study attempts to determine the effects of various dosages and frequency of administration required to produce optimum effects. In a Phase III study, the researcher tries to establish whether this compound is more useful and/or less toxic than already available compounds.

AGENTS USED IN CHEMOTHERAPY

Certain chemicals have the ability to inhibit the growth of proliferating cells. Not very much is known about the effect of chemicals on the cancer per se, but the ability of certain chemicals to influence the growth and development of cancer cells, and thus the growth of the cancer as a by-product of that activity, is known. This knowledge is what is exploited when chemicals are used in the treatment of cancer. Of course, the drugs' actions are also exerted on normal cells and organ systems, and this creates problems of toxicity.

The agents used in chemotherapy may be classified according to their different characteristics (see also the Appendix, p. 364):

1. *Polyfunctional alkylating agents*—agents that produce a biological effect by reacting intracellularly with DNA in such a way that cell division is interfered with. This group includes mechlorethamine (nitrogen mustard, Mustargen), chlorambucil (Leukeran), cyclophosphamide (Endoxan, Cytoxan), triethylene melamine (TEM), triethylenethiophosphoramide (Thio-Tepa), busulfan (Myleran), and melphalan (Alkeran).

They are useful in both slow-growing and rapidly proliferating tumors: the leukemias; Hodgkin's disease; myeloma and carcinoma of the lungs and ovary.

2. *Antimetabolites*—agents that closely resemble such normal physiological substances as hormones and vitamins. By virtue of a slight alteration in their structure, they can enter into metabolic processes but cannot fulfill the requirements for completing the process and, therefore, they inhibit the growth of cells that are dependent on that particular metabolic reaction. This group includes amethopterin (now called methotrexate), aminopterin, mercaptopurine, thioguanine, 5-fluorouracil, and Arabinosylcytosine (Ara-C, Cytarabine).

They are useful in various leukemias; cancer of the breast, testis, gastrointestinal tract, and ovary; and in choriocarcinoma.

3. *Antibiotics*—agents that resemble penicillin and streptomycin but which are too toxic for use in treating bacterial infections. They have been found to have some activity against tumors by being more damaging to the cancer cells than to normal cells. This group includes dactinomycin (Cosmogen, actinomycin D); and daunorubicin (Daunomycin). A new addition to this group is bleomycin which has different biologic effects and possibly more specific antitumor activity.

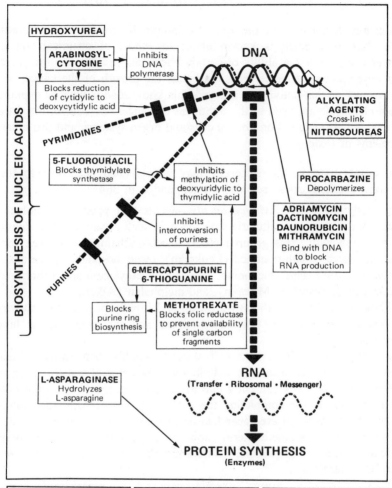

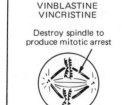

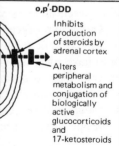

They are useful in choriocarcinoma; Wilms' tumor; neuroblastoma; acute lymphocytic leukemia; and carcinoma of the testis.

4. *Antitumor steroid hormones*—agents that act by changing the environment of the tumor thus antagonizing the growth-stimulating hormones that promote growth of cancer cells in certain tissues. This group includes the androgens, progestins, estrogens, and adrenocorticosteroids.

They are useful in breast cancer; metastatic endometrial cancer; prostatic cancer; lymphoma; multiple myeloma; and acute lymphoblastic leukemia.

5. *Miscellaneous agents*—agents (usually alkaloids) that are derived from natural plant sources or chemicals. The mechanism by which they affect cancer cells is not always known. This group includes vinblastine and vincristine.

These agents are useful in tumor of the testis; Hodgkin's disease and other lymphomas; choriocarcinoma; and acute lymphoblastic leukemia.

L-asparaginase, an enzyme which destroys the amino acid, L-asparagine, has been found to have definite useful activity in the treatment of acute lymphoblastic leukemia.

CHOOSING THE PATIENT AND THE SETTING
FOR CLINICAL TRIAL

The patient who is chosen for participation in the trial of a particular drug must be very carefully selected. It is important that he be one in whom the researcher can evaluate the effects of the agent. Hopefully, the agent may provide useful treatment for the patient while being sure that he is not denied conventional treatment that has proved successful in the past.

The setting for a study must be one with proper physical facilities for carrying on research. Laboratory facilities must not only be available but must be staffed with personnel capable of interpreting results of studies, thus supplying useful data for the researcher. Beds and financial support must be available for maintaining patients who are being treated with a drug on a trial or research basis, as well as for long-term treatment and follow-up care on an outpatient basis. Finally, research funds must be at hand, as well as research personnel expert enough to obtain meaningful data. "It is immoral to do a study when there is little possibility of getting useful information from it." Incidentally, it is also wasteful of money and facilities.

A "fallout" of the studies of effects of chemicals on cell growth in cancer is an increase in our knowledge of genetics, virology, immunology, and embryology, both as they relate to cancer and as they relate to the broad fields of medicine and biology.

In general, research chemotherapy is used when no other available measures are likely to be useful, when the patient can be evaluated, and when the patient knowingly and willingly accepts the new agent. Informed consent is mandatory for participation in a clinical trial of a new agent.

WHEN IS CHEMOTHERAPY USEFUL?

Chemotherapy is used in conjunction with, or instead of surgery and/or radiotherapy. In many cases in which there is only a slight possibility of producing a useful response, chemotherapy is employed because it is important for the patient's general support to exploit the chance that the agent might possibly produce such a response. However, this therapy can induce significant benefits and obtain some prolongation of life in a wide variety of cancers. These benefits are marked in some cases and less significant in others. Two types of cancer in particular, choriocarcinoma and acute leukemia, exemplify what can be accomplished with chemotherapy.

Choriocarcinoma is a rather rare but rapidly progressive tumor that arises in the placenta. It spreads very rapidly, metastasizes to other parts of the body, particularly to the lungs, and until about ten years ago was considered 100 percent fatal. This cancer may start early in pregnancy, result in a miscarriage, and be followed by the development of a tumor. It may also occur after the delivery of a normal child. The most gratifying results achieved with chemotherapy to date are in its employment in the treatment of this disease. The overall cure rate is 75 percent and, in a selected group, may reach 95 percent. The woman can become pregnant again, her pregnancy will be normal, and the child born of this pregnancy will be normal.

This type of cancer also occurs as testicular cancer in men. Microscopically, it is similar to choriocarcinoma in women, and it elaborates the same kind of hormone, but it behaves quite differently biologically.

The factors that predispose against recovery in choriocarcinoma are high levels of hormone production by the tumor, and involvement of the brain or liver.

Acute leukemia responds to chemotherapy by substantially lengthening the survival time of some patients. Before 1960, patients with acute leukemia had a 50 percent chance of surviving for 10 to 12 months. With each successive year, under different regimens, there has been a progressive increase in the survival rate. Recently, in one study, 73 percent of the patients were still surviving after 24 months and 70 percent after 36 months. Therefore, it seems reasonable to look forward to prolonged survival of a significant number of patients with acute leukemia.

CARE OF PATIENTS ON CHEMOTHERAPEUTIC REGIMENS

The term "chemotherapy patient" is rather ambiguous. Patients who are receiving anticancer drugs are as varied as the drugs themselves. They may be of either sex, any age, from any and every socioeconomic background, have any of the malignant diseases, and be in any stage of their illness. Each patient reacts to his disease in an individual way and responds to chemotherapy in an individual way. Thus the professional nurse must assess the nursing needs of each patient on an individual basis and deliver care and support according to that assessment.

Generally, the patient on chemotherapy is considered a medical patient, or at least is treated on the medical service. He may only recently have been diagnosed as having leukemia or lymphoma, or he may have a solid tumor that has become extensively metastatic. He may be receiving chemotherapy alone or in conjunction with surgery and/or radiation. Usually, however, chemotherapy is used to treat cancer when surgery or radiation can no longer be employed. Chemotherapy is used for the purpose of destroying or at least altering the reproductive ability of malignant cells. But, unfortunately, the drugs are not so selective as to act only on the malignant cells—they are equally toxic to normal cells. Therefore, the treatment plan may have to be to treat the patient to toxicity, because toxicity may be manifest before therapeutic effect can be obtained. The nature of the treatment demands the full use of the judgment, knowledge, understanding, and skills of the professional nurse. She must be aware of the drugs the patient is receiving, their modes of action, their toxic effects and whether these effects can be expected to manifest themselves immediately or will be delayed. When the patient is receiving conventional chemotherapy, the nurse must be fully aware of the side-effects and toxic manifestations that have been documented for the drugs being used. When he is receiving a research drug for which these effects have not yet been documented, she must be constantly alert for any sign or symptom of change in the patient.

In addition to this thorough knowledge of drug action and toxicity, she needs to be aware of the parameters of the therapeutic effect being measured in each patient. These may include bone marrow improvement, decrease in transfusion requirements, decrease in analgesic needs, change in size of lymph nodes or other tumor masses, or improvement in blood chemistry. Whatever drug the patient is getting, the role of the nurse is one of acute observer, and her creed must be "Take nothing for granted."

The nurse spends more time with the patient than any other person involved in his care. Thus, the observant nurse may be the first to note any signs of toxicity or therapeutic effect. Some of the drugs are toxic to the rapidly proliferating cells in the oral mucosa and the gastrointestinal tract. Patients receiving such drugs should be observed for mouth ulcers, vomiting, diarrhea, or bleeding. Stomatitis may be the first sign of toxicity; if observed and treated early, further toxicity to the gastrointestinal tract may be prevented. Severe nutritional deficiency may develop as a result of stomatitis or nausea, with or without vomiting, and all patients on chemotherapy should be weighed daily. Often these patients are hospitalized for a long time; the nurse should be attentive to their nutritional needs and spend time encouraging them to eat and assisting them at mealtime. Diligent and effective care must be given to prevent skin breakdown. The patient should be turned frequently in bed, helped to get in and out of bed as frequently as possible, and encouraged to ambulate when he is able to do so.

Drugs that are toxic to the proliferating cancer cells in the bone marrow also destroy the normal red and white cells and platelets. Peripheral blood counts are taken daily and the nurse should watch the reports carefully so as to be aware of any changes in the cell counts. When the red cells are being destroyed, the patient may become severely anemic and need frequent blood transfusions. If the white cells are being destroyed, the patient's normal defense mechanism against infection is destroyed also, hence any patient with a low white cell count must be observed carefully, in spite of the fact that he may be up and around on the unit, apparently feeling perfectly well and offering no complaints. His skin should be inspected for open or reddened areas that could be potential sites for infection. His temperature should be taken every four hours, or oftener if he seems lethargic or appears flushed or warm to the touch. A patient with a low white cell count may have a normal temperature at 8:00 A.M., have a chill at 10:00 A.M., and by noon have a temperature of 105°. The professional nurse must be cognizant of such change and report it immediately so that the patient can be treated early enough to prevent development of a generalized septicemia and/or septic shock.

The patient whose platelets are being destroyed is in as precarious a situation as the one with a low white cell count. Careful observation by the nurse can often prevent a disastrous situation. At any time, the patient may begin to bleed from the gums or nasal passages; ecchymotic areas that are unexplained by trauma may appear on the body; or a rash of petechiae may appear. In watching for these symptoms, the nurse often has to act as a sort of detective so she can note if any untoward sign appears but, at the same time, not alarm the patient. For example, she may note that his gums bleed when he brushes his teeth, or that he daubs at his nose with a tissue because he has a slight nosebleed, or she may see a slight rash on his body that he thinks is just the result of some slight irritation. Patients who are up and about on the unit must be asked to give stool and urine specimens so that regular checks can be made for bleeding from the gastrointestinal or urinary tract. Intramuscular injections are avoided. Prolonged and intensive pressure must be applied to puncture sites such as those resulting from venipuncture or bone marrow aspiration. Because these patients have so many blood studies, immunological studies, and intravenous infusions, the nurse becomes the coordinator of the patient's care—his advocate, so to speak—in order to reduce the number of punctures that must be made. Not only are all puncture sites potential sources of bleeding, but they also increase the risk of infection and thrombophlebitis. Male patients with low platelet or low white cell counts are discouraged from shaving to avoid infection or bleeding from slight breaks in the skin.

Many other side-effects and toxic effects accompany the use of both conventional and research drugs. Anaphylactic and allergic reactions are constant potential dangers. Neurotoxicity may result from some of these drugs, and somnolence or lack of coordination may be subtle enough initially that only the nurse, who is most acutely aware of the patient's daily activity level, may notice a change. Irregularity of the pulse may indicate cardiac changes resulting from the drug. Skin toxicity may develop as has happened with bleomycin, one of the newer drugs. Nurses who were caring for patients receiving bleomycin were the first to note the appearance of blisters and ulcerated lesions on the skin, particularly around the mouth and anal areas, and at pressure points. The nurse must be able to distinguish between these lesions and beginning decubiti or even herpetic lesions.

Some of the drugs are toxic to the kidneys; therefore a rigid intake and output record must be kept, and 24-hour collections are taken. Fluid retention may be a problem in some patients on chemotherapy. Many patients with cancer have bone involvement and must be handled carefully to prevent pathological fractures. Others have severe pain, and the nursing assessment includes seeing that they have received medication for this as often as needed, evaluating the effectiveness of the analgesics given, and requesting reevaluation of the patient's needs if his pain medications appear to be ineffective.

Close attention must be given to patients who receive various intravenous infusions. Some who receive frequent blood transfusions may become sensitized and must be watched for transfusion reactions. Others are on infusion therapy for electrolyte balance, fluid replacement, fluid balance, or antibiotic therapy and, in the latter case, must be closely observed for allergic reaction to the antibiotic drug. The rate of infusion must be carefully monitored in patients whose cardiac or pulmonary function is impaired because too rapid infusion can result in fluid overload or pulmonary edema, and too slow infusion can result in dehydration or poor kidney function. The regulation of fluid intake can be of particular importance in patients receiving drugs that are excreted through the kidney, since poor kidney function may result in accumulation of drugs in the blood and lead to toxicity.

The emotional needs of patients on chemotherapy vary with the individual. Many patients are completely knowledgeable about their therapy and know that they will be sicker before they are better. Others know that the drugs they are receiving are still in the experimental stage and that not all of their toxic effects, side-effects, and therapeutic effects are yet known. The nurse who works with these patients must give them complete assurance that she has full knowledge of their drug regimen and that she is aware of and understands their fears and anxieties. She must impart to the patient her own confidence that she will be competent and constant in her care, should any complications develop.

The nurses who care for patients on chemotherapy develop an exceptionally strong emotional commitment to their work and to their patients. They are the ones to whom the patient turns first when he needs help. One young man who had been receiving chemotherapy at Memorial Hospital and in the outpatient department for three and a half years once expressed his feelings about the nurses this way: "They are super people—just great! I have reached a point where I am not only dealing with these people in a patient-nurse relationship but I am very good friends with them. Now this could be a sticky situation you know, because there are certain boundaries that have to be dealt with. In other words, if I were to go up on the floor in the next few weeks and get into trouble it would be hard on me, of course, but it would also be hard on these people because they are my friends and they would be concerned. Now with a normal person you would never establish these relationships to begin with, but these people operate above that level. They look at everything, weigh everything, and react to everything at a higher level and that makes them just great people."

Speaking from the nurses' viewpoint, one of them described how they cope emotionally with the continuous strain of caring for patients with cancer. "Because many of the patients are in the hospital for long periods of time we become very close to them and their families. It is sometimes a very draining experience for us, but we support each other and are constantly invigorated by the support that the patients give us. Many of them are informed about their illness and their treatments, and the fact that we can discuss these things very openly with them puts it all on a very honest, open level that helps us all. On the other hand, I'm not ashamed to say that sometimes we cry."

The chemotherapy research nurse plays an important role in the clinical evaluation of a new anticancer drug. When the present intensive program of clinical investigation at the Memorial Sloan-Kettering Cancer Center first began, the investigators saw the need for a group of nurses, in addition to the unit staff, to assist them in this medical research. Several registered nurses on the adult chemotherapy research unit now provide this help and are responsible to the investigators in the division of chemotherapy research.

Before a new drug is tried clinically, the chemotherapy research nurses study all the available data on that particular compound. This gives them an indication of what to anticipate in patients who are put on the drug. They summarize this preliminary information and review it with the staff nurses on the research unit prior to the first patient trial. They then carefully monitor each patient who is started on a new investigational agent and observe him for both expected and unexpected reactions. Their experiences early in the investigation of L-asparaginase will illustrate how the chemotherapy research nurse functions.

The first preparations of this enzyme, which is derived from a strain of Escherichia coli, were not purified of contamination by the endotoxin. Patients routinely experienced fever, chills, nausea, vomiting, and hypotension. Because L-asparaginase is a protein, the possibility of an allergic reaction existed. The research nurses were able to remain constantly with the patients, thus freeing the staff nurses to care for the rest of the patient population of the unit. They were able, too, to record sufficient patient data to establish a pattern of expected acute toxic reactions to this drug. After the drug was purified, and they learned what the acute and delayed toxicity would be, the research nurses helped to evaluate a dosage schedule which ranged from a low of 10 units per kilogram of body weight to 5,000 units per kilogram of body weight. Also, they assisted in many protocol studies by coordinating the collection of specimens to determine L-asparaginase levels in blood and urine. This is an important function, because even one specimen that is not accurately collected can interfere with the analysis of a new drug.

The research nurses also perform the intravenous therapy required for the patient on investigational drugs, and prepare the drugs for administration on written order of the physician-investigator.

Close communication between the research nurses and the staff nurses provides for ongoing exchange of information so essential to their cooperative efforts. Patients receiving experimental chemotherapy benefit uniquely from the expertise of these two highly skilled nursing teams.

When a Phase I study of an experimental drug is completed and the agent is to be used in treating patients in other areas of the hospital, both a drug protocol and an individual patient care protocol are placed in those patients' charts. These two reports give the staff nurses who will be taking care of such a patient pertinent information about the compound, route and frequency of administration, and toxicity—both acute and delayed. They also provide the details of the course of therapy planned for each patient. In addition, for every patient who is receiving an investigational agent, the chemotherapy research nurse fills out an orange colored card that has pre-printed spaces for the patient's name, date, the research drug that is being given, and any pertinent information about any toxic effects that may occur. This orange card is placed in the Kardex. Whenever any new development is to be reported, it is entered on the card so that nurses on the next tour of duty will know about it. Changes in therapy or reasons for withholding therapy are entered; for example, a patient's blood count may be low on a certain day and the physician will decide to withhold the dose of the drug for that day. This procedure provides all nurses who deal with the patient with an up-to-date account of his therapy, reactions, and special treatments.

Occasionally, the medical board committee approves an investigational drug for safe administration by a professional nurse. These compounds, which are usually given orally, are sent to the nursing unit with a research label and drug information. In addition, every nursing station has a chemotherapy research data notebook which contains investigational protocols, reprints, results of drug trials, and new information. It is updated as new protocols and new details become available.

The nurses in the chemotherapy research unit at Memorial Hospital have also been involved with two experimental approaches to the prevention of infection in patients whose lowered white blood cell count makes them particularly susceptible to infection—the life island and the laminar air flow unit.

The life island is a patient isolation system in which a hospital bed is enclosed in a plastic canopy. Air inside the canopy is filtered to remove all airborn microorganisms, and materials that are placed in the unit are either gas or steam sterilized. Items are passed into and removed from the isolator unit through two ultraviolet-radiated locks at the foot of the unit which eliminate any surface contamination. Any contact with the patient by a nurse or doctor (for taking blood pressure, giving injections, starting IV's, etc.) is through a set of arm-length gloves built into the side of the unit. While the life island was in use at Memorial Hospital, it was found that a separate team of nurses in addition to the unit staff was essential to provide for 24-hour operation of this unit. Although the life island does reduce the risk of infection, it also creates an abnormal and limited environment for the patient. Among the reasons the use of the life island was discontinued at this hospital were the restrictions it placed on the patient's activities, the time-consuming and very complicated method of delivering nursing care, and the expense of operating the unit.

The laminar air flow unit concept originated in the aerospace and electronics industry and had its first medical application in operating rooms. It is, in reality, a self-cleaning unit based on the principle that a constant stream of purified air flowing across the width and height of a "clean" area will keep pathogenic organisms from coming into contact with a patient within this space. The unit consists of a rigid, three-sided enclosure that is installed in an already existing single patient room. A constant stream of germ-free air passes through the unit in a horizontal non-turbulent pattern and is propelled by fans located behind a bank of microfilters on one wall of the unit. The microfilters are fine enough to screen out organisms smaller than any pathogenic particle. The continuous air flow, which moves at about 100 feet per minute (about one mile per hour), prevents air-borne organisms from moving against the flow of air toward the patient. Anyone or anything that remains downstream of the patient cannot infect him. All personnel who enter the room and touch the patient wear a sterile gown, cap, mask, gloves, and shoe covers. Visitors must stay within a designated area but are not required to wear a gown since they will remain downstream of the patient and may not come in contact with the patient or any of the room equipment. This unit allows the patient more activity and a more conventional environment than the life island, and does not necessitate the employment of additional nursing staff.

The expectation is that the patients who are treated in this unit will be in good physical condition and will not require constant nursing attention. Obviously, in an emergency situation, common sense will prevail and techniques will be broken if it becomes necessary to give the patient immediate attention. A great deal of preparation and planning went into setting up this unit. The cooperation of many other departments was needed and readily forthcoming—dietary, bacteriology, central service, and laundry to name a few. Procedures had to be written, supplies ordered and then either gas or steam sterilized, cultures obtained, the room cleaned, a diet planned for the patient, and all possible needs of the patient anticipated. An important aspect of the first study of the laminar air flow unit was patient teaching. The first patient admitted to the unit was a woman with acute leukemia. To minimize the number of people who would enter the room, she was taught to make her own bed, to clean the sink with a germicidal agent, and to line the commode pail with a gas-sterilized plastic bag. She was shown how to remove, close, and place the plastic liners within the designated area from which the nurse could reach them for disposal without dressing in complete sterile garments. Before entering the unit, the patient had vigorous baths and was started on an antibiotic gut suppression protocol, that is, she received specific oral antibiotics to suppress the gastrointestinal flora. A schedule of daily activities was worked out with the patient so that all routines were coordinated. A copy of this schedule was posted both inside and outside the room, so that staff and patient knew when meal hours would be, when chemotherapeutic procedures and blood work would be done (in one visit), when the patient would do her housekeeping chores, and what the visiting hours would be. This schedule was modified as needed but it proved to be a very useful guideline.

Among the many items that were sterilized and passed in to the patient were pencils and pads of paper so that she could jot down questions and suggestions for us as they occurred to her. A television set and a radio that had been sanitized before she entered the unit provided some diversion. A curtain on the inside of the window of the door could be opened or closed, as the patient desired, and gave her privacy for bathing and using the commode. This woman had lost all of her hair from a previous course of chemotherapy and was very anxious to wear her wig while she was in the unit. She shampooed the wig just before she entered the unit and after that washed it just as she would have washed her own hair. She was very unhappy when she found she could not use cosmetics because they would not be sterile. However, her husband worked for a leading cosmetic firm and they rallied to this challenge by preparing lipstick and eyebrow pencils for her under completely sterile conditions. The result was a very happy and attractive woman who, when she was discharged from the unit, left a supply of these sterile items for the next female patient who might occupy the unit. She reported that the single most important item in the room was the telephone because she could make and receive calls and even direct the household activities for her young daughter at home. It kept her from feeling completely isolated; she knew that she could always reach a nurse immediately simply by dialing the nursing station extension. Before she entered the unit the patient had a psychiatric evaluation, and this was repeated periodically throughout her 26-day stay in the unit. After she left the unit, the psychiatrist found her angry and resentful at being removed from this very protective environment. Whether this will be a typical reaction of future patients remains to be seen, but the nursing staff now has an increased awareness of the need for a realistic discussion with these patients, while they are in the unit, about their return to routine hospital care, and to home and society in general.

This first study was not a true test of the value of the laminar air flow unit in preventing infection or of the nursing care problems that might have developed from it, because the patient's white blood cell count did not fall below 1,000 following her course of chemotherapy. However, it provided excellent opportunity for learning how to manage the unit and what the needs of a patient in it might be. In addition, it gave the nursing staff insight into the emotional and supportive needs of the patient who is totally dependent on others for an extended period of time.

The second patient to use the unit was a young man with lymphoma. For him, "clean" technique and supplies were used instead of "sterile" ones. Plans are under way for further studies of the unit using both "clean" and "sterile" techniques. If the laminar air flow unit proves effective in preventing infection, it may be possible to prescribe more aggressive chemotherapy for patients in this "clean" or "sterile" room and, hopefully, induce longer remissions.

The chemotherapy nurse is often asked how she feels about her part in experimental work with chemotherapeutic agents. It is sometimes very disappointing, as when a promising drug fails to show the expected antitumor activity, or when the toxicity of a new compound seems to outweigh its therapeutic effects. A patient who has become a dear friend may fail to respond to any further therapy. On the other hand, nurses working in a chemotherapy unit share an optimism and a hope that the next new drug will be effective and that the new patient just admitted will respond to the course of chemotherapy that will be planned for him. When an anticancer agent that the nurse has helped evaluate leaves the experimental stage and becomes available as a safe and effective treatment for cancer patients throughout the country, as the compounds procarbazine and Cytarabine did in 1969, she knows that all her efforts have been worthwhile.

PSYCHOLOGICAL REACTIONS TO MALIGNANT DISEASE

The usual first reaction of a person when he learns that he has a serious illness is one of shock. He is dazed or stunned, seemingly paralyzed with regard to rational thought and action. Denial and disbelief are often the initial reaction and response. "This can't be true. The laboratory must be wrong." Actually it is this response—denial— that, at various times during his illness, helps the patient to maintain emotional equilibrium. Denial, or lack of awareness, is really a defense mechanism that functions to reject or transform external reality so that unpleasant experiences are more or less done away with. Patients deny in many ways. If the denial is complete, the patient will say that he is not sick but is in the hospital for a few tests. Denial may also be manifested in the minimization of feelings and thoughts about the illness, and the patient will say, "What I have is not so bad." Denial sometimes utilizes projection too: "I'm not sick. It's that fellow in the next bed who is sick." Probably the most common form of denial is expressed in delay in seeking help. "Let's forget about it for now and wait till the doctor comes back from his vacation." Thus a long period of time may elapse before a patient actually seeks help. Refusal to take medications is another way of saying, "If I'm not taking the medication I'm not sick."

Depression or other emotional manifestations are disguises that patients may use to cover up somatic disease. For example, when a patient with leukemia is in remission he denies his illness even more, and this is appropriate. However, when he is sick, a greater awareness of the reality of his situation is important. If the sick person's denial is out of proportion to his illness, many problems can result. For example, a young person who has a serious disease, and who minimizes many of his feelings of anger, fear, and loss of self-esteem, may find it difficult to deny these feelings should his illness take a downhill course. If he cannot or does not deal with these feelings he may experience a serious emotional upset. Denial should be reinforced when it is appropriate but the reality of the situation must also be clarified for the patient after the treatment team has carefully evaluated how this person has handled previous stresses. Young leukemic patients, early in their illness, while they still feel well, may not need to know and probably could not assimilate all the facts of their disease. However, at some later stage, perhaps during a relapse, complete communication of these facts is necessary. Hence, it is appropriate to foster denial in the beginning, but not appropriate to do so when the individual should be dealing with the implications of his illness.

In addition to being generally nervous, seriously sick people have many fears which they may describe as tension, apprehension, "butterflies." What they really fear is anticipated damage to their bodies, dying, being alone, losing their place in society. Aside from the actual state of nervousness that it creates, fear presents itself in many disguised forms. The frightened patient often becomes angry, loud, and demanding. Or, he may become overly compliant and seductive in order to protect his relationship with the people who are taking care of him. Psychotic, bizarre, or unpredictable behavior often indicates a chronically ill patient's inability to deal with his fears. He may only be asking that someone be concerned and not abandon him.

Loss of his self-esteem and the capacity to function independently, together with the changes in his appearance tend to make him feel unworthy. For example, the effects of knowing that she faces surgery for some disease of the reproductive system may be disastrous to a young woman's self-esteem. Anger may be the response in young adults who view their serious disease as a brutal personal attack against the self-sufficiency and self-confidence they have worked, trained, and striven to achieve. Patients handle anger in different ways. Some become demanding and irritable. Others become so withdrawn that they dismiss the physician or the treatment protocol. When the patient turns his anger inward, he is likely to become depressed, or he may project his anger.

Guilt or guilt feelings are manifested in many ways. Many times a patient will consider his illness as a kind of punishment visited upon him for past sins and indiscretions. He may feel distressed about not making enough progress in his illness, about not getting better, about being a burden to his family, about expressing angry feelings toward the staff.

Dependency and helplessness are often fostered by illness and may be expressed in the tendency to regress when one is hospitalized, put to bed, and cannot engage in any activity without the permission of the professional staff. Often, too, the patient experiences feelings of helplessness when he knows he has a disease that might not be curable. How he responds to dependency is simply his response to having to be cared for by someone else. At one extreme, the patient may feel exceedingly humiliated, even angry about his situation. At the other extreme, he may actually bask in his dependency. Such feelings may result in a need to parentify nurses and doctors who then become very important to the patient, whether he be of the clinging vine or the non-cooperative type.

Loss and isolation also occur in patients who develop serious illnesses. They not only lose their self-esteem, but have premonitions that people will no longer respond to them as they did in the past and will not be as close. And it is true that, as a patient becomes more seriously ill, persons close to him do tend to move away. Young children, especially, feel the loss of their parents, their brothers and sisters. For all patients, the feeling of abandonment can be very real.

In the process of accepting and getting used to an illness, and in dealing with his various emotional reactions, the patient finds comfort in knowing that someone else cares, that he is not alone. It is important that his dependency needs not be fostered and that his dignity be maintained. An individual's ability to be realistic about his disease is often underestimated, and it can be quite disheartening for him to know that the staff knows as much as he does but feels too uncomfortable to share it with him. It is this sharing of knowledge about the situation that gives the patient dignity, hope, and an opportunity to become involved in the treatment of his disease which, actually, belongs to him. More specifically, the care team gives emotional support by tolerating and understanding the patient's angry feelings, by not indulging his dependency needs, and by allowing him some realistic control in the treatment of his illness; for example, by teaching him how to administer his own medication. Reducing his irrational guilt feelings and appropriately handling his denial will help an individual to feel better about himself and maintain his self-esteem. When the staff member and the patient work together to create a relationship that reduces isolation, the patient feels he has someone he can trust implicitly, and both experience a sense of accomplishment.

How does one accomplish all of this? Obviously, one cannot sit down with every patient every day for a long discussion. On the chemotherapy research unit at Memorial Hospital an attempt is being made to keep the patients functioning, feeling better about themselves, sharing thoughts and emotions with the staff members and other patients. The presumption is that patient care takes precedence in the total environment which involves the patient and his disease, the nurse, doctor, social worker, other staff members, and the family. When these components are in balance, a therapeutic milieu is created. Since the nurse is so important to the patient, the approach in a therapeutic milieu is focused on the nurse-patient relationship. The staff that cares for the patient may have feelings too. And, after careful examination of these feelings, staff members start to assume and accept more of the patient's emotional burden. They will then tolerate fear, anger, and bizarre behavior, get closer to the patient, and allow him free expression. Nurses soon become experts at predicting when difficult situations will arise and can take steps to prevent them. It soon becomes clear that verbalization is the therapeutic tool that should be used by the patient in dealing with his disease, by the nurses when talking among themselves, and by doctors and the family as well. When a person is quite sick and actually depressed about his illness, it is the obligation of the care team to allow the patient to sort out and verbalize his thoughts about being sick. In other words, the depression results from holding in one's feelings—realistic feelings that ought to be expressed.

THE SOCIAL WORKER AND THE CHEMOTHERAPY PATIENT

Some patients and some families seem to touch a raw nerve in all members of the care team. They ask the impossible of all staff members, and move from one crisis to another throughout the course of a long illness. By definition, a crisis is a hazardous circumstance that constitutes a serious stress because it jeopardizes such important life goals as health, security, and loving family ties. The story of an unforgettable family, who shall be called the Ricardos, embodies many of the crises experienced by chemotherapy patients and their families.

Mr. Ricardo, a 35-year-old Brazilian was verbal, bright, and manipulative. He had formerly been a professional soccer player, but later became a taxi driver in order to support his wife and their four children, all under the age of six. He had a fierce sense of pride and independence, was often uncontrollably temperamental and jealous, and ruled his family with an almost autocratic hand, very much in keeping with his cultural background.

Mr. Ricardo was well aware of the progressive nature of his colonic cancer, having already undergone a colostomy and radiation therapy at two other hospitals where he had been told that nothing more could be done for him. He was angry at the attitude of his former doctors, suspicious and distrustful of the doctors at Memorial Hospital as a result, and desperately afraid of pain, suffering, helplessness, and impending loss of function. When his physical condition had deteriorated to the point where he was no longer able to work, the family had to go on welfare. His illness became the central theme and focus of all of their lives.

All of these circumstances provoked Mr. Ricardo's sense of loss of control and power, which had been based upon his being the wage earner and the family spokesman. Now his position was in jeopardy, as his wife had to assume these responsibilities. His situation was one of tenuous balance and shaky equilibrium which could be thrown off by any setback in his illness or any difficulties with the welfare department.

During the Ricardos' frequent clinic visits, the social worker built up a strong and warm relationship with the family. She saw their need to recognize that Mr. Ricardo's actions antagonized and angered those around them. For example, he had thrown a crutch at the welfare investigator whom he thought was prying unnecessarily. He found it difficult to accept doctors' directions and constantly challenged medical advice, setting himself up as judge and childishly arguing with the medical staff. Questions he often asked were: Would it be worth it? Would he be making himself sicker if he consented to treatments? Was he being used as a guinea pig? The social worker encouraged him to ask the doctors questions that were legitimate, and prepared the doctors for the terrific anxiety and panic they would be faced with. She directly challenged his antagonistic attitude and tried to get him to see that his gloating and attempts to outsmart the staff were hurting him dreadfully and alienating the people who could help him the most.

At the same time, the shift in the Ricardo family roles was painful and complicated by cultural factors that supported male dominance. This adjustment was made even more difficult by the typical phenomena of relapse, remission, regression, and relative control of the disease. Patients often experience a concomitant mood swing that calls for constant and intense change and adaptation within the individual and the family. For Mrs. Ricardo to assume more responsibility, she needed her husband's permission, which he alternately gave and then withdrew when he was feeling better. By teaching his wife to speak English, and telling her how to handle family situations that involved such things as dealing effectively with the welfare department, for instance, he could stay in control indirectly.

The emotional stress of the situation was almost too much for the family to handle but, in addition, there were constant delays in receiving the welfare checks and frequent refusal of investigators to deal directly with the Ricardos because of Mr. Ricardo's explosive anger. The social worker was in frequent touch with the welfare investigators, who changed frequently, and tried to explain the situation to them. Some of her frustrations were understood by the Ricardos and this helped solidify her relations with them. As the weeks of treatment passed, the family became well known to the clinic staff, all of whom gave them much attention and encouragement.

When Mr. Ricardo complained about being restless at home, the doctor suggested that he take up a hobby. After some discussion, he decided to take guitar lessons which would be paid for out of a special fund held in social service. Again, because this man had to be independent and in control, the social worker gave him the responsibility for finding the best bargain he could, which included a teacher who would come to his home, and renting a guitar. He did this quite successfully.

The doctor honored Mr. Ricardo's wish to stay at home as long as possible. During this time he received his weekly chemotherapy at the clinic but, eventually, he became too ill for this and returned to the hospital. After his death, his widow began studying English at night school. She has answered her children's questions, made friends with neighbors, and is dealing confidently with the welfare department. As she now dares to find her own identity, she is eliciting from other people a warmth and concern that mirror her own.

The Ricardo story illustrates typical events in the lives of his relatives when the chemotherapy patient turns to familiar surroundings and people in order to retain his sense of mastery. He gets to "know the ropes." At other times, however, a patient may move beyond the stage of mastering and form a destructive relationship with the staff in which he manipulates, breaks rules, and demands special favors. When such a situation exists, the health team must work together and support each other to avoid frustration and backing away from this now abrasive patient, for such action can only contribute to a new crisis.

QUESTIONS AND ANSWERS

Q. What is the relation of radiation therapy to chemotherapy in the treatment of cancer?

A. Radiation therapy is effective in certain types of cancer—the lymphomas, for instance. It is also useful in Hodgkin's disease when it is still in Stage I.

Chemotherapy is especially effective in the treatment of choriocarcinoma, the lymphomas, and the leukemias, and moderately effective in certain other types of cancer.

Whether one uses radiation or chemotherapy depends on the disease, its stage of development, and the patient's general condition.

Q. What is the usual course of chemotherapy; how long does it last; and what does it cost?

A. It is impossible to generalize about a course of chemotherapy because the chemotherapist does not deal with an entity such as a cholecystectomy, for instance. He treats diseases as diverse as leukemia in one-year-olds and carcinoma of the prostate in 80-year-old men. So one cannot say what the usual course is.

Some drugs are given only once, perhaps by intravenous injection which takes about 30 seconds. However, the doctor may deliberate for weeks before giving such an injection, and then follow the patient's progress for six months afterwards. Some techniques involve continuous infusion over periods of a week or more, or intermittent injections that are given once a week for six months. So, again, one cannot say how long a course will last.

As to cost, that too is extremely variable. Vincristine, for example, costs about $11 for a single injection of one milligram. Other drugs are very inexpensive, almost negligible in cost.

Q. At what low in the white blood cell count do you discontinue chemotherapy?

A. One cannot be arbitrary about the point at which chemotherapy should be discontinued. It depends on the level of the white cell count when the therapy is started and the goal of therapy. For instance, when one is dealing with leukemia the goal may be to get the count much lower than 1,000.

Q. Does hepatitis often occur in patients who receive multiple transfusions as a supportive measure during drug therapy?

A. This occurs less often than it used to, perhaps partly because bloods used are now being screened for the hepatitis antigen and, while this is not foolproof, it is often possible to screen out infected blood. Why there is not more hepatitis in patients receiving multiple transfusions is a mystery.

Q. Is the 75% cure rate for choriocarcinoma applicable only to females?

A. Yes. Choriocarcinoma that occurs in the testis is an endogenous tumor, whereas that which arises in the placenta is a transplanted tumor, that is, it arises in the fetal tissue. Because the disease in the female arises from tissue that is not her own, chemotherapy enables her to reject it. This is not possible in the male and thus choriocarcinoma is not curable in nearly the same proportion of cases, the cure rate in males being probably about 5 percent.

Q. What, exactly, is a remission?

A. A remission is the return of a patient to a normal status from all the manifestations of a disease; that is, there are no abnormal findings in the blood count, the bone marrow examinations, and so forth. Remission is not regarded as a cure, because many patients who have complete remission with absolutely no symptoms of disease may relapse eventually. Some may remain disease-free for long periods of time and consider themselves cured, but the physician thinks of remission as disappearance of evidence of the disease.

Q. Are chemotherapy patients capable of administering their own medications?

A. Bleomycin is one of the newest antitumor agents. Over the past year, the drug has usually been given intravenously. But it is now evident that patients will respond to a smaller dose that is given either intramuscularly or subcutaneously. Obviously, some patients could be discharged from the hospital to home if there were a way for them to receive their medication daily. So a program was started at Memorial Hospital for teaching patients while still hospitalized to administer their own bleomycin subcutaneously. After they go home they return to the clinic once a week, or as often as necessary, for checkup. When the patient lives alone or is not ready to handle this himself, he is referred to the Visiting Nurse Association who sends a nurse to his home to supervise and assist him in giving himself the medication.

For a person who is very ill, the psychological effect of being able to give himself his medication is often very positive, since this gives him a sense of being in control of at least part of his treatment. Allowing him to do this is also one way to avoid fostering dependency.

Q. What percentage of Memorial Hospital patients treated by chemotherapy die from drug effects?

A. It is unquestionably true that some of the toxic side-effects of some of the antitumor chemicals are of such an extent that they are life-endangering and, occasionally, there is a clearly drug-related death, but they are gratifyingly infrequent.

In our recent experience with bleomycin, a compound that has been under investigation, we have treated approximately 175 patients, all of whom had advanced cancer, and have had only one clearly drug-related death. For an experimental agent, this is really a very small percentage, and a testimony not only to good experimental design, but also to scrupulous and agonizing attention on the part of every doctor, nurse, or other person who worked with these patients.

Until specific drugs that are useful against cancer and virtually non-toxic are developed, there will always be some hazard of serious, and occasionally fatal, toxicity.

Q. Are denial and depression normal reactions to knowing that one has a serious disease, or are they mental deviations?

A. To be angry, to feel depressed, to feel life is not worthwhile is very common. People should have these feelings at appropriate times. Denial becomes a problem when people should think realistically about their situation but cannot do so; that is a kind of deviation. But, other than that, anger, sadness, and depression are normal responses.

Q. When the patient has a long hospitalization what provisions are made for preserving family ties?

A. At Memorial Hospital every effort is made to get the family together as often as possible. If a husband has evening working hours allowances are made, and visiting hours are adjusted to his convenience. Children under 15 cannot visit the wards but often a patient is well enough to go to the lobby where the family can be together. Often, too, patients are able to go home on weekends. It is vital to keep communication open between the patient and his family who are very much involved with what is being done for their loved one.

The only rule that is adhered to strictly is that children under 15 are not allowed on the wards. The reason for this, of course, is to protect patients with lowered immune responses from viral infections which children are more likely to carry than adults.

APPENDIX

Specific Agents Used In Cancer Chemotherapy

Agents	Principal Route of Administration	Usual Dose	Acute Toxic Signs	Major Toxic Manifestations
Steroid Compounds				
Androgen				
Testosterone propionate	I.M.	50-100 mg. 3x weekly	None	Fluid retention, masculinization
Fluoxymesterone (Halotestin®)	Oral	10-20 mg./day		
Estrogen				
Diethylstilbestrol	Oral	Breast: 1-5 mg. 3/day		
		Prostate: 1 mg./day	Occasional	Fluid retention, feminization
Ethinyl estradiol (Estinyl®)	Oral	Breast: 0.1-1.0 mg. 3/day	N. & V.*	Uterine bleeding
		Prostate: 0.1 mg./day		
Progestin				
Hydroxyprogesterone caproate (Delalutin®)	I.M.	1 gm. 2x weekly		
6-Methylhydroxyprogesterone	Oral	100-200 mg./day	None	
(Provera®)	I.M.	200-600 mg. 2x weekly		
Adrenal Cortical Compounds				
Cortisone acetate	Oral	20-100 mg./day		
Prednisone (Meticorten®)	Oral	15-100 mg./day		
Dexamethasone (Decadron®)	Oral	0.5-4.0 mg./day		Fluid retention, hypertension,
Methylprednisolone sodium succinate	I.M.		None	diabetes, increased susceptibility
(Solu-Medrol®)	I.V.	10-125 mg./day		to infection.
Hydrocortisone sodium succinate (Solu-Cortef®)	I.V.	100-500 mg./day		
Polyfunctional Alkylating Agents				
Methylbis (β – Chloroethyl) Amine HCL		0.4 mg./kg.	N. & V.	
(HN2, Mustargen®)	I.V.	Single or Divided Doses		Therapeutic doses moderately depress peripheral blood cell
Chlorambucil	Oral	0.1-0.2 mg./kg./day	None	count; excessive doses cause severe bone marrow depression
(Leukeran®)		6-12 mg./day		with leukopenia, thrombocyto-
Melphalan	Oral	0.1 mg./kg./day x 7	None	penia, and bleeding. Maximum
(Alkeran®)		2-4 mg./day maintenance		toxicity may occur two or three
Cyclophosphamide	I.V.	3.5-5.0 mg./kg./day x 10		weeks after last dose. Dosage,
(Endoxan, Cytoxan®)		(40-60 mg./kg. Single Dose)	N. & V.	therefore, must be carefully controlled. Alopecia and hemor-
	Oral	50-200 mg./day		rhagic cystitis occur occasionally
Triethylenethiophosphoramide	I.V.	0.8-1.0 mg./kg. or		with cyclophosphamide.
(TSPA, Thio-TEPA®)		0.2 mg./kg./day x 4-5	None	
Busulfan				
(Myleran®)	Oral	2-6 mg./day	None	

Specific Agents Used In Cancer Chemotherapy

Agents	Principal Route of Administration	Usual Dose	Acute Toxic Signs	Major Toxic Manifestations
Antimetabolites				
Methotrexate® (Methotrexate, Amethopterin)	Oral / I.V.	2.5-5.0 mg./day / 25-50 mg. 1-2x weekly	None	Oral and digestive tract ulcerations; bone marrow depression with leukopenia, thrombocytopenia, and bleeding. Toxicity enhanced by impaired kidney function.
6-Mercaptopurine (6-MP, Purinethol®)	Oral	2.5 mg./kg./day	None	Therapeutic doses usually well tolerated; excessive doses cause bone marrow depression.
6-Thioguanine (6-TG, Thioguan®)	Oral	2.0 mg./kg./day		
5-Fluorouracil (5-FU, Fluorouracil®)	I.V.	12 mg./kg./day x 3 Smaller dose, 1-2 x weekly for maintenance	None	Stomatitis, nausea, GI injury, bone marrow depression.
Arabinosylcytosine (Ara-C, Cytosar®)	I.V.	1.0-3.0 mg./kg./ day x 10-20	N. & V.	Bone marrow depression, megaloblastosis, leukopenia, thrombocytopenia.
Antibiotics				
Adriamycin	I.V.	50-75 mg./m² in single or divided doses every 3 weeks	N. & V.	Stomatitis, GI disturbances, alopecia, bone marrow depression. Cardiac toxicity at cumulative doses over 600 mg./m²
Bleomycin	I.V. / S.C.	0.25 mg./kg./day x 5-7 / Maintenance: 1.0-2.0 mg./day	N. & V. Chills Fever	Mucocutaneous ulcerations, alopecia, pulmonary fibrosis in approximately 5% patients
Dactinomycin (Cosmegen®)	I.V.	0.01 mg./kg./day x 5 or 0.04 mg./kg. weekly	N. & V.	Stomatitis, GI disturbances, alopecia, bone marrow depression.
Daunorubicin	I.V.	0.8-1.0 mg./kg./day x 3-6 Total doses never to exceed 25 mg./kg.	N. & V. Fever	Bone marrow depression with leukopenia and thrombocytopenia, alopecia, stomatitis; cardiac toxicity at cumulative doses over 25 mg./kg.
Mithramycin	I.V.	25 micrograms every other day x 3-4	N. & V.	Bone marrow depression particularly thrombocytopenia, bleeding, hypocalcemia, hepatic toxicity at large doses
Miscellaneous Drugs				
L-Asparaginase	I.V.	200-1,000 IU/kg. 3-7 x weekly for 28 days	N. & V. Fever Hypersensitivity reactions	Anorexia, weight loss. Somnolence, lethargy, confusion. Hypoproteinemia (including albumin and fibrinogen). Hypolipidemia and (?) hyperlipidemia, abnormal liver function tests, fatty metamorphosis of the liver. Pancreatitis (rare). Azotemia. Granulocytopenia, lymphopenia, and thrombocytopenia (usually mild and transient.)
1,3-bis (β-Chloroethyl)-1-nitrosourea (BCNU)	I.V.	100 mg./m² every 6 weeks	N. & V.	Bone marrow depression with leukopenia and thrombocytopenia.
o,p'-DDD	Oral	2-10 gm./day	N. & V.	Skin eruptions, diarrhea, mental depression, muscle tremors.
Hydroxyurea (Hydrea®)	Oral	20-40 mg./kg./day	None	Bone marrow depression
Procarbazine (Matulane®) N-Methylhydrazine	Oral	50-300 mg./day	N. & V.	Bone marrow depression, leukopenia and thrombocytopenia, mental depression.
Quinacrine (Atabrine®)	Intrapleural	100-200 mg./day x 5	Local pain, Fever	
Vinblastine (Velban®)	I.V.	0.1-0.2 mg./kg. weekly	N. & V.	Alopecia, areflexia, bone marrow depression.
Vincristine (Oncovin®)	I.V.	0.015-0.05 mg./kg. weekly	None	Areflexia, muscular weakness, peripheral neuritis, paralytic ileus, mild bone marrow depression.

*Nausea and Vomiting

NEOPLASTIC DISEASES WHICH RESPOND TO CHEMOTHERAPY		
TYPE OF CANCER	**USEFUL DRUGS**	**RESULTS**
Prolonged Survival or Cure		
Gestational trophoblastic tumors	Methotrexate, Dactinomycin, Vinblastine	70% cured
Burkitt's tumor	Cyclophosphamide (many others)	50% cured
Testicular tumors	Dactinomycin*, Methotrexate* Chlorambucil*	30-40% respond, 2-3% cured
Wilms' tumor	Dactinomycin with surgery and radiotherapy	30-40% cured
Neuroblastoma	Cyclophosphamide with surgery and/or radiotherapy	5% cured
Acute lymphoblastic leukemia	Daunorubicin*, Prednisone*, Vincristine*, 6-Mercapto-purine*, Methotrexate*, BCNU*	90% remission; 70% survive beyond 5 years
Hodgkin's disease Stage IIIB & IV	HN2*, Vincristine*, Prednisone*, Procarbazine*, Bleomycin	70% respond, 40% survive beyond 5 years
Palliation and Prolongation of Life		
Prostate carcinoma	Estrogens, castration	70% respond with some prolongation of life
Breast carcinoma	Androgens, estrogens, alkylating agent*, 5-Fluorouracil*, Vincristine*, Prednisone*, Methotrexate*	20-40% respond with probable prolongation of life
Chronic lymphocytic leukemia	Prednisone, alkylating agents	50% respond with probable prolongation of life
Lymphosarcoma	Prednisone, alkylating agents	50% respond with probable prolongation of life
Acute myeloblastic leukemia	Arabinosylcytosine and Thioguanine	65% remission with prolongation of life
Palliation with Uncertain Prolongation of Life		
Chronic granulocytic leukemia	Alkylating agents, 6-mercaptopurine	90% respond with good control during most of course
Multiple myeloma	Alkylating agents	35% respond objectively; 50% have subjective relief of symptoms
Ovary	Alkylating agents	30-40% respond
Endometrium	Progestins	25% respond, chiefly pulmonary metastases
Uncertain Palliation		
Lung	Alkylating agents	30-40% respond briefly
Head and Neck	Alkylating agents, methotrexate	20-30% respond briefly
Large Bowel	5-Fluorouracil	10-20% respond
Stomach	5-Fluorouracil	10% respond
Pancreas	5-Fluorouracil	<10% respond
Liver	5-Fluorouracil	<10% respond
Cervix	Alkylating agents	<10% respond
Melanoma	Alkylating agents, VLB**	<5% respond
Adrenal cortex	o,p'DDD	Relief of Cushingoid syndrome
Soft tissue and Osteogenic sarcoma	Adriamycin, Methotrexate	20% respond
Local Chemotherapy		
Technique		
Intracavitary injection for recurrent effusion	Alkylating agents, Fluorouracil, Quinacrine	50% of effusions controlled
Intrathecal injection for meningeal leukemia	Methotrexate, Arabinosylcytosine	80% improved 2 months
Extracorporeal perfusion for cancer of extremities	Alkylating agents	Irregular and uncertain
Continuous infusion for cancer of head and neck, liver and pelvis	Methotrexate-Leucovorin, Fluorouracil	Irregular and Uncertain
*May be used in combination		**Vinblastine

SUGGESTED READINGS

Books

Bradshaw, Isidore and Benham S. Kahn. *Cancer Chemotherapy; Basic and Clinical Applications.* New York: Grune & Stratton, 1967.

Brodsky, I., S. B. Kahn, and J. H. Moyer. "Cancer Chemotherapy; Basic and Clinical Applications," *The Fifteenth Hahnemann Symposium.* New York: Grune & Stratton, 1967.

Burchenal, J. H. and M. R. Dollinger. "Chemotherapy of Leukemias and Lymphomas," in *Chemotherapy of Cancer,* edited by W. H. Cole. Philadelphia: Lea & Febiger, 1970.

Clark, R. Lee, Jr. (Ed). *Cancer Chemotherapy.* Springfield, Ill.: Charles C Thomas, 1961.

Cole, Warren H. (Ed.). *Chemotherapy of Cancer.* Philadelphia: Lea & Febiger, 1970.

Dowling, M. D., I. H. Krakoff, and D. A. Karnofsky. "Mechanism of Action of Anti-Cancer Drugs," in *Chemotherapy of Cancer,* edited by W. H. Cole. Philadelphia: Lea & Febiger, 1970.

Freireich, E. J., G. P. Bodey, D. S. DeJongh, J. E. Curtis, and E. M. Hersh. "Supportive Therapeutic Measures for Patients Under Treatment for Leukemia or Lymphoma," in *Leukemia-Lymphoma,* pp. 275-284. A Collection of Papers Presented at the 14th Annual Clinical Conference on Cancer, 1969, at the University of Texas M. D. Anderson Hospital and Tumor Institute. Chicago: Year Book Medical Publishers, 1970.

Greenwald, Edward S. *Cancer Chemotherapy.* New York: Medical Examination Publishing Co., 1967.

Karnofsky, David A. The Guy H. Heath and Dan C. Heath Memorial Lecture: "Problems in the Evaluation of Chemotherapy for Lymphomas," in *Leukemia-Lymphoma,* pp. 13-25. A Collection of Papers Presented at the 14th Annual Clinical Conference on Cancer, 1969, at The University of Texas M. D. Anderson Hospital and Tumor Institute. Chicago: Year Book Medical Publisers, 1970.

Nealon, Thomas F., Jr. (Ed.). *Management of the Patient With Cancer.* Philadelphia: Saunders, 1965.

Nichols, Major Glenadee A. "Isolation in a Regulated Environment for Safety," *A.N.A. Clinical Sessions 1966.* New York: Appleton-Century-Crofts, 1967.

Periodicals

Ager, Ernest A. "Current Concepts in Immunization," *American Journal of Nursing, 66*:2004-2011, September, 1966.

Bottomley, R. H. "Problems Associated with Chemotherapeutic Agents," *Cancer Bulletin, 20*:29-30, March/April, 1968.

Clark, R. L. et al. "Rehabilitation of the Cancer Patient," *Cancer, 20*:839-845, May, 1967.

Crate, Marjorie A. "Nursing Functions in Adaptation to Chronic Illness," *American Journal of Nursing, 65*:72-76, October, 1965.

Dollinger, M. R., R. B. Golbey, and D. A. Karnofsky. "Cancer Chemotherapy," *Disease-A-Month*, April, 1969.

Donaldson, S. S. and W. S. Fletcher. "The Treatment of Cancer by Isolation Perfusion," *American Journal of Nursing, 64*:81-88, August, 1964.

Easson, W. M. "Care of the Young Patient Who Is Dying," *JAMA, 205*:203-207, No. 4, July 22, 1968.

Fox, Shirley A. and Louis C. Bernhardt. "Chemotherapy via Intra-Arterial Infusion," *American Journal of Nursing, 66*:1966-68, September, 1966.

Fracchia, Albert A. et al. "Intrapleural Chemotherapy from Metastatic Breast Carcinoma," *Cancer, 26*:626-29, September, 1970.

Geisler, H. E. "Young Cancer Patients Require Special Counseling," *Hospital Topics*, 46-60, August, 1968.

Geller, W. "Hodgkin's Disease," *Medical Clinics of North America, 50*:819-832, May, 1966.

Grant, R. "Nursing of the Cancer Patient," *Nursing Forum, 4*:57-58, No. 2, 1965.

Hall, Thomas C. "Chemotherapy of Cancer," *New England Journal of Medicine, 266*:129-34, 178-85, 238-45, and 289-96, January, 1962.

Hilkemeyer, R. "Intra-Arterial Cancer Chemotherapy," *Nursing Clinics of North America, 66*:295-308, June, 1966.

Karnofsky, David A. "Cancer Chemotherapeutic Agents," *CA, 18*:72-79 and 232-34, July-August, 1968.

Klagsbrun, S. C. "Cancer Emotions and Nurses," *American Journal of Psychiatry*, March, 1970, pp. 1237-1244.

Kohle et al. "Psychological Aspects in the Treatment of Leukemia Patients in the Isolated-Bed System Life Island," *Psychotherapy Psychosomatics, 19*:85-91, 1971.

Krakoff, I. H. "The Management of Myeloproliferative Disorders," *Medical Clinics of North America, 50*:803-817, May, 1966.

Lacher, Mortimer J. "Long Survival in Hodgkin's Disease," *Annals Internal Medicine, 70*:7-17, January, 1969.

Levitan, Alexander A., and Seymour Perry. "The Use of an Isolator System in Cancer Chemotherapy," *American Journal of Medicine, 44*:234-42, February, 1968.

Livingston, Barbara M. "How Clinical Progress Is Made in Cancer Chemotherapy Research," *American Journal of Nursing, 67*:2547-54, December, 1967.

Livingston, Barbara M., and Irwin H. Krakoff. "L-Asparaginase: A New Type of Anti-Cancer Drug," *American Journal of Nursing, 70*:1910-15, September, 1970.

Lunceford, J. L. "Leukemia," *Nursing Clinics of North America, 2*:635-647, December, 1967.

Lunceford, J. L. et al. "Nursing Care of the Patients in the Laminar Air Flow Room", USDHEW Publication No. (NIH 72-93), *Nursing Clinical Conferences,* 1-16, December, 1971.

Mathe, G. "Immunotherapy in the Treatment of Acute Lymphoid Leukemia," *Hospital Practice, 6*:43-51, December, 1971.

McFayden, Iain R. "Choriocarcinoma," *Nursing Times, 64*:793-94, June 14, 1968.

Meinhart, N. T. "The Cancer Patient: Living in the Here and Now," *Nursing Outlook, 16*:64-69, May, 1968.

Metka, Ruth J. "Nursing Care of Patients with Acute Leukemia," USDHEW Publication No. (NIH 72-94), *Nursing Clinical Conferences,* November, 1971.

Poi, D. M. "Who Cared About Tony?" *American Journal of Nursing, 72*:1848-51, October, 1972.

Rodman, M. J. "Anticancer Chemotherapy Against the Leukemias and Lymphomas," Part 3, *RN, 35*:49-50, April, 1972.

Ross, Walter S. "Leukemia: We're Starting to Use the Word Cure," *Today's Health,* October, 1970.

Schmale, A. H. "Importance of Life Setting for Disease Onset," *Modern Treatment, 6*:643-655, No. 4, July, 1969.

Senescu, R. A. "The Development of Emotional Complications in the Patient with Cancer," *Journal of Chronic Diseases, 16*:813-832, 1963.

Vernick, Joel, and Janet L. Lunceford. "Milieu Design for Adolescents with Leukemia," *American Journal of Nursing, 67*:559-61, March, 1967.

Verwoerdt, Adriaan, and Ruby Wilson. "Communication with the Fatally Ill Patient; Tacit or Explicit?" *American Journal of Nursing, 67*:2307-2309, November, 1967.

Whitehouse, J. M. "The Leukemias: Acute Leukemia," Part 1, *Nursing Times, 68*:703-6, June 8, 1972.

Appendix A

Participating Agencies—Regional Medical Program

ONCOLOGIC NURSING SEMINARS

October, 1970—March, 1972

	Seminars Attended
R.M.P. Hospitals	
Memorial Hospital, New York, N.Y.	10
Adelphi University, Garden City, N.Y.	4
Alexian Brothers Hospital, Elizabeth, N.J.	1
American Cancer Society, New York, N.Y.	7
American Cancer Society—Chester County Unit, Chester County, Pa.	1
Ann May School of Nursing—Jersey Shore Medical Center, Neptune, N.J.	2
Babies Hospital, New York, N.Y.	1
Bayonne Hospital and Dispensary, Bayonne, N.J.	1
Bergen Community College, Paramus, N.J.	2
Beth-Israel Medical Center, New York, N.Y.	9
Bird S. Coler Memorial Hospital, New York, N.Y.	1
Bloomfield College, Bloomfield, N.J.	2
Boulevard Hospital, Long Island City, N.Y.	1
Bridgeport Hospital, Bridgeport, Conn.	1
Bronx Community College, Bronx, N.Y.	2
Brookdale Hospital Center, Brooklyn, N.Y.	8
Brooklyn Jewish Hospital School of Nursing, Brooklyn, N.Y.	2
Brooklyn State Hospital, Brooklyn, N.Y.	2
Catholic Medical Center, Jamaica, N.Y.	4
Central Islip Hospital, Central Islip, N.Y.	2
Central School for Practical Nurses, New York, N.Y.	1
Children's Hospital of Philadelphia, Philadelphia, Pa.	1
Christ Hospital, Jersey City, N.J.	3
Clara Maass School of Nursing, Belleville, N.J.	2
Columbia Memorial Hospital, Hudson, N.Y.	1
Elizabeth General Hospital, Elizabeth, N.J.	4
Englewood Hospital, Englewood, N.J.	3
French & Polyclinic Hospital, New York, N.Y.	4
Flushing Hospital Medical Center, Flushing, L.I., N.Y.	3
Glen Cove Community Hospital, Glen Cove, N.Y.	6
Greenwich General Hospital, Greenwich, Conn.	5
Horton Memorial Hospital, Middletown, N.Y.	1
Hospital for Special Surgery, New York, N.Y.	6
House of Calvary, New York, N.Y.	6
Interboro General Hospital, Brooklyn, N.Y.	6
Leroy Hospital, New York, N.Y.	1
Mountainside Hospital, Montclair, N.J.	2
Nassau Hospital, Mineola, N.Y.	2

New York Hospital-Cornell University, New York, N.Y.	10
Overlook Hospital, Summit N.J.	1
Phelps Memorial Hospital, North Tarrytown, N.Y.	4
St. Barnabas Medical Center, Livingston, N.J.	6
St. Francis Hospital, Hartford, Conn.	1
St. Luke's Hospital, Newburgh, N.Y.	5
St. Vincent's Hospital, New York, N.Y.	7
Stamford General Hospital, Stamford, Conn.	7
Staten Island Hospital, Staten Island, N.Y.	3
Vassar Brothers Hospital, Poughkeepsie, N.Y.	7

Other Agencies

Altro Workshop, Bronx, N.Y.	1
Columbia Presbyterian Hospital, New York, N.Y.	9
Columbus Hospital, New York, N.Y.	2
Cooper Hospital, Camden, New Jersey	3
Doctors Hospital, New York, N.Y.	1
Downstate Medical Center, Brooklyn, N.Y.	8
Dunlap Psychiatric Hospital	1
Dutchess Community College, Poughkeepsie, N.Y.	2
East Orange Hospital School of Nursing, East Orange, N.J.	7
Elm Hospital	1
Family Nursing Service of Hunterdon Co., Hunterdon, N.J.	1
Farmingdale State University, Farmingdale, N.Y.	1
Flower & Fifth Avenue Hospital, New York, N.Y.	2
Forest View Nursing Home, Forest Hills, N.Y.	1
Francis Find Insurance Company	1
Fulton Montgomery Community College, Johnstown, N.Y.	1
Governeur Health Service Program, New York, N.Y.	1
Grassland Hospital, Valhalla, N.Y.	1
Hackensack Hospital School of Nursing, Hackensack, N.J.	1
Harlem Hospital Center School of Nursing, New York, N.Y.	6
Harlem Valley State Hospital School of Nursing, Wingdale, N.Y.	1
Hartford Hospital, Hartford, Conn.	3
Hartwick College, Oneonta, N.Y.	1
Helene Fuld School of Nursing, Trenton, N.J.	3
Hemotology Associates,	1
Holy Name Hospital, Teaneck, N.J.	5
Hospital for Joint Diseases, New York, N.Y.	7
Hudson River State Hospital	2
Hunter College-Bellevue School of Nursing, New York, N.Y.	9
Jamaica Hospital, Jamaica, New York	3
Jewish Hospital of Brooklyn, Brooklyn, N.Y.	2
Julia Richman High School, New York, N.Y.	5
Kings County Hospital, Brooklyn, N.Y.	1

	Seminars Attended
Kings Park Community Hospital, Kings Park, N.Y.	2
Kingston Hospital Tumor Clinic, Kingston, N.Y.	1
Knickerbocker Hospital, New York, N.Y.	1
La Guardia Hospital, Forest Hills, Flushing, N.Y.	1
Lehman College, Bronx, N.Y.	1
Lenox Hill Hospital, New York, N.Y.	8
Long Island College, Brooklyn, N.Y.	1
Long Island Jewish Medical Center, New Hyde Park, N.Y.	7
Mabel Dean Bacon High School, New York, N.Y.	5
Manhattan EENT Hospital, New York, N.Y.	5
Manhattan State School of Nursing, New York, N.Y.	1
Marcy State Hospital School of Nursing, Marcy, N.Y.	1
Marsan Manufacturing Company, Chicago, Ill.	3
Martland General Hospital, Newark, N.J.	1
Mary Immaculate Hospital, Jamaica, N.Y.	4
Mary Manning Walsh Nursing Home, New York, N.Y.	5
Mercer Hospital, Trenton, N.J.	1
Meriden-Wallingford Hospital, Meriden, Conn.	2
Mercy Hospital, Rockville Center, N.Y.	1
Methodist Hospital, Brooklyn, N.Y.	5
Metropolitan Hospital, New York, N.Y.	2
Middlesex County College, Waltham, Mass.	1
Misericordia Hospital, Bronx, N.Y.	6
Molloy College, Rockville Center, N.Y.	2
Montefiore Hospital, Bronx, N.Y.	5
Morristown Memorial Hospital, Morristown, N.J.	3
Mount Sinai Hospital, New York, N.Y.	8
Mount Vernon Hospital, Mount Vernon, N.Y.	3
Mulhenberg Hospital, Plainfield, N.J.	2
Nanticoke Memorial Hospital, Seaford, Del.	1
Neurological Institute, New York, N.Y.	2
New Jersey State Department of Education	1
New York City Community College, Brooklyn, N.Y.	3
New York City Department of Health, New York, N.Y.	1
New York Infirmary, New York, N.Y.	7
New York Medical College, New York, N.Y.	3
N.Y. Medical College Graduate School of Nursing, New York, N.Y.	2
New York University, New York, N.Y.	1
New York University Hospital, New York, N.Y.	9
New York University Research Unit, New York, N.Y.	2
Newark Beth-Israel Medical Center, Newark, N.J.	1
Norwalk Hospital School of Nursing, Norwalk, Conn.	7
Orange County Community College, Middletown, N.Y.	1
Orange Memorial Hospital, Orange, N.J.	1
Our Lady of Lourdes School of Nursing, Camden, N.J.	1

Pace College, Pleasantville, N.Y.	1
Parkway Hospital, Flushing, L.I., N.Y.	1
Peninsula General Hospital, Far Rockaway, N.Y.	1
Perth Amboy General Hospital, Perth Amboy, N.J.	1
Point Pleasant Hospital, Point Pleasant, N.J.	1
Prospect Heights Hospital, Brooklyn, N.Y.	1
Queens General Hospital, Jamaica, Queens, N.Y.	3
Queensboro Community College, Bayside, N.Y.	2
Ramampo Manor Nursing Center	3
Rockefeller University Hospital, New York, N.Y.	2
Rockland Community College, Suffern, N.Y.	2
Rockland State Hospital School of Nursing, Orangeburg, N.Y.	6
Roosevelt Hospital, New York, N.Y.	2
St. Clare's Hospital Sch. of Nursing, New York, N.Y.	2
St. Elizabeth Hospital, New York, N.Y.	1
St. Francis Hospital, Jersey City, N.J.	1
St. John's Episcopal Hospital, Brooklyn, N.Y.	2
St. John's Hospital-Cochran Sch. of Nursing, Yonkers, N.Y.	3
St. John's Hospital, Elmhurst, N.Y.	1
St. John's Queens Hospital, Long Island City, N.Y.	3
St. Joseph's Hospital, Paterson, N.J.	2
St. Joseph's Hospital, New York, N.Y.	1
St. Luke's Medical Center, New York, N.Y.	8
St. Mary's Hospital, Passaic, N.J.	4
St. Mary's Hospital, Brooklyn, N.Y.	2
St. Mary's Hospital, Waterbury, Conn.	3
St. Mary's Hospital School of Nursing, Orange, N.J.	3
St. Peter's General Hospital, New Brunswick, N.J.	2
St. Raphael's Hospital, New Haven, Conn.	1
St. Rose's Home, New York, N.Y.	2
St. Vincent's Medical Center, Staten Island, N.Y.	1
St. Vincent's Hospital, Bridgeport, Conn,	4
Samaritan Hospital School of Nursing, Troy, N.Y.	1
Seton Hall University, South Orange, N.J.	1
Skidmore College, New York, N.Y.	1
Somerset County College, Somerville, N.J.	1
Staten Island Community College, Richmond, S.I., N.Y.	2
Strong Hospital, Rochester, N.Y.	1
Suffolk County College, Selden, N.Y.	2
Teacher's College-Columbia University, New York, N.Y.	6
Tuxedo Memorial Hospital, Tuxedo Park, N.Y.	1
Ulster County College, Stone Ridge, N.Y.	1
United Hospital—School of Nursing, Port Chester, N.Y.	1
University of Bridgeport, Bridgeport, Conn.	4
University Hospital, Boston, Mass.	1

	Seminars Attended
Upstate Medical Center, Syracuse, N.Y.	1
Villanova University, Villanova, Pa.	1
Visiting Nurse Service, New York, N.Y.	9
Wagner College, Richmond, S.I., N.Y.	4
Waterbury Hospital, Waterbury, Conn.	3
Westchester School of Nursing, Westchester, N.Y.	2
Wickersham Hospital, New York, N.Y.	1
William Paterson College, Wayne, N.J.	1
Wilmington Medical Center, Wilmington, Del.	2
Woman's Hospital, New York, N.Y.	1
Yale-New Haven Hospital, New Haven, Conn.	4
(Affiliation Not Stated)	2

Appendix B

Regional Medical Program—Oncology Nursing Seminars
Evaluation

Data about the number of seminar participants from Memorial Hospital (intramural) and from other agencies and institutions (extramural) which are reported in Appendix A indicate that a total of 4,923 persons attended the 19 seminar sessions. However, it should be noted that some of these people attended only one or two series, while others participated in most of them. The latter was particularly true of Memorial Hospital personnel.

To keep this portion of the evaluation report brief, we will not present detailed data pertaining to the precise number of series which each of the participants attended. Rather, we will note some of the comments and suggestions made by participants which might be of more interest to the reader.

Considering the pressure of time felt by the participants at the end of the sessions, we were gratified to receive a total of 3,369 completed evaluation forms; this represented 68 percent of the total attendance. This relatively large number of evaluations seemed to indicate a high degree of involvement on the part of various participants in the program. Over two-thirds of the professional nurses (68%), one-fourth of the student nurses (25%), and 96 of the licensed practical nurses who attended completed the evaluation forms. The majority of the 865 student nurses attended one or two of the seminar series (that is, two or four of the seminar sessions).

If one were to measure the relative popularity of the various seminar sessions only in terms of the number of participants who completed evaluation forms, it would readily be seen that some sessions elicited greater post session response than others. Similar variations occurred in the ratings given to the different aspects of each session as well as to a particular aspect of the different sessions. For example, in one particular session, the majority of the evaluators noted that "Content and Ideas" were very stimulating (rank # 5); the "Speaker Presentations" were seen to be only moderately stimulating (rank # 4) or adequate (rank # 3); and the "Panel Presentations" were considered either adequate (rank # 3) or left something to be desired (rank # 2). By and large, the 3,369 evaluators indicated that they were very pleased with the information that was presented, particularly when patients, or former patients, were among the resource personnel serving on the panel.

Since this particular program of seminars was exploratory in nature, one of the principal advantages of the session evaluations was their usefulness in suggesting modifications of aspects of the program that the evaluators felt needed improving, so that each succeeding seminar group benefitted by the comments of participants in earlier sessions. Moreover, as is the case with many evaluation tools that employ both scales and open-end questions, responses to the latter were both highly informative and useful. We did not attempt to quantify the qualitative data obtained from the open-end questions, but the composite sample of participants' responses that follows indicates that the responses may be considered as either general, didactic, or social in nature.

375

TABLE 1: Relationship between the number of participants who completed evaluations by position or discipline

	Colon or Rectum	Head and Neck	Breast	Chemotherapy	Gynecology	Lung	Radiation Therapy	Liver	Urology	Pediatrics	TOTAL
Registered Nurse*	132	202	149	250	259	263	293	152	286	312	2298*
Nursing Student	13	99	108	55	151	36	70	33	145	155	865
Licensed Practical Nurse	2	15	9	10	9	13	9	2	9	18	96
Nursing Instructor	0	0	6	4	4	8	8	0	8	0	38
Social Worker	4	1	3	5	3	0	11	4	1	6	38
Nurses' Aide/Technician Other Technician	0	0	0	0	1	4	3	0	0	1	9
Graduate Nursing Student	1	1	1	0	0	0	2	0	1	0	6
Public Health Nurse	2	0	0	0	0	0	3	1	0	0	6
Director/Asst. Director Nursing Education	1	0	0	0	0	1	0	0	1	1	4
Hospital Administrator	0	1	0	0	0	1	0	0	0	1	3
Physical Therapist	0	0	1	1	0	1	0	0	0	0	3
Volunteer/Playroom	0	0	0	0	0	0	0	0	0	2	2
Recreational Therapist	0	0	1	0	0	0	0	0	0	0	1
Total Evaluations Completed	155	319	278	325	427	327	399	192	451	496	3369
Total Attendance	228	502	446	574	629	498	508	252	615	671	4923
Percentage of Participants who Completed Evaluations	68%	64%	62%	57%	68%	66%	79%	76%	73%	74%	68%

* Figure may include some directors, instructors and others who did not indicate their specialty

Seminars extremely well planned, the informal approach very stimulating.

Excellent format; topics well presented; slides most helpful and informative.

Much valuable and informative knowledge disseminated.

Seminars have all been excellent.

Excellent planning and organization. Congratulations and thanks for a job well done!

Good balance between scientific knowledge presented by doctors and nursing care presented by nurses. It is difficult to motivate a staff as well as yours appears to be.

Glad to see nurses had audiovisual material prepared.

Patients on panel gave insight into their sensitivities and fears. Added a more humanistic outlook to activities performed.

Good techniques and skills presented (rectal and colonic cancer).

Panelists were informative, had good audiovisual aids, and presented latest methods (head and neck cancer).

This seminar (pediatric oncology) would have been very educational for the lay public.

Full team approach very enlightening.

Optimistic attitude of staff and patients inspiring.

Psychological aspects of cancer nursing were well explored.

Appreciated focus on nursing care.

Hospitality was warm and thoughtful.

Liked panel discussions best.

Patients on panels were great! Continue patient participation.

Reach to Recovery volunteer was excellent. Have more participation by volunteers who once were patients. It is more stimulating to hear it from one who has been through it all.

Speakers discussed facts that helped me to function on my unit.

Answered many questions on a distressing type of cancer which involves too many women in the world today (breast cancer).

I became familiar with the side-effects of drugs being used today in cancer treatment and research.

Stimulated good discussion and controversy (gynecologic cancer).

Question and answer session most informative and interesting.

Cleared up outdated concepts re treatment of lung cancer.

Presented a field unfamiliar to me (radiation therapy).

Helped me in my postoperative care of patients (rectal and colonic cancer).

Clarified techniques I use every day with thoracic cases.

Refreshed use of Pleur-evac and significance of blood gases.

Discussed respiratory system—important in every phase of nursing.

Afforded much information on principles and practice of nursing. Also good case studies.

Felt most personally informed.

The idea of a day hospital was interesting.

Individual participants expressed a desire for more time to discuss the following topics in any future seminars on oncologic nursing:

Team members' experiences with patients.

Psychological approaches to patient care.

New patient care techniques.

Postoperative complications.

Post-mastectomy nursing care.

Nursing care for each type of cancer.

Preoperative care information.

Leukemia.

Crisis intervention and psychological problems.

Case histories.

Detailed examples of psychiatric care.

Problems of parents and children.

Coping with the critically ill child and dying children.

Nursing care of the patient after discharge from hospital.

Hodgkin's disease. Importance of physical therapy and encouragement to carry on activities of daily life.

Plastic repair work available.

Chemotherapy and radiation used in conjunction with or opposed to surgery.

Psychosocial and nursing care aspects, especially with regard to radical surgery.

Rehabilitation of patients—modes and methods.

Nursing care of patients undergoing chemotherapy, radiation therapy, and transplant.

The family's role while patient is hospitalized.

Diversional activities used to relieve patients' anxieties.

The theory and physical aspects of the disease, prognosis, therapy.

Pediatric oncology.

The need for understanding of and support of parents and children.

Projected future theories, medications, treatment.

The nurse's role in intra-team departments.

Financial problems of patients and costs of illness.

Chemotherapeutic drugs.

*   *   *

Other suggestions made by participants included:

Some of the content was too technical for the nursing students present.

Perhaps a tour of the hospital facilities first would familiarize students with some of the problems and techniques used.

Perhaps more could be said about the realistic picture of cancer—face up to the tragic side of the coin as well.

Hand out information on the slides and speakers' topics before the session.

Have a parent on the pediatric panel.

Use more slides, fewer statistical slides, and perhaps movies—of nursing content if possible.

Have more panel participation by teachers and recreation specialists to complete the picture of the child in the hospital.

Include public health nurse on all panels to emphasize importance of continuity of care.

Include a husband, family member, member of industry or the community on panels. Also, if a patient who has undergone transplant could shares his experiences with us, that would be wonderful!

Allow for more exchange between panelists—would make for a greater depth and broader overall view.

Cut down on straight lecture time. Formulate one or two case studies to cover nursing care. Have speaker present topic briefly and then open the meeting for discussion.

Allow more time for questions and answers.

Use animated demonstrations.

Distribute literature packet to members of the staff unable to attend sessions.

Make printed matter on chemotherapy available to participants since many of the drugs discussed are used only at Memorial Hospital.

Appendix C

Sample Forms Used for the Seminars

The following three pages provide samples of the announcements, programs, and the evaluation form used for the various seminars. The contents and format of the pocket folders that were distributed to the participants as they registered for each seminar series varies according to the subject under consideration. For example, the folder for the series on Nursing Management in Pediatric Oncology contained a tastefully and artistically designed illustrated program. Suggested readings, reprints of published materials, and other pertinent illustrative materials were also included in the folders.

MEMORIAL HOSPITAL *for* CANCER *and* ALLIED DISEASES

N E W   Y O R K ,   N E W   Y O R K   1 0 0 2 1   T R A F A L G A R   9 - 3 0 0 (

DEPARTMENT OF NURSING

ANNOUNCING...

September 21, 1971

REGIONAL MEDICAL PROGRAM - ONCOLOGIC NURSING SEMINAR
on
"NURSING CARE MANAGEMENT OF PATIENTS
WITH TUMORS OF THE LIVER"
* * * * *

*TUESDAY - OCTOBER 12, 1971
1:00 - 4:00 p.m.
*(There will not be a repeat of this program.)

MEMORIAL HOSPITAL - AUDITORIUM
424 East 68th Street
(between York & First Avenues)
* * * * *

Joseph G. Fortner, M.D.
Chief, Gastric & Mixed Tumor Service
Chief, Transplantation Service
Seminar Leader

Seminar Highlights:

The program will focus on:

....Overview of current surgical interventions for liver tumors -

HEPATIC LOBECTOMY
HEPATIC ARTERY LIGATION
LIVER TRANSPLANTATION

....The complexities of preoperative studies and postoperative management

....The challenge of nursing practice and clinical nursing expertise

....The utilization of immunosuppressive drugs in the control of host
resistance to organ acceptance

....New developments in the use of ALG and tissue typing

....A film describing new techniques of hepatic surgery

Additional speakers will be:

David W. Kinne, M.D., Clinical Assistant Surgeon, Gastric & Mixed Tumor
Service and Clinical Assistant Surgeon, Transplantation Service
and...
Members of Memorial Hospital Nursing and Medical Staff

*Registration from 12:30 p.m. Program commences promptly at 1:00 p.m.
and ends promptly at 4:00 p.m.*
CLINICAL UNIT OF MEMORIAL SLOAN-KETTERING CANCER CENTER

RMP ONCOLOGIC NURSING SEMINAR
EVALUATION

TUESDAY - MARCH 28, 1972

Please circle the number which exemplifies your reaction to each category:

Speaker Presentations: 5   4   3   2   1
          Stimulating   *Adequate*   *Unsatisfactory*

Content & Ideas: 5   4   3   2   1
          Stimulating   *Adequate*   *Unsatisfactory*

Panel Discussion: 5   4   3   2   1
          Stimulating   *Adequate*   *Unsatisfactory*

Question & Answer: 5   4   3   2   1
          Stimulating   *Adequate*   *Unsatisfactory*

Entire Seminar Session: 5   4   3   2   1
          Stimulating   *Adequate*   *Unsatisfactory*

Please circle past seminars you have attended:

RECTAL & COLON   HEAD & NECK   BREAST

CHEMOTHERAPY   GYNECOLOGY   THORACIC

RADIATION THERAPY   LIVER   UROLOGY

Are you interested in attending future Oncologic Nursing Seminars?

(*please circle*)   YES   NO

Do you have any helpful comments for future seminars?

_____

_____

_____

_____

_____

_____

Please check your current status: ( ) R.N.
                        ( ) Nursing Student
                        ( ) Social Service Worker
                        ( ) Other:_____

Please indicate your Agency Affiliation
and Agency Address: _____

    _____

383

MEMORIAL HOSPITAL *for* CANCER *and* ALLIED DISEASES

NEW YORK, NEW YORK 10021   TRAFALGAR 9-3000

DEPARTMENT OF NURSING

REGIONAL MEDICAL PROGRAM - ONCOLOGIC NURSING SEMINAR
on
"NURSING CARE MANAGEMENT OF PATIENTS
WITH TUMORS OF THE LIVER"
* * * * * * * * * * * *

Tuesday - October 12, 1971 - 1:00 p.m. - 4:00 p.m.
Memorial Hospital - Auditorium
* * * * * * * * * * * *

P R O G R A M

Welcome
Mrs. Beatrice A. Chase
Chairman, Department of Nursing

Dr. Guy F. Robbins
Director, Memorial Hospital RMP

Liver Tumors: Incidence, Diagnosis, Treatment, Prognosis
Dr. Joseph G. Fortner
Chief, Gastric & Mixed Tumor Service
Chief, Transplantation Service
Seminar Leader

Hepatic Artery Ligation
Dr. David W. Kinne
Clinical Assistant Surgeon, Gastric & Mixed Tumor Service
Clinical Assistant Surgeon, Transplantation Service

Film: "Isolation-Perfusion Technique for Hepatic Lobectomy"
Narrator: Dr. Joseph G. Fortner

Pre- and Postoperative Nursing Care Management
Mrs. Donna Vermes, R.N., Assistant Head Nurse

- *REFRESHMENT BREAK* -

Nursing's Response to Transplantation Surgery
Patricia Mazzola, R.N., B.S.N., Clinical Instructor, Special Care Unit

Liver Transplantation
Dr. Joseph G. Fortner, Chief, Transplantation Service

Immunosuppression
Dr. Sandra Nehlsen, R.N., Ph.D, Assistant Immunologist, Transplantation Service

Nursing Care Management of the Liver Recipient
Noreen Byrne, R.N., Head Nurse, Special Care Unit

AUDIENCE INVITED TO PARTICIPATE IN OPEN DIALOGUE

/ps 10-7-71

CLINICAL UNIT OF MEMORIAL SLOAN-KETTERING CANCER CENTER

384

INDEX

385